Heartlines and the Web

The *Amanita rubescens* Experience

Stuart Deeks

AYNI BOOKS

Winchester, UK
Washington, USA

First published by Ayni Books, 2013
Ayni Books is an imprint of John Hunt Publishing Ltd., Laurel House, Station Approach,
Alresford, Hants, SO24 9JH, UK
office1@jhpbooks.net
www.johnhuntpublishing.com
www.ayni-books.com

For distributor details and how to order please visit the 'Ordering' section on our website.

ISBN: 978 1 78099 328 7

A CIP catalogue record for this book is available from the British Library.

Design: Stuart Davies

Printed and bound by CPI Group (UK) Ltd, Croydon, CR0 4YY

CONTENTS

Acknowledgements

All the provers and supervisors who boldly took part in the proving.

All those involved in the case examples.

Sarah Keays for her help typing up some of my text.

Sam Goodchild and Roberta Young for working on rubrics. Roberta for her drawings. Lindsey and Stephen and my family for their constant support over these last six years. Pauline Black for her encouragement in directing me to O-Books.

Introduction

Some thoughts about illness and wellness. The effects of toxic substances and toxic thoughts.

Readers unfamiliar with homoeopathy and its terminology can refer to Part One for explanations.

This book records the impact of a fungus, *Amanita rubescens,* on several people's lives, mine included – experiences and sensations. This influence has been far reaching and may even seem far-fetched. Some of it is truly weird. We begin to recognize that this mushroom and the homoeopathic remedy's territory is nothing less than the interconnectedness of everything – the matrix.

The matrix. The web. The wyrd.

In Old English the word 'wyrd' as a noun suggests the web of interconnections. A web links many parts.

Weird – odd, uncanny. *Wyrd* is a concept in Anglo-Saxon culture roughly corresponding to fate or personal destiny. The word is ancestral to the Modern English adjective *weird. (From Wikipedia.)*

'*Wyrd* is too vast, too complex for us to comprehend, for we are ourselves part of *wyrd* and cannot stand back to observe it as if it were a separate force.' *(From Brian Bates' documentary novel about the spiritual wisdom of Anglo-Saxon England* – The Way of Wyrd, Tales of an Anglo-Saxon Sorcerer.*)*

Some things that defy words turn up in this book.

It is a book woven from three main threads, with the influence of *Amanita rubescens* as their common origin.

- I describe my experiences over a period of six years, as episodes. An unfolding tale of discovery and change, in diary type entries.
- The information from the 2006 homoeopathic proving tells of

the varied experiences of a group of second year students at the South Downs School of Homoeopathy in the UK, at the time and since.
- The cases give examples of the remedy's use in homoeopathic practice, over five years – evidence of benefits.

It is the nature of the wyrd's web of influence to be non-linear. Webs operate that way. For this reason the material in this book cannot be presented in a simple A–Z fashion. You will find reviews and retrospective comments attached to the story as it goes along. Also lateral references to related areas, to ideas, books and contemporary events. Individual inner journeys are interwoven with outer conditions and incidents.

Much of this is personal. I for one have been deeply stirred up, as if woken up by the power of this mushroom, since I first ate it in 2005. Impressed by it, amazed and awestruck at times. Like you, I move along in life with a collection of references and associations, received and acquired – ways of looking at things. Several books read during this period have been useful and inspiring, resonant with me in some way, and timely. They are listed in the bibliography. Some of this may be unfamiliar, even foreign to you. I hope this doesn't get in the way. Your individual experience of life offers you points of access to these human issues. There is common ground here, connected, by way of the web, the matrix, the wyrd. Universal matters.

Illness – some considerations

Feelings of Connection	**vs.**	**Feelings of Separation**
The connected feeling		The separated feeling
Qualities –		
At one		At odds
In the flow		Out of sorts
On track		Lost the plot

On form	Off the mark*
In the now	Absentminded
Aware	'Out to lunch'
Centred	Off his head
Grounded	Space case
Inspired	Bored
Engaged	Loss of will
In the groove	Going against the grain
Open	Shut down
At ease	Disease

* The original and true meaning of the word 'sin' is to lose the way, to miss the mark.

And along the same lines –

Truly in control	vs.	Needing to keep things under control

An example –

A client came. Her presenting complaint was vertigo. In the conversation she spoke of nothing doing by way of her sexual aliveness. With the gesture of both hands palms holding down she said, 'I keep all that *under* control.' Cut off from part of herself? After taking *Conium maculatum,* the giddiness was gone. She says, 'I feel so much more *in* control.'

To 'control' a vehicle well means being in touch (and not only literally) with how the machine functions. Then it will get you where you want to go. Intimate with purpose.This requires being in touch with what is going on.

The body – the vehicle. Listen to the body. It never lies.

Maybe illness simply follows a separation of one kind or another. There might be a loss of connection with the body, the vehicle, not listening to its messages. Ignoring symptoms. Signals. Symptoms draw our attention, flagging up a condition, a dis-ease. We may then respond to resolve the situation, one way or another, in order to return to a state of ease, symptom-free again. The smooth-running connected state is simply how it is meant to be.

> Like light, this connected mode is of the essence.
> Like darkness in relation to light, separation is felt in the absence of connection.

At ease
– the state of being at one with everything, at one with the body and so symptom free.
Disease
– the absence of the at ease state, symptoms indicating that something is up.
Symptoms can be subtle or obvious.

Not connected

- unaware, not fully present. Accidents can happen in this state: tripping on a step, slipping with a kitchen knife, burning your finger.
- not paying attention or blocking out the body's messages, bodily sensations, symptoms, e.g. finding stimulants to keep going when you are tired and in need of rest.
- alienated feeling, from your true self. This could be from suppression of emotions, or will: blocked aliveness.
- feeling separate from others, from the surrounding life on the planet, from universal energies.

Connected

- sense of belonging, ease in the body and in relation to everything. As if 'in tune' with everything. At one. Atonement as a part of this. Full sense of being an aspect of creation, a spirit in a form, vehicle for a spirit. Connected to source, the divine felt within and without. Flawless flow betwixt and between.

An example – A small baby, affected by an abrupt separation from its mother, has breathing difficulties. Placed skin to skin with Mum and the breathing comes easily again.

We might have a feeling of separateness from our source, like a river that has lost its upstream part. So we feel separate from others, and within we are cut off from true realization of our potential.

As outside, so within – If the free optimum movement of energy of my body is blocked in any part, the whole system is not connected up.

Turns of phrase reflect this nicely –

Mind/head – Off his head, eyes bigger than his belly, big-headed. Severed head = heart not engaged.

Throat – Choked with emotions, lump in the throat, something he can't swallow. Something unspoken.

Heart – Hard or cold-hearted. Heartbroken. Affected from behind the heart – a stab in the back. Positive aspect – Heartfelt.

Belly (solar plexus) – cut off from feelings. Like being kicked in the stomach. Lily-livered. No guts. Or 'He has the gall' to do/say such a thing. On the positive side – Fire in the belly. Full of spleen.

Sex centre – emasculated, hysterical.

Base (foundation) – Scared shitless. Undermined. Positive aspect – Down to earth. Solid, dependable.

Any separations, blockages, disconnections within me will be reflected in how I perceive the world around me.

An example – One day I am fed up, withdrawn. I go out and no one seems to notice as we pass in the street, to say hello. The next day my mood has lifted. I am greeted with an open smile from a stranger.

And another – Try on the crumpled posture of dejection and you can almost feel that mood. Then if you are truly able to expand to think tall, and open out in the chest, you feel brighter and lighter.

Any loss of easy connectedness within and in relation to the outside contributes to unwellness, disease. Symptoms of our dis-ease are there to draw our attention, so that we look for a way to recover that basic experience of well-being and fluent interconnectedness, free of such distractions.

In relation to four elements

Earth – grounded   Water – flowing
Fire – aligned   action Air – inspired

The mix
Thou earth, thou sun, thou sky, thou sea,
Be thou mixed equally in me.

Toxicity – All Sorts

Toxin – any substance that accumulates in the body which is harmful or poisonous to the system.

External toxins have an impact on an individual's health. It might be chemicals used in food production, pollutants in the water, nicotine, alcohol, from vaccines or dental procedures. Many things impact us. Invisible forces like background radiation or electromagnetic frequencies have an influence too, on everyone. However, the nature and extent of any reaction and symptoms depend on a person's susceptibility.

Internal toxins. My thoughts and attitudes may be toxic too, firstly to myself, and then spilling out into the world around me. Negative thoughts about myself: not good enough, unworthy or whatever else. This toxic mind-set imprints in each body cell. As a symptom of this we may notice negatively charged thoughts about others, life and the universe. Between me and my perceived outside world – a separation, and loss of ease. This contributes to disease.

Clearing and transformation

HEAL = WHOLE

Clearing and cleansing requires awakening to what is going on and its impact. The dark poisonous side is recognized; then things can change.

Food poisoning gives a physical example of this – Some rotten food affects us. We notice the discomfort. The intensity of response is individual in nature and extent. Vomiting and diarrhoea may take over. These are vital and involuntary processes. We await the return of appetite and easy digestion.

Trouble. Response. Awareness.

Surrender.

Release. Relief. Equilibrium.

Another example of this sequence – I am tired, maybe need a break. I get a cold. It will stop me in my busy tracks, if I can let it. There comes a time when I feel it's going on for ever, this feeling lousy; also these feverish or chilly sensations, runny nose and so on. It takes over; nothing else exists for that time. Then somehow, and outside of my control, a subtle surrender takes place. Sleep is a likely part of this. I begin to recover; the symptoms subside.

What we notice in a brief illness applies over a longer period in chronic disease states. Here 'chronic' means extending over a long time. A patient and probing awareness is called for. More is at stake, and there will be more to deal with.

Heart

Heart centre.

The heart of the matter.

My connection with *Amanita rubescens* centred around my heart, physically and in other ways. In the proving and cases we read about sensations felt around the heart as well as emotional hurts.

Matters of the heart.

The heart is central.

There is interesting research being done on heart states and energies: observing situations that affect the state of our hearts, and ways in which our heart states emanate out from us.

Both Princess Diana's death in 1997 and the destruction of the World Trade Center buildings in 2001 brought on a massive surge of emotions. This was seen to have an effect on the electromagnetic field of our planet.

I was deeply moved and inspired to learn of this, and began to acknowledge this weird web of interconnection. Hearing about this work warms my heart.

(See www.heartmath.com The HeartMath Institute, and especially www.glcoherence.org the Global Coherence Initiative. Also notes and quotes section of Part Six.)

This initiative is both congruent and contemporary with the work we have begun on *Amanita rubescens*. You will see this illustrated in the proving text and the case examples.

Part One

Homoeopathic principles described. Specialist terms and abbreviations explained.

Homoeopathy

Homoeopaths are people who prescribe medicines according to the principles of homoeopathy. This word was coined by Samuel Hahnemann early on in the nineteenth century. He was a German chemist and physician.

Here are two examples of the homoeopathic principle:

- Something heavy, a brick maybe, falls on your foot, or you stub your toe. As first reaction you might well shout OUCH! loudly, or some other more vigorous expression, then press hard on the place of impact, for relief of the pain.
- Eating something poisonous will bring on symptoms. If it is a lethal poison, you will die. However, the symptoms in their sequence of stages will vary considerably depending on the nature of the poison. For example the toxicity of the common foxglove, *Digitalis* includes certain effects on heart function. The homoeopathic principle is seen in useful action when much smaller doses of that same dangerous poison relieve particular kinds of heart conditions. It is generally acknowledged, and not just by homoeopaths, that poisons are an essential medical resource; hence the symbol known as the Caduceus. This symbolizes the dual aspects of a poison: what can kill or harm as poison can relieve or 'cure' as medicine.

Proving

The word itself. Homoeopaths' use of this word reflects Hahnemann's pioneering work. In German the word 'prüfung' is used for a trial, a test, an investigation into, or examination of something. In English we have the saying, 'The proof of the pudding is in the eating.' Hahnemann conducted clinical trials of the medicines of his day, and our use as homoeopaths of the word 'proving' as the name used for this method of investigating medicinal effects came directly from the German 'prüfung'.

A Prover. Someone who takes part in a proving.

How is a proving done?

Anyone might discover the properties of a potentially medicinal substance on their own. Accidental as well as deliberate poisoning can be like this. The symptoms provide useful indicators of the field of action of the poison. However, deliberate provings are undertaken as a reliable way to provide homoeopaths with a thorough and detailed understanding.

Homoeopathic pharmacy

For a proving, tablets are prepared, usually, by a homoeopathic pharmacy, from the substance to be tested. This preparation involves sequential dilution and succussion of the original. This has to be preceded by trituration if the original material is insoluble in water. The sequence of dilutions renders an originally poisonous substance by degrees less fiercely toxic, down to the level where it can be employed appropriately as a medicinal agent. This was done by Hahnemann to reduce the intensity of experience when taking a medicine, albeit chosen homoeopathically. Along with the dilution he established the use of succussion, which he realized as essential to retain the characteristic field of action and potency of the medicine. Succussion involves striking the phial with the liquid inside it against a hard surface, originally a leather-bound book. The medicine is made and preserved in a high alcohol medium, and this is then used to medicate blank sugar/lactose or sucrose tablets.

Potency

All potencies used in the proving of *Amanita rubescens* are centesimal. This relates to how the remedies are prepared at the pharmacy. The proportion of dilution is 1–99 parts at each stage. This starts with one part of the original to ninety-nine of the liquid ethanol medium. This is succussed a set number of times. One part of this mix is kept for the next stage of adding 99 parts of ethanol, and succussed again. When this is done thirty times, for example, it is known as 30 C, or 30 CH: the thirtieth centesimal potency. Another type of preparation is called decimal, because the dilution proportions are 1–9 at each stage. The sixth decimal potency would be called 6X or 6D. In this book all potencies are of the centesimal kind, unless indicated.

Taking part in a proving

One person can do a proving as a trial or test to learn about a medicine, but usually and more usefully a group will be involved. One could say that there is no such thing as perfect health, but provers are required to be clear of any obvious illness at the time of the proving. Starting on the same day at an agreed time each person takes a tablet by mouth, probably repeating the dose at intervals over a few days, stopping the dosage when they begin to experience changes. Their symptoms indicate these changes. These experiences are recorded in detail for as long as evidence of the changes continues. Some changes may be immediate, others later on.

Bringing the information together

Then, after a time, the provers' information is collated. At this stage comparisons and similarities emerge, serving to clarify the scope and territory of the medicine.

As can be imagined, each prover reacts to the stimulus, in part, according to their individual sensitivities and susceptibility. For example a person, who may at other times get skin eruptions or cracking, especially in cold weather, in the proving experiences beneficial changes to his cracked fingertips. Such changes relieve an already existing condition. This indicates that the person has benefited from testing the medicine, and 'needed' it in this aspect. More commonly, experiences of change will show as new and possibly uncomfortable sensations or feelings. These stay for a while and then fade away, once the initial stimulus has 'worn off'. As indicated already, tablets are only taken until changes or symptoms are noticed, and in any case only for a few days.

The group effect

It has been frequently observed, and is very much the case with the proving of *Amanita rubescens*, that others involved in the process get affected without even taking the tablets; hence the contributions to the text from supervisors. Each of our provers had a 'supervisor', a student colleague, as a support, to talk to each day and describe experiences as they arose.

States and Symptoms listed

Once most of the effects have died down, the symptoms can be sorted under headings – states of mind or spirit, emotions, as well as physical symptoms. You will see that the text of the proving in this book is laid out this way.

To match each section rubrics are found. These might already exist in homoeopathic repertories, in connection with other remedies, or devised freshly to match symptoms of this proving. A rubric is a means of directing someone to a particular medicine. It derives from the gained knowledge of the medicine – from poisoning, proving and confirmed clinical use. It serves as a two-way signpost – pointing to and originally coming from the medicine.

Rubrics of different medicines are brought together in repertories. A repertory is a 'store or collection of information, instances etc.' The word comes from the Latin reperio = I find.

This gathered and collated information tells us of states and symptoms experienced by the provers since taking the tablets.

In Practice

The medicine is ready for homoeopathic clinical use. It goes like this: a patient comes to a homoeopath in a particular state, with symptoms. The homoeopath observes closely and goes into the detail of the symptoms. Then he or she chooses a remedy according to the homoeopathic principle. It will be one that is known from its proving to have produced/induced states and symptoms similar to those presented by the patient. All this requires skill and enough time. The chosen medicine is given. If the patient's state and symptoms begin to change and improve, it is considered that the medicine was a good one. (The term remedy is now justified!) The choice is confirmed and the workings of the homoeopathic principle are witnessed.

Materia Medica

Once we had experience of this remedy in clinical use, we could begin to confirm the Materia Medica. In Latin this simply means 'medical material'. It represents a synthesis or distillation from the study of a particular medicine, to indicate and assist its possible uses.

It is worth adding that this whole process of proving a medicine through to materia medica can be repeated with another group. This has been done with long established remedies like *Sulphur*, one of those that Hahnemann first proved 200 years ago. Repeated provings verify and enrich the body of information: similar threads and themes emerge, with each prover's individual nature as a colouring factor.

Other terms used

Use of the words Medicine, Drug and Remedy can be confusing.

Dictionary definitions:

Medicine – 'drug, etc. for the treatment or prevention of disease, especially taken by mouth'.

Drug – 'medicinal substance'. A word with other uses and connotations.

Remedy – 'medicine or treatment', or 'a remedy for a condition' As a verb, to remedy = 'to rectify or make good'. (Latin remedium from medeor = heal.)

Homoeopaths tend to use the word 'remedy' to refer to one of the substances that they might prescribe to a patient. Other disciplines are more likely to use 'medicine' or 'drug'.

The remedy names are mostly in Latin and are printed in italics. For example – *Natrum muriaticum* is the remedy made from Sodium Chloride, common rock salt.

Abbreviations

Am. rub. = *Amanita rubescens,* the remedy

b.d. = dosage – twice a day

s.s.d. = 'single split dose.' A term used when three doses of a remedy are taken in a 24-hour period.

amel. or > = ameliorates, symptom improves.

agg. or < = aggravates, symptom gets worse.

Rx. = remedy given or taken.

5/7 = remedy taken daily for 5 days.

4/52 = remedy taken weekly for 4 weeks.

Part Two

My *Amanita rubescens* experiences. How it brought me into a time of severe illness, exposing dark places for attention.

The *Amanita rubescens* story

This part of the book tells of my experience of the past six years in connection with this mushroom.

Setting the Scene

(Written in the winter of 2005/6)

This is the third year that I have been responsible for co-ordinating a proving with second year students, as part of their course at the South Downs School of Homoeopathy in the UK. Around the time of the Autumn Equinox 2005, I was looking for two things: a substance suitable for the next proving, and some resolution of an issue that I felt stuck with.

As it happened the two came together.

Episode one – Late October, Halloween and to the end of that year – 2005.

Meeting (and eating) *Amanita Rubescens*

It had been a warm and moist October, ideal for fungus growth, and I had a new interest – finding edible fungi. Driving past a roadside public park grassy area, I spotted the bright red-with-white-spots *Amanita muscaria,* known also as Fly Agaric. This is the typical toadstool of children's storybooks, renowned for its hallucinogenic effects. Near these were a few of another species, similar in size. I was interested, so picked a couple of these sturdy, thick-stemmed fungi. I identified them at home to my satisfaction as *Amanita rubescens*. This fungus is also known as 'The Blusher' because the white gills become spotted with pink-red when old or damaged, and the same is true of the stem base. That evening I cooked the two samples, for an hour as advised, and ate them as part of a pasta sauce. The following day I finished off the leftovers.

What began to happen the next day was entirely unexpected.

I experienced a marked sensation as if of a 'board' from my solar plexus upwards, in a V shape, at least as far as my shoulders. It was as if this part of my body was firmly fixed and contained. This limited my breathing, constricting the expansion of my chest when breathing in. I 'read' this as an indicator of the area of influence of this fungus, energetically and medicinally, i.e. from the solar plexus in an upward direction. From this, and what followed, I knew it had potential as a medicine.

During this second day I noticed myself becoming unusually hot, almost breaking into a sweat, any time I exerted myself or became anxious about something. It would come on with cycling, or walking up a hill; or once when I was parking for five minutes on a double yellow line with no traffic warden in sight. Even the slightest anxious thought would bring on this heat.

I was mildly alarmed by what was happening to me, having read that, if eaten raw, it had haemolytic properties, which could cause anaemia. I had cooked it thoroughly but I had no way of knowing what was going on.

The heat was how I imagine hot flushes are for women in menopause. It came on in similar circumstances for around a week; then stopped. It has not returned since, except that I am feeling generally warmer than before.

By now it was clear that this fungus had significant medicinal properties, and that it could serve well for the coming year's proving at the South Downs School. It was down to me to choose something for this. It turned up this way. Ideal timing.

On Halloween I returned to the same spot and cut another, enough to send to Helios Pharmacy. They would make it up to the 30 CH potency for the proving. Passing by this patch of grass two days later there was none to be seen. The council mower had cut them all, probably the last of the season.

As far as I know, there is no record of any medicinal use of this Amanita. *(For toxicological and chemical information see Part Seven.)*

November 2005

Three weeks after this all began I went to stay in a place familiar to me from childhood, a weekend break. It is a centre for retreats and, as I found, of a healing quality for me at this time. I had thought that something good might come of it, concerning the issues that had been bothering me; I already suspected that coming across and eating the Amanita was somehow playing a part in this process of resolution. While I was there I found a liberating and new perspective on the problem. This made such a difference to me that I felt able to go to a family birthday meal that I had previously decided not to go to. I had been feeling uncomfortable around most of the people who would be there. The family scene was connected to my (second) ex-wife, and she was to be there. This discomfort faded during the weekend away, and I did go to the meal after all.

As a result, I began to have a different attitude to those with whom I had previously had difficulties. Up to that time these difficulties had seemed insurmountable. It was my feelings about my ex that I was hoping to address during the winter months. I now could begin to 'increase the good' rather than be judging and 'fighting' what I thought of as bad. There has been a radically transforming and beneficial outcome from all of this. *(September 2011. Still wrestling and working with these issues.)*

Episode two – January 2006. Before the proving begins.

Early in the New Year the pharmacy sent me the tablets of this new medicine for the college proving. There were twenty phials in all, and three potencies: 6, 12 and 30 CH. I begin to keep a diary.

Night of January 6th. I place the phials, wrapped as sent, by my bed, wondering what might happen from having them close to me as I sleep.

Wake at 3 a.m. Not unusual. I feel very calm and relaxed, a glowing warmth around my heart centre/chakra. Also warmth from solar plexus upwards, seeming to reach right up to the level of my ears and further, like a big letter **Y**. This was where I had the fixed-like-a-board sensation after my pasta supper some months before. I wonder what the Y form holds in its associations in Rudolf Steiner's work and Eurhythmy? *My association with the Y form – On the glyph of the Kabbalah Tree of Life: the path up the central pillar from Malkuth, moving on up to Tifaret, then out in a Y shape to Gevurah-Chesed and to Binah-Chockmah. (See Part Six for Eurhythmy/Steiner parallels.)*

Then, still laying awake – a vivid recall of kingfishers I had seen a few days ago – the iridescent blue/green, and the way they fly at such speed horizontally just above the water level. *Bird flight in association with this remedy? Later some provers had dreams or images of kingfishers.*

Heat again, but not to such an extent as after eating the fungus. Then for a while a less settled state before falling back to sleep. No remembered dreams.

Waking in the morning I feel well rested and generally well, despite weariness when I went to bed. Yesterday was busy and unsettling. I have lots of energy, despite not taking vitamins or mineral supplements since eating the mushroom. I haven't missed them at all. *(This is still the case two months later.)*

I feel very calm and easily able to make the final preparations for this proving. As I type this, there is a warm glow in and behind my heart centre and a strong feeling in my solar plexus, a firm sense of purpose along with a balanced containment of the excitement of bringing this new medicine out.

January 7th, a week before the proving is to begin.

I set off to go to the college. Tablets are to be given out to the provers with final instructions. On a train replacement bus service, as part of my journey to Chichester, I sit upstairs behind a boy (four years old?), and his mother. He was lively, but not over the top. He gets up to look out the window. His mother is stern with him, saying, 'Behave! Sit down and keep quiet!' and 'This is supposed to be a treat for me, and you are spoiling it.'

At first, and characteristically, I am irritated by her style – critical and judging, even thinking for a moment that I might say something to her about it. I don't. Then I realize that my attitude is making *me* uncomfortable. Mother, child and now me, all having an unpleasant time on this bus.

A small voice says to me, 'Step out of it! Try something different!'

I set about an experiment, with an archangel meditation that I use *(from the book* God is a Verb *by David A. Cooper)*. First for myself. A minute or two. Then I imagine it around mother and child. Within two minutes he asks to sit on her lap. She agrees. 'As long as you are good,' but not as sternly as before. For the rest of the journey there are no more harsh looks. They're smiling together and he's singing *Jingle Bells*!

A change!

I had been critical and wanted to counter what I judged as bad parenting. Then humility, followed by a kind of playfulness. 'Try this,' the small voice said. Going for something that could have a good effect – to 'increase the good' rather than be preoccupied in 'fighting' something judged as bad. This bus journey was a test for me. It was the first time I had tried such a thing, and I was quite amazed to see it apparently working. I had wondered at the assertion that thoughts can change the entire unfolding of the universe. I had tested this out in a small way. They appeared to be more content and happy too!

This kernel experience illustrates what I would test out over the following years.

Six days to go before the proving begins. I sleep right through the night, unusual for me. Deep sleep. Normally I would have woken in the early hours, with thoughts of yesterday's events and sense of excitement buzzing around in my head. I feel a close and warm connection with my partner.

My hair has been more greasy than usual, in the last two days.

Five days to go. I had a very long sleep – nine hours, very unusual. I woke briefly at 5 a.m. with a warm upper chest. It reminded me of the heat I experienced during those first eight days after eating the mushroom.

Dream – I get on a London bus with my daughter and her mother my ex. *(Association with my father, a Londoner.)* The bus is going to a part of London connected with the first childhood home that I remember. My daughter is sitting next to me and her mother has a seat a bit further up. We are in the downstairs part and the bus is pretty full. *An image of connection and going somewhere together – out in the world at large. This felt good, and as if something had resolved between my ex and myself, along the lines of my autumn quest.*

After waking up I notice a pink/red mark in the middle of my forehead – at the third eye place. I feel warm all day. Despite sleeping lots, I am tired again by 4 p.m., as if I could sleep more, but it is a very mellow and comfortable kind of tiredness.

Again hair greasy.

Four days to go. Long sleep again. Third eye patch less pronounced.

Afternoon. Slept for twenty minutes.

Three days to go. Nine hours sleep again. Third eye patch less pink/red, but now there is a change of skin texture compared with the surrounding skin, more smooth and slightly harder. Today I feel settled and mellow in myself, and not so tired in the afternoons as on the previous two days. In fact, I have lots of productive energy, working at various things till late.

Fire. Some music I was writing out got burnt by placing it above a nightlight candle that was on the table. The candle was behind something else and I had forgotten about it. I realized I was working too late! *Later on I read of the association between the solar plexus chakra and fire, and became aware of the connection with Amanita rubescens, from the proving and the cases.*

Two days to go.

Dream 1. Water. I am in Edinburgh, crossing Princes street. *(My mother was from Edinburgh.)* The green man is showing but traffic is still coming. I point to the green man, indicating it to the car drivers, and carry on crossing over. *I do sometimes realize I'm crossing roads dangerously when there is traffic about. It also reminds me of my uncle who had depressive tendencies, and died this way in a road accident. (Syphilitic miasm.)* Then I go into a church-like building. The stone floor is covered in water, which came from a nearby stream. The water is clear and clean, like spring water. People (mostly young backpackers) are taking it easy there. The water is not at all cold. There are sofas on the dry bits. A young guy is leaning back towards the water and falls into it. There is a light-hearted feel to it all.

Dream 2. I am in a house with many rooms, like a hostel. My first wife is in front of me, naked and beautiful, and our adopted son is around too. *(It is his birthday today as it happens.)* I can touch her and be with her. She is standing there straight in front of me. But then I think, how can I do that since I have a new partner in my life now? She will be around later, perhaps, or maybe she is somewhere else. However, it is a good feeling with her, and a sense of reconciliation. *Generally I have a sense of unresolved issues around her.*

Dream 3. I am in Oxford Street in London, again crossing a wide and busy road dangerously. I am looking for a bus to get me back to Hackney. *I used to live there with my first wife.* It is all very realistic, and I think of the various numbers of the buses that could take me there.

Themes running through the dreams: Reconciliation in respect of unresolved difficult issues from my past. Returning to previously familiar places: Edinburgh with family associations, especially in my teens, London/Hackney where I lived in my twenties and thirties. Also childhood home link. Father–Mother.

Third eye 'patch' is now not there at all.

The day before the proving. Not such a long or settled sleep at all. The effects of last weekend, having the remedy with me and being with the group at college have worn off. I woke at 3 a.m. overstimulated by late night conversation.

January 14th 2006. The proving begins.

Here you could take a break from my diary to check out the proving record in Part Three. It brings together the students' accounts of their experiences from taking the tablets. I never did take it in that form, until November 2011. Apart from the effects of eating it in the beginning, what has happened for me since seems to have come from just thinking or writing about it. This strangely strong influence continues through the following years. It still goes on. (September 2011)

The Proving is strand two in the three-part weave of *Amanita rubescens* experiences.

Episode three – My diary during the time of the proving. Fifty days.

Day 1. Sleep again unsettled. Later in the day a mellow feeling comes on and I am sleepy with it.

I decide to have a phial of the remedy with me in my shirt pocket, with the intention of supporting and connecting with the provers. Also during the first weeks of the proving, if I was awake in the night, I did the archangel meditation, first for myself, then 'sent' it to each member of the college group in turn, imagining them asleep in their homes. I suppose it was prayer, as well as astral travelling for a beginner?

When two of the provers said that I had appeared in their dreams as if in their room, I decided to 'stay at home' at night. I was impressed, even surprised but cautioned. It did seem that what I had been doing was effective, but risked overstepping boundaries via the energy web/matrix. I stopped it.

I wonder if it is a remedy for the adrenals. It seems to change the likelihood of my daytime thoughts/stimulus/excitement spilling over into early morning wakefulness (at 3 or 4 a.m.). Often, and before contact with this remedy, I found these night times necessary for me to 'integrate' these active thoughts.

My partner is unwell today. We have been talking about old emotional hurts. Maybe she is affected by me carrying the remedy around, and I did have it under the pillow.

Day 2. Sleep better. Nine hours again.

A day of feeling not at home, of still waiting for the time when my domestic situation is more settled. Eventually I will leave this rented accommodation and move in together with my partner. Long time waiting.

Day 3. *Dream* – A small car is on fire. There was a tiny child nearby. It is the child of a close friend of mine from my twenties. My first concern is to take the child to her. This friend of mine is young and very pretty. *This I associate with those times, when I found her very attractive. A car of hers did go on fire once.* She is lying next to and amongst lots of other people of a similar age.

Woke early and refreshed. Sitting meditation, and felt clear and ready for the day.

Day 4. Long sleep again. Awake 3 a.m. for half an hour, maybe from the effects of laptop electricity? *Had been typing till late last night.*

Dream – At a 'personal growth' seminar *(directed by someone I worked with some years ago and would like to contact again)*. The task is to make a drawing of a black place. I haven't done it yet. I see one of the others' drawings. My partner is there too.

Today my hair is parted on the right side, and the way it lies is markedly different to anything it has ever done before. *Generally my hair seems to reflect my mood and energy, parting in different places, or sticking up when I'm feeling especially lively.*

Day 5. Long sleep again. Slight tickle/dryness in my throat. My voice is deeper – more relaxed. My hair is still greasy, this is unusual.

Review five days into the proving – This has been a period of having less to do by way of working with/for others, fewer homoeopathy clients, and violin pupils off sick or away, but still earning. The school I teach at was closed unexpectedly, but I was still paid for the day's work. Life was working out fine without me having to make so much effort. This feels consistent with my more settled and slightly sleepy, non-adrenalin state. I find I am taking my time with things more, and doing things in larger blocks without breaking off in the middle to do something else.

Day 6. I am thinking that the remedy has an operating 'base' in the adrenals/kidneys area, already an area of susceptibility for me. Again I am reminded of the wedge shaped 'board' that I experienced after eating the mushroom, extending upwards from my solar plexus up to my shoulders.

I am feeling mellow and warm. Perhaps the remedy is warming my kidney energy?

Day 9. I slept with the tablets under my pillow again.

Dream – Of somehow managing to make it across a big chasm *(the abyss of the Tree of Life in the Kabbalah?)*. I am on a bike and swing across holding a rope, but I only just make it.

An insight. This came near the time that I woke up; it was not a dream. It came in the form of a 'message', giving information about this remedy, perhaps? It went like this: Healing and being well is a radical step, more radical than not being well or not healing. It is a radical way of life, because you go to the root of issues, and things change radically. *I had been talking in this vein with a homoeopathy client the previous day.*

Hair still greasy

Day 10. Yesterday and today I have felt strong and able, staying with one activity to see it through.

Day 12. *Dream 1.* Of reconciliation with an old friend in the cathedral where he is bishop. Organ music is playing. I am holding a wooden staff. *I have been feeling the loss of our friendship, and would like to see this resolved.*

Dream 2. A familiar dream of going down a steep hill in a car without seat belts on.

Feeling generally warmer despite the cold weather.

Day 14. Visited an aunt, a wise woman in her eighties. Lively, not stuck in any way, interested in things, accepting of people's different ways, e.g. different choices for healing. *She is someone who sailed through the menopause. I thought of the aspects of this remedy that may relate to menopause, especially the hot flushes.*

Day 16. Generally: More energy and it sustains well through the day. I drove a long distance without tiring.

Day 19. Greasy hair still. Nasal sinuses unusually clear and open, and with this a tendency for my nose to be watery, especially when outside in the cold air. *This has been the case for the past four weeks, not noted down until now.*

Day 21. Put the remedy phials near my bed again last night. Awake at 4.30 a.m. Meditative breathing. What might I learn tonight? I imagine 'being the mushroom', and start the archangel meditation. While I am breathing and in a receptive state, I have a clear sensation – energy coming from above the crown of my head, flowing into and through my body, simultaneous with a similar energy rising through me, upwards from below my feet. The two meet and pass smoothly at the level of my heart – from above going down to the base and further, and from below rising up to the crown and beyond. I thought now of the letter **X**, following on from my earlier encounter with the **Y** form.

Some time later I realized the connection between this experience, the **X**, *and the Star of David. In this symbol one equilateral triangle points up, the other down, with an implied centre as they intersect to form the hexagonal shape. (See symbols section in Part Six.)*

Review – at three weeks: From this experience of simultaneous movement, upwards and downwards – further thoughts about *Amanita rubescens* and its medicinal properties, with the heart as centre.

Physical symptoms
Heat and hot flushes. Element – fire. Rising flames.
Watery nose. Element – water. Downward flow.
A model of the potential action of the remedy?
Up and down simultaneously.
The meeting place is the heart centre.

This idea appears in the book *Talking with Angels*. The task for the human is to reach upwards, as a flame of fire, towards the angels; conversely the angels need the downward pull, as of gravity and the downward flow of water to enable a meeting with human energies. The heart centre is the bridge where this can take place. *(See Prover 9's text in Part Three, Page 95.)*

The connection with the third eye. I have more clarity of thought and perception since I came across the mushroom. Along with this – clear sinuses. Catarrh as a reflection of the various 'bodies' (astral, emotional, physical) being out of alignment. This remedy assists to align those bodies.

A remedy of alignment?

Chakras. Sacral, rising to Brow and Crown by way of the Lower Heart where clearing may be necessary. 'The lower heart is susceptible to corruption, very susceptible to negative attack from outside' From *The Elements of the Chakras*, by Naomi Ozaniec.

Anxiety and sleep. Not so anxious about things – hence more settled sleep. The healing of the past and what is behind, with clarity ahead into the future. Previous familiar anxieties and discomforts were related to this need for resolution and healing.

Strength and focus. Staying solidly with one thing. Able to focus in meditation – much easier to bring my mind back if it wanders.

The diary continues –

The night after the first college meeting with the proving group.

Day 23. *Dream:* I am going on my bicycle to a friend's house. The house is up a hill somewhere out of the centre of the town where I live. Then, as I am going down again on the short stretch of road to my own house, I pass by a group of dustmen doing their round. They are clearing a great load of rubbish from a fisherman's place: nets, old shells and ropes mixed together, and all wrapped in a big synthetic sheet, like a tarpaulin. It takes three or four of them to lift it and get it into a skip before taking it away. They are working in the road so I stop to wait. Then one of them comes down the road in the direction I was going in. Just then I remember that my partner wanted to change the day the rubbish was collected from her house, so I begin to speak with this dustbin man about it. I ask him if his firm also collected from Brighton. 'Yes,' he says. I tell him the address but then, as I am speaking, I can't remember, however hard I try, which day she wanted to change it to, or why she wanted to make the change in the first place. So I have to break off talking to him about it, saying I was sorry, I can't remember etc. Then I realize that I have mistakenly come away from my friend's house on a scooter (non-motorised). It is an enlarged bicycle length version of the children's scooters that first became popular in the 1990s. I have left my own bike at my friend's house and haven't realized till now that I am on a completely different type of machine, that isn't mine or at all familiar to me.

I awoke at 4 a.m. excitedly thinking about everything to do with the provings I am working on, almost wanting to get up and start writing, to get on with it urgently. It took a while to settle back to sleep.

Day 24. *Dream – Not a familiar kind of dream; more an experience halfway between sleeping and waking.* I am on my bike, going where I plan to go today, but it is in the night time – as if I am in two places at once – 'shape-shifting?' – in my sleep and cycling along – not like a dreaming context, more a sense of actual, real travelling. *(Is this what they call astral travelling?)* Then a double-decker London style bus passes me and begins to drive where I am cycling – to the left across me. I am aware of the danger and have to stop to avoid the bus colliding with me or running me over. I have no distinct sense of a bus driver, but the bus is not taking any notice of me being there. It turns a full 180 degrees round and ends up on the pavement.

I woke and remembered this vision-journey-dream, with bodily sensations that connected with the sense I had of being in two places at once.

Then I slept again, deeply, and woke refreshed and not overexcited. The day started well.

Later in the day. I realize how much I have been affected by the time together with the provers two days ago, as if the group energy was too much for me to take on? I needed 'grounding', so I put off my planned cycling circuit, and do everything on foot instead.

Day 25. *Dreams* – (more like my usual dreams.)

- I am on an extremely high stepladder up alongside a very tall building. I think that I might topple off and fall but I manage not to. There are other people at the base of the building, and they are trying to unsettle me. Then there is something in the dream to do with the violinist Nigel Kennedy – his skill and energy that I admire.
- Of getting to play in a concert *(a very familiar type of dream).* There are people in the way. I have to walk up and over a dinner table. My white, baggy trousers (for the concert) drag in the sauces on the table – tomato etc. staining them red.

The proving (or the effects of the mushroom) seems to be coming to an end now with the return of more familiar dreams. However, beneficial effects were still being felt a week later.

I still feel unsure of myself, especially wary of buses on my bike, and there was a moment where a car came a bit close for comfort. The whole episode served to bring me 'down' to a safe place, without having to lose access to some new areas of experience.

Day 26. *Dream 1.* Again a familiar theme – of missing a rehearsal and then being late for a concert. *The musicians in the dream are ones I used to play with twenty-five years ago. I think, 'These people are still playing music together and I'm missing out on it.'*

Dream 2. Of someone I was attracted to at music college, again many years ago. Holding her fondly, I kiss her and say, 'It's been such a long time since I saw you.'

Dreams again about the past, in association with musicians and friends from that time. Maybe this relates to the theme of unresolved matters that has come up in this proving?

Day 27. *Dream 1. (Old style)* Problems getting to a rehearsal and not having the right clothes for the concert; again musician friends from the old days.

Dream 2. (A more unusual one) People are bringing grains to a place where you could mill them. There is a building next to a very tall tree. The tree is set in a wall-like cut in the land; you can see its roots. Across the yard is the place for milling the grain, an old-fashioned mill. I remark to the others there how unusual it is for such a place to exist these days. It was like a piece of living history.

Other symptoms. Still sleeping deeply and long. Warmer generally than before. Greasy hair. Stools more formed than before. Haemorrhoid bleeding less frequently?

Day 28. Still very clear sinuses. Also consistent thirst – not extreme but definitely have to drink (water). *I have noticed this extra thirstiness right back to when I ate the mushroom.*

Day 29. *Dream.* I am back at the boarding school I went to, wearing the uniform. I am taller and older than the others there, as I am now. Each of the boys gives me an item of clothes, part of what the school provides. A teacher and the boys speak with very posh voices. Then something in a different scenario to do with cancer and a medicine for it.

Associations – During my time at boarding school I felt unsettled in respect of where I felt at home, as I often do these days. Then I had glandular fever, aged 20. Homoeopaths have noted this disease as a possible precursor to cancer.

Afternoon. Tired from the week's work, and not feeling at home, not settled, > after a short nap.

August 2011. As I edit this, I am struck by the congruence between the themes of these dreams and experiences and what took place for me over the intervening years. As if a presentiment of what was to come; also, the parallels with both the proving content and the cases that followed.

Other observations during these four weeks. With heightened energy I have been walking faster than usual, stronger in my belly area. It has also been easier cycling up hills. Also a few times I have looked down, for example at things on a table, and had a sensation of the table top and the things on it appearing to be further away than they 'really' are – disconcerting for a moment.

On reflection – I have learnt again, this time more deeply, how medicines can show up for using. This one had my name on it, for sure! I have heard about animals in the wild finding medicinal plants or roots when they need them. Now I had come by the medicine that I needed. This has been an experience of Grace, and I am grateful. Also I have been shown a way out of a stuck place within myself.

I have had a new but clear experience of a kind of two-way traffic: giving to and receiving from the world/the universe; and for the first time, as direct experience, awareness of the potential of prayer-directed thoughts.

'A single thought can change the unfolding of the entire universe.'

Day 33. Saw Martin Miles, my homoeopath. (I don't know what remedies were given.) However, symptoms and states that I by now associate with the Amanita continued to turn up after taking other remedies.

Day 34. *Dreams*: again of family members, my daughter and mother in one dream. (My mother died about a year ago.) *Again places associated with the past.*

Day 39. Today I felt very clear and confident cycling in busy traffic, rather than the feeling I had two weeks ago that I had to be wary in case of a possible accident.

Day 41. Talking to provers seems to connect me again to the power of this mushroom. I feel very relaxed and settled with everything, ecstatic and solid at the same time.

It is interesting to see how my themes from the proving time continue to show up after being given other remedies. One of the provers told me that she took *Nux vomica* recently for a hangover and it worked very well; previously, in a similar situation, she had hardly any benefit from it. Perhaps this remedy clears the way for others to be more effective, in the same way as it brought me mental (and nasal) clarity?

Day 49. Lying awake in the early hours, I 'enquired' in order to know what a new left side mouth ulcer was there to tell me. It was to do with receiving strength/courage. At this time, I was feeling a bit overloaded with many tasks – the provings and other projects in hand at the same time. The mouth ulcer sensations began to change with this realization, and I had a feeling of renewed strength to keep going. I fell asleep and woke later with a dream: this time of my father. (He died 18 years ago, with a cancer.)

I think of my personal issues of power, strength and physical development in connection with my father. Again a reminder of past issues and the need for reconciliation.

Afternoon. After a short but deep nap, I got up, feeling a bit dopey, and trod on my glasses. I had (unusually) left them on the floor. They were broken beyond repair. I had been putting off buying a lighter pair; now I would have to get on with it. An accident with a meaning? Still acute sense of smell, and general clarity: I seem to know in advance when clients are not going to show up for appointments

During this time I reread *The Elements of the Chakra*, by Naomi Ozaniec, Element Books, 1996. An extract follows. Reprinted by permission of Harper Collins Publishers Ltd.

The Solar Plexus Chakra

Sanskrit name: Manipura, meaning 'lustrous gem' or 'city of jewels'.
Element: Fire.
Function: Will, power.
Inner state: Intense emotion – laughter, joy, anger.
Glands: Pancreas.
Body parts: Ulcers, diabetes, eating disorders such as anorexia and bulimia, hypoglycaemia
Colour: Yellow.
By meditating on this navel lotus,
the power to destroy and create is acquired.

Manipura can be translated as 'lustrous gem', 'city of jewels' or 'filled with jewels.' In Tibet this chakra is known as manipadma or 'jewelled lotus.' This chakra radiates its fiery energy like a bright sun. Its colour is yellow, its element is fire.

The abdomen contains the digestive system, which transmutes food into energy. Food provides fuel for the body. Just as the physical digestive system extracts energy from food, so the solar plexus chakra extracts and stores prana.

Prana is the energy that pervades all life; where there is prana there is life. Each of the chakras is a centre of prana, but it is generated and distributed by the manipura centre.

This centre is given great importance in traditional Japanese teachings. It is called the hara, which literally means 'belly.' It is the centre point where all things both visible and invisible find their balance. The hara is traditionally located three fingers' width below the navel. When this chakra functions as the gravitational centre of being, emotions are both felt and expressed. When the powers of this centre are repressed, serious discrepancies between true feeling and action can arise. Anorexia is a disorder in which the gut feelings are overlaid instead with a false self-image. When the hara is operative, unified expression through word, action and body language follow. In Japan a person is judged to be untrustworthy and insincere unless the voice comes from the hara.

The solar plexus chakra is our place of empowerment in the world. It is the personal fuel store. If the fuel store is low, we lack the driving force to project ourselves into the world with much impact. We become victims of fate and circumstance when we lose touch with willpower, which is a direct expression of inner being. The will is fundamental to well-being and personal fulfilment, translating our innermost nature into outer expression, enabling us to overcome difficult life circumstances. If an individual is weak-willed, the qualities of self-determination and self-direction are undeveloped. They are easily swayed from any given course by the influence of others. If someone is wilful, they exercise power with total disregard for others. It is through the expression of will that we create our own reality; our power in the world is an expression of our sense of will. The human will has been seen by many esoteric writers as a reflection of a divine attribute, the Primal Will, which brings creation into being. It is through the human will the change for good or evil comes into being in the world. We have free will; this gives us the choice and teaches us the value of discrimination. It is through the conscious use of will that our lives are forged.

When the will is blocked we experience a sense of frustration, which is often accompanied by a tightening of the whole solar plexus area. When we lose our sense of power, the stomach seems to turn to water. Our strength vanishes, our fire has been extinguished. Ideally there should be a free flow of energy between the personal will and the freedom to project in the world, but this is often blocked. It can be a temporary obstacle created by a personal dispute or it can be a longer-lasting situation of repression. Accord between inner comprehension of personal will and outer freedom of expression allows the energy of the third chakra to flow evenly. When the will is blocked, either at source or externally, the chakra cannot release and energies begin to impact. The chakra acts like a dam holding back feelings, energies, needs and drives. There is inner turmoil, repressed anger and contained force. Eventually something snaps and there is an emotional scene, a crisis, even a breakdown. This chakra contains our raw emotions. When our emotions are freely expressed they pass easily from us into the appropriate situation and become integrated as part of our total being. When emotions, for whatever reason, are not expressed but turned inwards, they remain lodged in this chakra until catharsis takes place. Anger especially can remain trapped here for many years.

This chakra represents an important step in the development of human consciousness. It carries no trace of our shared animal ancestry, unlike the base and sacral chakras. Some tantric teachings regard it as the starting point for higher human development for this very reason. Satyananda calls it the place of 'confirmed awakening', indicating that when this level is reached the Kundalini force will not sink back into the lower centres.

Traditionally the awakening of this chakra is said to bring the power to locate hidden treasure. The name of this chakra, lustrous gem, may also have a symbolic meaning indicating that spiritual reality itself is the hidden treasure.

Increased psychic sense comes with the awakening of this chakra.

When the energies of this chakra are active and balanced, the individual enjoys well-being and has a clear sense of personal self-determination.

Materia Medica for *Amanita rubescens*

First ideas

March 2006

This represents a synthesis of my experiences between October 2005 and the beginning of April 2006. *(For a later Materia Medica see Part Five.)*

THE LINE
THROUGH
SOLAR PLEXUS – HEART – SHOULDERS – THROAT – THIRD EYE.

Spleen (and kidneys?): Heat, warmer than before. Hot flushes, < anxiety, exertion. Energy good, strong in 'hara'.

Bowels: Stools more formed. Bleeding haemorrhoid >.

Sleep: Sleeping 15% longer. Generally mellow, slowed-down feeling, combined with greater focus and mental/intuitive clarity. Less likely to wake in the early hours with excited thoughts. Not adrenalin-driven.

Sexual energy/rising Kundalini: Strengthened, with further ease of internal rising of these energies; linked to third eye centre.

The 'Lower' Heart and issues of reconciliation, in relation to past unresolved issues; the main one for me was characterised by my attitude of critical judging of someone with whom I had unresolved issues. Within myself I feel the potential for full reconciliation with this person, as well as to my own past experience that connects me with her. Nothing has been said or discussed between us; rather an internal change has taken place within me. This is having good results. It has been an important issue, and it had been bothering me. The anxieties and discomforts, as felt with the hot flushes, were connected to the previously unresolved matters.

Dreams: Mostly set in places associated with my past, involving family members or previous relationships, several to do with unresolved difficulties. Reconciliation. In one of these dreams a fire, and in another, water. Healing of the past and what is behind, and clarity ahead.

Relaxed shoulders: this as a direct result of the strengthened solar plexus/spleen/kidney energy.

Thirsty for water.

Opening of third eye centre: Nasal passages very clear and dry, with watery nose when I am out in the cold air. Keen sense of smell.

Increase in ability to 'see' and choose remedies for clients. Ease of focus in meditation, and a new found ability to focus my mind. With this an ability to complete tasks without petty distraction.

Strange visual sensation when looking down.

Need to remain 'grounded': not to get unbalanced by the benefits of the rising energy. Stay aware of the physical environment. Watch out in case of accidents or danger!

A remedy for radical healing

Episode four – April 2006 to June 2007
The Heart

April 1st. (April Fools' Day in England!)

Day of the final proving group meeting. I did loads. Crazy! In addition to the final college proving group sessions I performed a difficult violin solo in the lunch hour, then extended my journey home to try and resolve an unresolved issue about an instrument that I had leant to a somewhat remote family member. *I was like a bike with no brakes on, speeding downhill.*

April 4th. Energy increased.

April 6th. Very low voice today.

It was as if my voice was dropping, comparable with puberty time. I think, 'I'm in for some big change.' Since then this lowering has carried on, and as I came through what follows it became very important to me to discover my new voice, singing.

April 9th. Perform as violinist with others in a church concert – Stabat Mater by Rossini. Hands are almost paralyzed and incapable of playing the violin. What is going on? *Causticum 30* taken. Just about managed the performance.

April 11th. Sudden, unanticipated, excruciating pain in one particular rotten tooth. *Hepar sulph 50M*. Got me through the night and to the dentist for extraction next morning. The dentist said that mine was the worst case of gum disease that she had seen.

I was wiped out, completely. Pain in all of the other bad teeth.

I had foolishly not taken proper care of my teeth, during the previous fifteen years or so! That started when I was indignant about a sudden increase in National Health Service dental charges. Bits had chipped off various back teeth, but I did not go to the dentist. Illusion of eternal youth, alongside something self-destructive. Tubercular/Syphilitic in homoeopathic speak. Till now, I had had no pains to speak of, except after eating something sweet, so thought I could get away with it!

Now the pain was intense and persistent. No respite. No escape. Continuous pain, morning and night from that April day until late September, first in my teeth then in my jaws and bones around my ears. I was in a bad way.

One night, awake as usual, I asked in a receptive meditative kind of way for some understanding. A message please, from Archangel Michael perhaps? Then a little fellow, a few inches high, stepped out towards me from the woodwork and said, 'You won't die. You will experience a transformation.' Then began to scuttle off in his generally speedy way. 'Hey, hold on. Thanks, but how do I do that?' I said. 'I will help you,' and off he went. I was reassured to have this information. It stood me in good stead.

Even at this time I knew/sensed that all this had come out or been exposed under the influence of the Amanita. It was so sudden and out of the blue, as well as being connected with what I had been asking for when I came across the mushroom six months previously. Other provers had teeth things stirred up, and this was confirmed later on in cases as a feature of the remedy – the exposure of toxic states.

May 2006. The worst month for pains. Now spread into my ears. Foul smelling, brown discharge from my left ear. Could not sleep from the pains. << Laying down.

Was this a proving of the Amanita? My version. Should keep a record.

Now that it was centred around my left ear I couldn't but be reminded of my father's latter-day illness. He had cancer in the bones around his left ear. It was cut off. He was a priest, and I was well aware of a biblical resonance – the story of a disciple, Peter perhaps, cutting off the ear of a high priest's servant, at the moment of Judas' betrayal. 'Jesus said to him, "Put your sword back into its proper place. All those who take the sword die by the sword". And in Luke 22, 'He touched his ear and healed him.' And in John 18, 'Jesus said to Peter, "Put your sword back into its sheath. Am I not to drink the cup that my Father has given me?" Fate.

Reserve your judging attitude

+

accept what is in front of you.

I thought I would be better by midsummer. It took a lot longer even to begin to recover. Bit by bit I cancelled all commitments and then all summer travels. Only, and optimistically, a planned week away in September stayed in the diary.

Exhausted with the constant pain.

Heart began to show signs of serious trouble. Link with gum disease. Could hardly get about, especially up stairs or hills. One night in May my heart went really dodgy – losing beats, it felt like. It was the one scary time – urgent. I propped myself up against walls and banisters to get down the stairs to my remedy collection and took a dose of *Syphilinum 1M*. It was good. Relief. The heart condition began to improve from then on.

In June I had a severe episode of cystitis. Kidney chills with it.

This was an already familiar area of susceptibility. *Cannabis indica 30* prescribed by Martin Miles, my homoeopath, was the remedy. I was beginning to sense the connection between my kidneys and my teeth/jaws/ears.

The continuing constant pains in my head were always worse at night. I had to sit up in a chair to have some partial relief, then I would become so flaked out from pain that sleep came – laying down, an hour at most, before waking again to the pain.

The pain would lessen relatively for some days, then increase again like a screw turning to a heightened pitch, exactly in parallel with me having to look at another one of my unresolved (toxic) issues. These were my stored hurts 'in the lower heart chakra'.

By the end of July I had the eight other rotten teeth out. I remained weak and weary with the constant pain. Pain saps energy. In a resigned way I dreaded the nights. I knew what I was in for every night. Mostly awake. Five months.

There were phases, stages. Like on a wave I come to a point of maximum pain intensity. At first I would think I could fix it, to ease it with remedies, meditations, breathing etc. Then such thoughts left me. All no use. Surrender. Unconditional. Letting go of proud ego control, most often with a paroxysm of weeping in the dark hours. Then a shift: a release for a while of the level of pain along with a sense of clearing that particular hurt. Grace experienced. A plateau of relative calm. A brief respite.

Trouble. Response. Awareness.
Surrender.
Release. Relief. Equilibrium.

Then after some days another similar sequence would begin.

As I edit this (Autumn 2011) I am reminded of the Rumplestiltskin type of tale. An extreme task is set to do through the night, by morning: to spin straw into gold for the King, and the pile increases over the three nights. The young girl gives up trying, weeping with the impossibility of it. An elf-like character jumps in. 'Who are you?' she asks. He won't give his name, but reassures her. He takes on the spinning. She is amazed to wake in the morning to see it all neatly done, and no sight of him.

All the time I was in a clear state of mind. Observing. There was nowhere to go, no avoiding. There was numbness in and around my jaws, like after an anaesthetic. I'd had quite a few of those with the teeth extractions. There was bone pain in my face, jaws and up both sides of my head. There was nerves-pressed pain down from by my ears to my neck, and both arms affected. Pressure on the same nerves affected my vision for a while – saw everything double, horizontally. Two lampposts, two cars side by side. So not feeling at all safe out in the street. The skin at the top of my ears began to itch and peel off – a good sign, I thought, of something reaching the surface. There was numbness and tingling in my hands and arms, especially if lying on my back with arms stretched out.

I couldn't raise my arms above my head without severe increase of pain. I might stand in the Indian style of heart prayer position and begin to move the joined hands upwards. As I came to throat level I felt I could not go any further. Uncomfortable, as if I might topple over. I just could not go any higher. I read this to mean that I have to stay close to the ground and find healing in the heart area – physical as well as the held hurt in lower heart aspect – before I could see resolution in the jaw/face/head area. Such was my slow and painstaking journey towards finding a connection (reconnection) with the higher aspects – call it the higher self, the sacred, mediated by angelic forces and all that kind of thing.

Whether I could reach up turned out to be a reliable measure of a progressive sequence. As I became well I could reach right up and painlessly. This ease was not complete until the spring of 2011.

As it is with any illness, I was alone with it. Had loving support, but still alone – and taking a hard look at my issues around separation and connection. The times of feeling left, incubator after birth, sent to boarding school. A sense of un-connection with my father. The heart of the matter was a feeling of having been hurt by someone, others; and separated.

The most urgent example and central to my autumnal quest was the break down then breaking up of my connection with the mother of my daughter. This had occurred five years previously. She came out as a lesbian.

These days I was judging her, and by association all homosexual people as sick for being that way. I felt uncomfortable having these thoughts. I could not let go of them. For me it was like this: I had been hurt. I had held on to that hurt. These thoughts arose from that place of held hurt, as from a swamp. Now I was the one most suffering from the thoughts, my attitude, my held hurt. My thoughts and attitude were like a poison to me.

Later on, in Eckhart Tolle's book A New Earth *I found further understanding from his term 'pain body'. Pain body = Held hurt. It bolsters and is maintained by the ego. (I do have a big head!) Kingfishers and Kookaburras become associated with this remedy and they have large heads too.* *(See Part Three, Page 286.)*

The pivotal example of my reoccurring sequence happened on the day of the Pride parade in Brighton. In hindsight what took place that day was the crux of my quest for resolution that had begun nine months earlier.

I was living at the time in a flat overlooking Preston Park, which is used for the festivities of the day. I walked out into the park that morning. It was a phase of great pain, physical, and I felt equally pained by my toxic attitude – my judging and critical attitude to gays as a whole. Watching those people making the final preparations for the day simply heightened my troubled state.

I came back into my room. There were several hours of great discomfort, familiar by now. Then I said to myself, 'This has gone on long enough. I can't bear it anymore.' I pleaded for healing of this in me, weeping and completely at a loss.

Surrender

As I type this word (September 2011) my laptop has 'responded' by going into a red text colour and underlined! Weird. Nothing I do will get it back to the normal black, or clear the underline. I have to start a new document to reinstate ordinary black type.

A feeling of release began to soothe me and expand my heart area as the desperate tears waned.

By now the parade had arrived and was filling the park. Still a fresh atmosphere in the place. I decided to go out there again. I thought, 'I will look for signs of love and affection between these people.' Almost immediately, as I walked around I became warm, and wet-faced with heart-felt tears. A joy in what I saw, and such different tears. I came home again, hugely moved and relieved, pains dwindling too. A turning point. I slept like after a long trek, having arrived at this place.

Heart healing

At this time and until the following May I was treated homoeopathically by Martin Miles. He reckoned only Anadin as OK for me to take for the pains. I did this a few times, and then left off. It made a marginal difference. As far as my alcoholic and rather eccentric GP was concerned, I was an awkward customer for not taking his recommended antibiotic for my 'ear infection' as he called it. Slight heart murmur, congenital. Nothing to justify any further investigations.

Understandably family and friends were concerned. Some pressed me to take the antibiotic. I was in such a poorly state I reckoned that I would not do at all well on them. Instinct maybe. It was not until much later that I could justify my choice, in hindsight. I did know that there was more than an ear infection going on. The bad state of my teeth and gums had to be connected (if only to my mind) by proximity to jaw and ears. The GP did not concur. Anyway I had been told in no uncertain terms that I was not going to die from this. I knew that. A conviction and maybe courage too, which some saw as stubbornness. I was acting and choosing from a sure place. Is that courage?

Episode five – September equinox 2006 to Midsummer 2007
Gathering Clues

Made it to Italy for a week in September. Travelled still in constant pain. First break from pain while there, thanks to *Sulphur 200*.

With this change slowly other possibilities returned. Mid November I took on a few of my previous homoeopathy clients, and did some violin teaching. Still weariness and pain but not constant now. So, better sleep at night. I continued treatment with Martin Miles through to the spring, until he became ill. I remember talking of my Dad and how I thought what I had been dealing with was cancer, like he had. Martin said, 'You are probably right.' Not long after this he was no longer able to work himself.

At this time I began to self prescribe. *Symphytum* made a big difference to the bone pains. Then I read of its use in bone cancers. This contributed to a growing realization. And there was another clue – the possible link between earlier experiences of uncomfortable separation and cancer emerging later on. A client had spoken of an awful feeling of having to start at a new school after a family move. *Carcinosin* was a good remedy for her, at that time.

The strands were beginning to come together and make sense.

Bad gum disease affecting my heart, the toxic state contributing to developing cancer. I had no fear around cancer, not least because by now I was well past the time of greatest pain and debility.

Realization

June 2007

I went to visit Doctor Jim Runcie. He was an old family friend, ninety-five years old now, and living in Tain in the northeast of Scotland. As a doctor homoeopath he had been practicing for seventy years! He had been linked to the Glasgow and London Homoeopathic Faculties. For me, and since my childhood he was Uncle Jim. He had treated my parents and elder brother and sister since way back and continued for years sending packets of powders and pills in little white boxes to my mother.

I hadn't met up with him since I became involved in homoeopathy. Recently I felt drawn to visit him, to reconnect. Some curiosity about how he worked, and hoping to absorb something from being with him, by osmosis, I suppose. I had read that Tain had been a place of healing and pilgrimage in earlier times. So it was to be for me.

One night while I was there, the pain rising strong again, I 'asked' for information, inviting a message from one of my previously useful quartet of archangels. Suddenly it all clicked. In this place of pilgrimage and healing I was linked strongly to my parents and early childhood. All my experiences of loss of connection, separateness flooded my whole being, weeping through me.

Awareness and physical sensation meet

I now knew for sure that it was cancer that I was recovering from. Then it was that the pain in my left ear stopped. Just like that. Never returned. This in itself confirmed my realization.

'The truth always leads to peace.'
From *A Course in Miracles*

I had come to this place for healing. A pilgrim blessed.

Around this time news programmes would often talk of murderous acts, in Iraq for example. I had a vivid dream. I am an Iraqi fighter in a hot sandy desert type place. I am armed with a gun. There are others there, in similar combat gear, not civilians. I come through this doorway in a roofless ruin of a building. I let rip and shoot them dead. That pleased me. End of dream.

In connection with this dream I acknowledge that during this time of being very ill I had this thought – You all out there, you have treated me badly and pushed me away. So I would have you all dead. I want to destroy everyone. Like in the dream.

I was reminded of Martin Miles' writings about cancer. He makes an analogy with terrorist acts within a society:

> In a larger context than that of the individual, cancer can be seen to be a consequence of a malignant society and its morbid components. Remember, that what is true on one level is also true on other levels.
>
> The analogue within society can be seen with the many breakaway groups prevalent today. These may be self-interested to the point of no longer serving the society within which they exist. The extreme example is the terrorist group prepared to destroy to get its own way.
>
> The physical body and the higher vehicles of human expression work together to produce the peace and harmony of natural good health so rarely experienced by human beings today. A bodily organ works successfully by its component cells cooperating harmoniously. Weakness in one will in time put stress on others. The human body functions through the proper balance and working of its component organs. Society works by the cooperation of all its members.
>
> From *Homoeopathy and Human Evolution.* Martin Miles, Winter Press, 1992.

Symptoms connected with *Carcinosin,* a homoeopathic remedy associated with cancer and cancerous tendencies include the following:

> Morbid impulses. Fanaticism, extremism, bigotry. Cruelty, brutality, barbarity, inhumanity. Also mildness, gentleness, considerateness masking violence, and censorious, critical, condemning, rebuking. From *Carcinosin, A Compendium of References.* Compiled by RD Micklem. 1998.

I could see these all in myself. The presenting surface and the dark side.

The dark side is to be faced, acknowledged, to know what is there in the murky waters. As others have noticed, this brings benefits, and marked increase of energy. Paradoxically it serves to increase the good, and not by fighting the evil.

I am not my thoughts.

I have heard it said that while there are people on the planet being violent or destructive in any way, this represents the same tendencies in each of us. If I acknowledge and bring light into my own dark corners, two things follow and simultaneously – firstly I experience an enlivening increase of energy, secondly the whole organism of life on our planet is affected for the good, or so they say.

Added here in November 2011

Colonel Gaddafi has been hunted down and killed. This is the very day that I decide on a name for this book. Such a person mirrors to us our own darkest aspects.

In parallel with his eventual demise there have been wilful uprisings of passion and fire against restrictive authorities, and a consistent tendency towards the healing of hearts and long-held hurts. As this develops and spreads through the web of interconnected humanity there is less need for the overt and extreme mirror that he and the like provide to our dark side. So he is no longer with us. We need less of all that out there.

Episode six – Midsummer 2007 to Halloween 2010 Repair Work

Repair and restoration – of the physical as well as the inner aspects.

At first I thought – that's it. Made it. Realization and pain shifts. Now on a simple track of recovery. It was recovery but not that simple or speedy. After the midsummer realization I had the pieces of my jigsaw. Even so there was repair work to do. *Symphytum* was good if the jawbone pain came on, and I used *Thuja* from time to time. I could get on with things again, able to work etc. I had been through something and was now coming out the other side – a vehicle with a new motor.

July 31st. Appointment with an ENT specialist.

Told by him that there was nothing to see in my ears, except a slight inflammation of the eardrum, and excess wax. 'If it had been cancer,' he said, 'you would not have got better.' The conversation could go no further!

Still blocked Eustachian tubes. If only I could clear it like blowing my nose. My previous GP who had got annoyed with me for not taking antibiotics suggested that that was all I had to – 'Hold your nostrils and swallow. That will do the trick.' Clearly I was at some distance from mainstream medical wisdom.

> 'Follow your own path. Any other way is straying.'.
> From *Talking with Angels*

I did not see Martin my homoeopath again. Later I learnt that he had cancer. The date he died was 27.09.2007. Something in that run of numbers, I'm sure. He was valued by many, as a person and homoeopath. For me it was poignant that he had helped me at my most difficult times, even when he was unwell. So grateful.

The lesson to me from the time of his passing is 'Do your work in homoeopathy, but not in a way that kills you!' So during this time I began to make sure of this for myself. I decided on regular days for practising the violin and making music. I set a daily calling in hour for clients. Better for everyone. Also gardening, walking and meditation.

August 2007 onwards. Well back into work.

October 2007. A time of continuing improvement and working on collating the Amanita proving material.

Diary entries –

October 17th. Read through proving notes, some for the first time. After a while needed a break from this because of disoriented state coming on, also renewed pressure in left side of head. Felt a bit better and less disoriented after a short walk in nearby woods.

Forgetting things on gas cooker. Today I left a saucepan lid on a gas ring with a low flame – forgot to turn the gas fully off. And realized that in the past year I have been forgetful about pans or kettles in this way. On one occasion I left a kettle on so long that it melted completely and was in flames, the smoke alarm ringing. It was a gas cooker type kettle with a whistle, but I had not put the whistle on. This was the most extreme of my forgetful burning.

What did it mean or have to tell me? I came to recognise that the fire was misplaced. I should learn and allow myself to have it within me, the fire in the solar plexus, and then it would not be happening out there.

By evening: sensation of something stirring in one of my teeth – one that has still been giving me concern.

October 18th. *Two dreams. 1.* With my elder sisters (or certainly one of them) at a place – somewhat derelict, associated with my mother. It had the air of an untended allotment. There was a thick cloud of midge-sized flies. I looked and saw that they were coming from/breeding in an old torn piece of cheap blue synthetic carpet that was half rotting in a dug hole. It had been my mother's carpet. I said I would take it to a tip – to clear it away, thinking that that would stop the flies hanging out there. I was aware that the flies were doing their bit to clear up this old piece of rubbishy carpet – also that there were other things I was meaning to take to the tip. In fact I already had quite enough to deal with, but I was willing to take on this as well. It felt like it had to be done. It was important to clear it. *Compare my earlier dreams of dustcarts, before proving began, and clearing of old stuff coming up in the proving. Also quote no 497 in Part*

Six. Page 382.

I was not at all surprised that I felt the Amanita effects from re-engaging in the collation work. I wonder. Maybe it is working on the same lines as other external effects on me? EMF (Electromagnetic Frequencies) for example.

Dream 2. In a B and B breakfast room. Only me there. Grey, undecorated, unadorned walls, dull minimal and utilitarian furnishings – just tables and chairs – metal legs, Formica tops, dull grey-brown. Strange man (who runs the place) serving breakfast. White sliced bread (I associate this with childhood), pappy, sticking to roof of my mouth. Cup of tea – white Pyrex-type cup and saucer and he tried to clear it away before I was finished; I had turned my back and he was taking the tea – even trying it himself.

Shaving this morning – skin felt tougher, less likely to get cuts even with a new razor blade.

Morning. Generally feeling stronger and more settled than yesterday but also clearer and stronger than before the day of starting working on the proving.

Evening. Feel clear-headed, well-orientated, clear 'vision' of third eye centre. Have felt as if I am enlarged, full of steady energy and with more space for it. As if I am expanding in my energies to be who I can be – a definite physical sensation of this. Also more comfortable in left side of head. Still some rubber-like numbed muscle feeling there, but not painful. Lots of energy, and able to be very still. Not tired from what was a full day with a late night yesterday. Greasy skin on face, and hair getting greasy also. This I associate with the time when I was very unwell – again 'under the Amanita influence'. By bedtime the 'raw' sensation inside my left cheek had lessened considerably in extent – a quarter the area compared to recent days.

October 19th. This morning, at first, the raw inside cheek area was as extended as ever, then less again after an hour. Yesterday and still today I feel stronger and well co-ordinated – handling things well in every sense. I have not played my violin these last two days but I expect that my recent violin-playing aches and nerve-end discomforts would either not be there at all or else less in degree. Also, and from yesterday, a marked improvement in my recent tendency to a slight dribble after urinating. Bladder muscles feeling competent again.

October 22nd. Good energy consistently through the weekend. Able to sustain more activity than usual – cycling daily into town etc. No feeling of weariness in hands and fingers. Will test this today when I play the violin for a couple of hours.

October 23rd. Waking frequently in night. 4 a.m. awake for long time. Yesterday only slight discomforts from violin playing – perhaps 10% of how it had been recently.

Dream of extremely vertiginous – dramatic mountainous area, just where my home is (in dream). Think of throwing myself into a big drop – at first looking like I would not survive the fall, then seeing that there was a way down there by which I could return. Decide in any case not to go there. *Association: The Abyss in the Kabbalah.*

Today rawness sensations inside mouth subsiding. Less pressure within ears.

October 24th. *Dream* – Cycling as it gets dark – urban – familiar feeling (but not in real life) – stopped by policeman in a van re no lights on my bike, or so I thought. Expected an on-the-spot fine, but then I found I was next to a van that I had bought – or it was mine anyway – it was like a Land Rover. Somehow the policeman was more interested in this than giving me a fine. Others were looking at it saying – 'You've got a good van there.' It didn't look completely smart but it has a good engine and was otherwise in excellent condition mechanically. Could I get my bike into the van? Policeman and others thought I could and helped me find ways to do that. *Bicycle to van sequence – reminds me of what I have said since I began to feel better – 'It's as if I have a new motor.'*

Sleep – woke 12.30 and 4 a.m. but not awake for long at all – less wakeful than previous night. Violin playing yesterday pain-free.

Evening report – spent several hours today working on the Amanita proving and talking to provers and supervisors about it, their experience since April 2006, and possible connections with the proving. Effects: gain in clarity of mind and from this felt able to make significant steps in the collation process. Walked out on the Downs for an hour with a feeling of strong solar plexus energy – as if propelled vigorously by that energy when walking. Enjoyed being out in the northeast wind despite it being quite cold.

Able to eat sweet cake without any long-lasting adverse effects. For several years now and until recently I would avoid sweet things – my sleep would be affected by the stimulus.

October 25th. When I was awake after a dream I felt a discomfort in my rectum – as if a place of tension and blockage – the plug referred to in the remedy *Anacardium* perhaps. This sensation has become familiar from other times in the past eighteen months when I have been going through an Amanita phase, as I call it; those times when I have been affected by being around the medicine, i.e. prescribing it to clients, or during the proving. At such times, and last night too it would be painfully difficult to pass a stool.

I muse on blockages in my energies. I have a vasectomy. Maybe my teeth/ears/jaws and heart symptoms and the cancer, too, are all somehow related to this elected blockage in my body's natural flow? Martin Miles had advised me against having the operation. A big question.

It has been typical of the sequential influence of *Amanita rubescens* on me that an area needing attention would become as if highlighted, exposed and thoroughly seen in all its aspects. Nothing escapes its rigorous scrutiny – as if a light is being shone to expose these darkened places.

October 31st. Effects again set in motion by giving the remedy to a client. Also my association with this date, the date of first picking the mushroom to send it to the pharmacy, three years previously.

November 4th. Unsettled in myself and in stomach and intestines – not taking care of things – get chilled and eat foods that upset me when already unsettled. Tired.

November 5th. Clear out of bowels. Begin to feel better. Feeling of being ready for the start of a new phase. Solar plexus as important area of influence of this remedy. Aware of this. Giving a client the remedy has a further effect on me.

November 7th. Energy increase. Clarity of purpose and action. That night's sleep broken every one to one and a half hours. Lively mind and body – as if speeding. Heat in body. Heat < thinking of something of only minor importance I had forgotten to say to a client, but still feel extra hot from the guilt.

Question – Where can I best place this heat/energy in my body, safely?

Answer – In my heart. Heart centre, heart chakra.

I think of the wide spreading aspect of *Amanita rubescens.* Fill myself with this energy – as if 'all the energy of the universe, all of it, is looking to find its place within me.' Have to allow expansion to accommodate it. Expand the chest with the breath. Then the heat goes. I am able to settle and sleep. Wake refreshed in the morning despite reduced hours of sleep.

I have known for a long time that this is a remedy with the heart chakra as a primary zone.

(August 2011. This has grown for me – learning bit by bit what it is to become heart centred, consciously and literally; and the feeling connected, in tune, aligned with the matrix of energies, those larger 'out there' forces.)

↑ and ↓ meeting in the centre +

November 8th. More settled, grounded, solid than I felt yesterday evening. The next night waking again, another night of slices of sleep. Dreams of practical things being resolved/sorted out, also of meeting with a friend/musician colleague from whom I have become estranged. A situation still waiting for reconciliation.

Some minutes of complete immobilized heaviness on the bed as I had at the beginning soon after eating the mushroom. It is as if I have been landed/thrown down with some force on the horizontal, into the hold of gravity.

November 9th. Links/connections: Pranayama – circle of breathing in connection with heart centre, this remedy, and the cradling arm circle that one person made after taking it. Heart cradled by earth, and all attuned to the larger energies. *(See illustrations in Part Six.)*

November 10th. Return of super-clear nasal sinuses and clarity of thought.

Clearing. Cleansing.

March 2008

Met with the proving group at South Downs School, now their last year. Some couldn't be there, expecting their uncomfortable issues to get stirred up again if they came. Just a mention of Amanita would be enough to set things going. *(I still have to be wary of contacting them. Autumn 2011.)*

May 2008

Vipassana ten-day silent retreat. Pains still severe in jawbones. Numbness as well. Much benefit from this time.

September 2008

Concerned about general increase of pain, especially from ears down to neck on right side. Checked out by a bio-resonance practitioner. Cancer active. Time to do something intensive in a therapeutic way.

- Rigorous pro-alkaline diet. Did this for six months.
- Follow Ramakrishnan's Plussing Method for taking homoeopathic remedies.
- Bio-resonance treatments, and Rife machine.

Improvements begin, felt in symptomatic changes and confirmed monthly by the bio-resonance device.

March 2009

Now only marginal evidence of cancer – like a pre-cancerous state. Clearing. Keep going. Gradual re-introduction of some foods.

May 2006, now three years ago, was the most painful and critical month. Since then I had been repairing. Repairing the damage. I remained feeling much better in myself but there were still physical symptoms, as well as lurking toxic thoughts. As I understand it these serve as companions, reminders to keep me alert and aware of the remaining task.

Episode seven
Halloween, end of October 2010 to Candlemas, beginning of February 2011, and up to the present time.

Decide to focus my attention again on preparing the proving material for publication. The three darkest winter months.

Tuesday 26th October 2010. Nine days' diary. The effects on me, again, of re-engaging with the *Amanita rubescens* material.

Day 1. Voice lower, richer, deeper especially early evening.

Head and jaw pains << again. Waking up the places of toxicity remaining in the jaws and teeth.

Lot of bright eyed energy. Light-hearted feeling. Skipping energy. Heartbeat stronger, pulse faster?

Post-urine dribble <.

Warmer – whole body.

That night woke 3.15 – 5.15 a.m.

After peeing, less dribble.

Alert. Not at all sleepy. Have slept four and a half hours so far.

Sinuses clear, thoughts too.

Warm, evenly through whole body. Jaw and teeth >> compared with yesterday. Now more a smooth sensation, i.e. less differentiated pain/numbness areas.

Heart chakra – feeling of centre to it and vibrant. Like the pin and a whizzing Catherine wheel.

Hand numbness on lying with arms extended, palms up much

improved. Only fingers numb, not palm of hand. Athlete's foot lots better.

Day 2. Feeling warm, despite damp weather. Spirits undampened.

3.30 p.m. Lots of energy. Not sleepy, despite being awake last night. Calm and centred. Through day with lightness – no drudgery feeling/weariness. Singing 9 p.m. Strong and open.

That night. 3.20 a.m.

Feeling of very still and deep sleep.

Ears, especially left side, very liquid and mobile feeling. Loosening, opening. Warm general feeling. Less speedy buzz than twenty-four hours ago, but very good sensation overall – the settled side of the Amanita experience. Breathing as if at thymus gland. In breath clockwise, out breath anti-clockwise. Gentle now, not racing like previous night's Catherine wheel.

Day 3. Spoke to one of the provers, who had offered to help with the selection of rubrics. She had been observing things of spirals, breathing and universal energy in last two days. Influence restarting in parallel.

Lot of energy.

Coincidences: After Catherine wheel association (mother's name) to a Spencer Street in London (father's name), and passed by his school too, on the way to see a play. Kookaburra on the front of the programme for the play.

Day 4. And more: Australian woman staying, from eastern Australia. Same part as the home of the playwright of last night's play.

Day 6. Then, a change: nothing easy, can't decide what to do or feeling of too much to do, losing things, not focussed easily. Thrown by change of clocks/rhythm, also by reports of 'terrorist' attacks in Yemen. Fears of uncertainties. The opposite state to before the weekend. Then cleared and cleaned the flat. Felt necessary and better for it – connecting with the physical, and found some previously lost things.

Day 8. November 3rd · I'm informed that time is speeding up, by 30 %. The feeling I get in the following weeks and since is that things are going fast (faster than before?), and that there is a lot of energy available. Can do a lot, swiftly but not in any kind of hurry.

October 2011. Nobel prize for physics awarded to Saul Perlmutter, Brian P. Schmidt and Adam G. Riess for proving that the expansion of the universe is accelerating, not slowing as previously thought. Are these things connected?

Day 9. Spilling vase of water. WAKE UP! Frightened about changes going on in the world. Didn't work on the Amanita material yesterday. Lying with arm out – right arm numb again. Doubts about the work that I am doing. Self doubt. Things not working out.

Lost feeling. 'Stay with the feeling'. Very tired, so slept in the afternoon, and felt lively the rest of the day. Then – things working out well, and in unexpected ways.

Halloween 2010 to Candlemas, early February 2011
A parallel strand
Knowing by now the spreading, cleansing effect of the remedy I thought of a somewhat playful experiment. I was living in a shared family house at this time, along with two other lodgers. I was curious to see if my renewed working on the Amanita material would have any kind of synchronous impact on those I lived with. So I asked them to keep note of any changes during the coming three months, without saying what I was up to.

In February I checked in with them one by one, a general enquiry as well as questions along the lines of what I knew as Amanita states and symptoms.

Lodger 1. 'It's been a roller coaster – like life and death. A feeling that something has to change. Time of high energy then 'burnt out. Switching, like a plug is pulled.' Intuition shift – trusting more and a sense that she can 'tune in' anytime. Not needing to set time aside especially for this, in meditation for example. Links. Picking up on things happening elsewhere. Receivings of this kind all the time, dipping in and out. Turning up in friends' dreams. Speaking up for myself more about domestic issues in the house.

'In myself, the kept in fire is moving now. That has been the focus of my Tai Chi work these months. Previously blocked sacrum area is beginning to move. As if the blocked energy can go down though to the ground now.' I showed her the **Y** position. *(See Part Six Page 385.)* 'Doing this feels like being born upwards – brain petals opening.' Watery feeling in head. Woozy like seasickness. Forgetting things more than usual. Dental issues have come up.

More aware that her craving for sweet foods is connected to emotional tension. Food as protection, for feeling safe. Need to keep lower back warm. There was a sudden change to sleeping on a mattress on the floor. Safe there. Aware of need to protect throat area in the night. Links have been with her early childhood.

Overall a pulling in of my energy. Looking after myself. Stop running around doing this and that. Looking after others. Look after yourself.

Lodger 2. Nothing at all to report. Everyone else in the house spoke of something that matched the Amanita themes and issues. From knowing him, I deduced that held hurt in the lower heart, the need to speak out to release it, judging others who had hurt him; none of these applied to him. So no resonance, no effect.

The family members.

1. Sense of impending big change within myself, without knowing what it is. Have had abdominal and left shoulder tensions. Lying on the floor in an X-shaped position there is tension in my solar plexus, but without the acute adrenalin spurts that used to come on. Now there is a lower level of anxiety expressing itself. I have been judging myself for how I was bringing up my children in their teenage years.

Have felt tired and forgetful. Crowded in by what's going on. Fusing lights – unaccountable.

2. Noticed changes beginning in early November. Things spoken of that have needed to be cleared within the close family circle, and noticing the others doing that too. Reconciliation following. Clearing out old clothes and other things. Judging others – past hurts, and feeling bad about the judging thoughts. Need for protection – having to mind my back. Solar plexus – new sense of drive there. Creative will and passion. Craving sweet foods.

3. *(Recalled in January 2012.)* 'This period of time was very significant for me; it was emotionally turbulent and thus exhausting. Having always been of the firm belief that what I experience emotionally and what I experience physically are inextricably linked, it was no surprise that what I went through emotionally was directly affected or mirrored in both my physical energy and my surroundings. I live in a communal household and was aware, through both observation and direct interaction, that those around me were experiencing something equally as momentous. (If not similar then of equal significance.)

One of the most prominent things during this period of time was the amount of energy I had. Not necessarily a life-force energy, but an uncontrollable forceful energy that would leave me feeling burnt out and depleted. My physical awareness was such that I felt 'out of sync' with my own body. I found myself knocking things over, tripping up, and forgetting the proximity of things that I've been around for years. This is all coupled with the feeling of being out of control of my own body, having always been very self-aware. It was as if I couldn't physically contain the amount of energy I had, but it could quickly diminish to leave me feeling exhausted in every sense.

Another prominent experience of that period was the urgent need I felt to clear out and detox my mind and my immediate environment. I have the natural tendency to want to sort/organize or clear my surroundings when I feel a loss of control in any aspect of my life, but this was to a whole new degree. I not only felt a sense of panic and urgency to clear my emotional baggage, but I desperately needed to confront the issues I had within my relationships with my closest family and friends. Suddenly, things I had been avoiding addressing for years bubbled to the surface so strongly that it became impossible to ignore, and imperative to act on. This, coupled with the amount of panic and high energy I had, just fuelled my need for all of these issues to come to fruition; to have a mass clear-out of my relationships, my surroundings, my mind.

Through avoiding confrontation in the past, I had inevitably avoided reconciliation, but the desire to start afresh and detox far outweighed my fear of confrontation. This had never happened to me before, and although it was an uncomfortable time to go through, things were moving that had been static for a long time.

During all the turmoil of this time, I was so emotionally preoccupied and physically out of sync. I became very absent-minded. Yet again the routine that was so ingrained previously suddenly felt foreign and difficult. Simple things around the house made me feel like I was losing my mind. I could forget my house keys, leave the stove on, completely blank out arrangements I had made with friends. These might not seem out of the ordinary for anyone, but it is extremely out of character for me.

Throughout this period of time I also had vivid, confusing and extremely convincing dreams. Often they were so realistic that I would wake feeling like I hadn't slept at all, exhausted both mentally and physically, and always left with an uncomfortable lingering feeling. I think my desire to re-evaluate and clear out my life evoked these tiring and disorienting dreams. Often about my relationships with friends and family, and always involving me having to run and rush either away from something or toward it. There was often an acute sense of panic and anxiety to help someone. Whenever I awoke, the lingering feeling could trigger the need to contact the people I had dreamt about, so life-like were the dreams that I was convinced they needed me in reality.

During this time I felt very vulnerable and out of control of my mind and body, leaving me with a sense of helplessness. I'm a very independent person, sometimes obsessively, so this sudden want to find protection and comfort in others was new to me. Because it was a foreign feeling, I was unsure how to deal with it and it left me feeling very disconnected from those closest to me. Almost as if I isolated myself as a means of self-defence. When I could try to connect with the people closest to me I found that there was an unbelievable amount of confrontation going on from all angles. My dearest family and friends were calling on me to help put out emotional fires all over the place, but I felt so disconnected from them and myself that I didn't feel equipped to help. The amount of energy I had and the lack of rest meant that I felt incapable of distinguishing what I was feeling and what it was that I needed.

Since then I have felt more balanced and level-headed. There has not been any more of that roller coaster, hectic emotional time. Even things that have happened since then that seemed more monumental, emotionally disturbing and tiring haven't been because I have been more balanced about it. I feel more able and equipped to deal with things. Now, when there are emotional things to deal with I don't get the wired feeling I used to get, which became so intense during those three months. Then I would feel a turmoil and angst running through my body all the time, relentless and wired. Even if I was tired I could not get a break, so restless.'

Other parallels during these three months

- Mayan calendar insights. Time speeding up.
- Arab countries uprisings. Demonstrations in many other countries.

And later – Urban riots in England. Things long held in. Suppression and oppression of individual will in relation to a constraining force.

Fire. *(See Part Six.)*

Dictator. Repression.
Uprising. Demonstration.
Transition. Fire. Spring.
Open communication. Connecting individuals.

Review and Synthesis

May 2011
Nearly six years now since I crossed paths with this mushroom. I found something that I needed. Things began to change. About time. I'm a slow learner.

Transforming. Aligning.

A tentative growing in awareness, in evidence and experience of connectedness – the quantum effect, the matrix, the world = universal wide web, in the 'as above, so below', the six pointed Star of David. In the heart as centre, as the radiant sun is central in our galaxy. In the tuning of the diamonds, alignment with all that is. Tune in.

This is a curriculum of the present times, as this phase in the Mayan calendar might suggest. An alignment time – Earth in relation to the centre of the galaxy. Each being with a sense and recognition of place in relation to above and below, the heavens and the earth. Informing/transforming influences coming our way across the universe in the form of electromagnetic flares, space weather, winds of change: prompting, requiring, impelling an evolution.

Previous cusps of radical change are recorded in the polar ice cap records, with the evidence of contemporary electromagnetic influence.

Shifts. Transformations.

Clarification. Clean up time. Cleansing. Water cleanses. Purification. Fire purifies. Detox of body and mind. Clearing negativity. Toxic planet. Fungi serve by clearing ambient toxicity. Clear the held effects of past wounds. Speak out what has been held in for so long. Arab spring. Civil unrests. Eruptions with regained vital will. Awareness of what has become toxic, release and relief from the load.

Amanita rubescens, the remedy is a hard taskmaster. Gives no quarter, no hiding place. Shines a light on the darkest corners, to expose what is there. Time to face it. It has an effect just by naming it. Impact at a distance – via the web, the energetic matrix. Those students most deeply affected by the proving who would not come to the review session at the college, I wonder what has come to them by now of resolution and reconciliation.

It repeatedly brings things up from the dark place, below under the water, to the light of day – and to an extreme degree where surrender is the only way forward. This means it's not to be fixed, sorted, resolved, avoided with medicines, remedies or remedial strategies, meditative modes, breathing techniques, praying etc., however useful these may have been before. The requirement for me was to give these up. To give up. Is this what sacrifice means? Nothing will make a difference until I give over. 'Hands up!' I surrender.

Grace follows.

May 2011
The most recent phase.
Nearly five years since this fateful mushroom crossed my path. Impact. Can this be conveyed in words? I continue to be impressed by the potential of this remedy. Familiar by now, and still amazed. Resonant with it as I am – just to talk of it with others is enlivening, invigorating, healing for me.

Move in to house, chosen together with my cherished partner. Long awaited after previous rented places. I knew they were all short term, waiting for the right time.

Colin Griffith *(The New Materia Medica,* Watkins, 2007*)* suggests that bone cancers can be linked to not having a home. 'It always turns out to be representative of the loss of fundamental structure and security in the life of the patient.' I can vouch for that.

June 2011

A surprise – more to deal with

Tiring business moving house. Weary again. Sharp pricking pains on both sides of my tongue drew my attention. Felt swellings there. Checked and cancer showing again. Concern – when will I be through all of this? A sense of 'something radical has to change in me' before these cancers stop recurring. Still some judging of others and myself. Less now, but acutely aware when it happens – and don't like myself for it.

Amanita rubescens still supporting/obliging me to go into those places that need clearing, for the detoxification of mind and body. Took immediate steps to refine my diet. Checking all foods by dowsing. Drinking own urine over a period of three weeks. All for a few days, then mornings only. Tongue pricking sensations cleared within a week, energy gradually better. Again facing issues, needing my attention.

Midsummer 2011

I came across this question in the book *Sand and Foam* by Kahlil Gilbran: 'Is there a greater fault than being conscious of the other person's faults?' This stopped me sharply in my tracks. Deeply sobering.

A turning point/learning time when on a walking holiday on Arran, Scotland. This poem indicates this –

Rocks fall
stumbling blocks
path changed
changed me
–
Wise cracks!

I had been noticing my judging attitude again, not liking it, and separated from people by it. As if the people were getting in my way. We were on a path where there had been a disruptive rock fall. I was shaky after crossing the boulders, stepping across big gaps.

Then I saw the connection to me in everything and in everyone I came across. The hostel, the roads, the ferry, the bus service, the shops that we depended on – all there and maintained because others were there to use them. Even the rocks supported me. Interdependence. Much easier to be with others now. No judgments, no self-righteous swords.

Peace again

Less pain

From time to time during these years I would look at all the things in my home, imagining who had made them, when and where. I would consider the places where foods had grown or come from. All available for my use. The surrounding evidence of supportive connection. Also the connection to trees and plants via the oxygen/carbon dioxide exchange.

Gratitude

Healing trends

The dark places and thoughts of separation clearing bit by bit. Experience of interconnection emerges. Don't fight the evil, the dark. Increase the good. All kinds of getting in tune, aligned. Times of attentive breathing, noticing sensations, any blocks. To allow the flow of energy through the whole body.

Connecting with sun and moon motions. Moon cycles, tides, waking with the sunrise. Sleep – more in the darker winter months, less need for it in the summer.

Imaging the polarity of energies from the skies to the earth. The vibration, the frequency. Imagining being in tune with it. Tuning the diamonds. Linking this way to all sources of 'exterior' energy – like the train or tram or trolley bus with its arms overhead, linked to its necessary power supply. How could I ever be short of aliveness and good energy if I am truly and properly linked up, lined up, aligned?

There has been an alternating interplay between 'I'm alone in the world', judging others and a slowly emerging sense and experience of the interconnectedness of energies. I'm included, connected, in the loop.

These five years have seen me go into and through illness, with prolonged pain and weakness, not previously experienced. All accompanied and influenced by *Amanita rubescens*. This influence comes over as strong, and many other people have felt it; still it is difficult to describe. There is something elusive and boundary-less about it. Defying any exact description, it gets everywhere, it influences lives through the energetic matrices – the 'quantum' effect.

As I strive to complete the preparation of the material for publication I sense the parallel nature of the journey over these past five years: as I work on it, it works on me, to heal and grow.

October 2011

Symptoms continue to clear in my jaw. Not taken any homoeopathic remedies these last months. Exactly as I edge towards that state of all working as one, symptom-free, I find myself at one with everything out there. Non-duality settling in.

Calm Being Ease
In place Connection
Ready energy
Lots going on, and able to match the pace without any hurry
At one
Getting to be like the trolley buses of my London childhood, with its upraised connecting arms – on track below and connected above.
Aligned
Connected
More and more so

October 31st 2011

Anniversary (6 years) of first collecting the specimen of Amanita rubescens.

Tested by bio-resonance practitioner. No more indications of cancer.

11.11.11 Submit text to O-books. 90% completed now. Nice date.

18.11.11 Given a favourable contract. Blessed to be included. Honoured.

20.11.11 Delight and swift enthusiasm to be at this stage with the various remaining tasks.

21.11.11 Dream. I am on a bike with no right-hand brake cable. It is a basic bike with no trimmings – mudguards etc. just like the one I made up in my teens. I am my teenager with the youthful abandon and exhilaration of speed. I come sliding off from a hill slope path on to a fairly busy road in open country. Passing car has to avoid me, suddenly arriving. I realize I have to watch out for traffic.

I cycle along thinking to stop at the next town's bike shop to get a new brake cable put on. Location – not exact, but resonances of being near Newhaven. *That's where the settled home I had until 18 years ago was. In 2012 it will be sold and the proceeds divided – an eventual resolution coming before long now.*

First thing I come across at the roadside is a bag with two-inch plain metal nails in it, not brand new but not rusty either. Then a large straw bale falls on to a field on the right side of the road. It is charred from burning, smouldering. Soon after an outsize bull falls through the air to land next to the straw pile. It is also burnt and perhaps still burning? Still alive, I think. Its burning had come from the burning straw. The smell of the animal burning comes my way. I imagine what the smell would become if it was to carry on burning.

There are several people around looking on. I see a couple of farming men in dark green uniforms – the holders of convention and tradition with knowledge of what to do with the animal in such a situation. I talked about this with them, but there was no conclusive outcome or action taken. End of dream.

Associations with Amanita rubescens

Brakes missing on a bike. This time there is one good one but that meant that riding is somehow unbalanced between left and right sides. Teenage vital style and energy. Fire.

Qualities/stages represented.

Mineral – The metal nails, sourced from the earth and made with fire.

Plant – The straw, growing before, now cut and dried.

Animal – The bull.

Human

This reminds me of the writings in the book *Talking with Angels* by Gitta Mallasz. Einsiedeln, Switzerland 1998.

I quote from it. By permission of Daimon Verlag, publishers. Page 301.

The Seven Souls are your dwelling.
Your foot rests on the first.
Six enfold you from toe to head.
And the Seventh is your crown.
Each of the Seven Souls acts:
Truth *is*.
Love *grows*.
Rhythm and Harmony *move*.
New awareness *creates*.
Peace *reposes*.
Joy and bliss *radiate*.
The primal source is a great mystery.
Unspeakable, inexpressible ecstasy: fulfilment.

Then a few pages later: Page 304.

- The first level *of being is the MINERAL, the stone, the crystal. Its animating soul is the truth, the number and the law.*
- The second level *is the PLANT. Its soul is streaming love and the*

capacity to grow.

- The third level *is the ANIMAL, enlivened by harmony, movement and rhythm.*

These three levels are contained in the fourth, *the HUMAN. But we – the so-called humans – are still not the HUMAN. The Four.*

It is our task to live on the fourth level and become a conscious link between the created and the creating world.

- The fifth level *is that of the ANGELS, where peace and silence reign.*
- *On* the sixth level *dwells the SERAPH, with burning power and joy.*
- The seventh level *is the mysterious, the highest degree of all life.*

And a little further on: Page 305.

> *All of these forces join in the middle, on the fourth level. They unite and give birth to the new Child, which is God* and *human… Creator* and *created… Light* and *matter.*
>
> *But the first step towards this evolutionary* universal *accomplishment is to become conscious of your own* individual *task and live it. This is the only gateway leading to the Four and it is also the only one to which we ourselves have the key.*

22.11.11. Having this dream I considered it might be time to take a tablet of our remedy. I dowse. Yes – to take the 100 potency, one at bedtime, one in the morning.

I have another dream –

I am outside a motel type place, not homely. A parking area at night time. Deep dark sky and clouds. A strip of rainbow colours rises in a bright arc from the earth. Brilliant against the dark sky. Also up above in the sky fantastic coloured strands and shapes, reminding me of the colourful sea creatures I saw in a recent nature program. There were several of these, like light energies, showing themselves above me out from the dark background. Exquisite and exhilarating.

A few others are around but nobody I know. Alone. I wanted to see my partner there. Didn't know if she would come. Suddenly she ran in to where I was and we could be together under that sky. This has a joyous significance for me. New outcome. Arrival. Connection. Deep delight.

Next days, some strong sensations in my still repairing jaws. Energy up. Vital feeling. Working and playing well.

25.11.11. Accept publishing contract. Time to publish our findings.

21.12.11. A dream the night of the solstice. I am the observer watching two figures, one male, the other female. They are neither clothed nor naked. The man has a shiny sword. He is about to embed it into the chest of the woman. She will die, I think. 'No, no, no,' I shout out, and focus all my thought powers to prevent this happening. He approaches her, but just to make a precise nick in her lower lip with the tip of the sword. Blood starts to drip on to her chest. He leans forward to lick that blood, and at the same time she does not recoil from him, rather moves willingly to meet his approach.

Associations of vampires. Is that me sucking energy from others? including homoeopathy clients? Even readers of this book. Self-questioning and self-doubt. What greater fault is there than to know the faults of others? A sobering thought for me.

Then I considered the significance of how the female figure meets the male in the dream.

Cleared the self-doubt. Deep resolution.

I am reminded of the following section from the book *Heart*, 1932, 169:

> It happens that people are so savage of spirit that they can only live by condemning each other. This is not an inspection of

> another's armour with the view of helping; on the contrary, condemnation becomes the meaning of life. If one deprives such a condemner of his tongue, he will perish and wither like a plant without water... One can see in this condemnation a kind of obsessive vampirism, when the possession of more active vital fluids is needed to nourish the obsessed one.

Feel deeply blessed by this dream, coming at this stage. A dream of redemption.

Postscript. 20.01.2012. A dream. The night after submitting the 'final' manuscript.

I am in a place something like a railway station waiting area. I am there and my mother is too. We look down and see my father is slumped on the floor. Some talk of 'he's too heavy' to lift him from the floor. Couple of men around, like paramedics or nurses who might do this. I bend down to him. His face goes all white. He is dying. I hold him in my arms. Feel him die with my left hand on his belly.

Sense of completion, in relation to the book and my personal *Amanita rubescens* experience.

Part Three

The account of the test or 'proving' of *Amanita rubescens*. The second strand.

The provers describe their experiences. Also a record of the effects on their colleagues and others more remotely connected. In addition, a complete list of rubrics to assist prescribing.

Contents

- Proving Text with Rubrics interspersed
- Provers' reviews
- Supervisors' experiences
- Rubrics complete list, mainly for homoeopaths

Participant's ages and birthdates and potency taken.

	Provers		Potency	Supervisors.	
1)	33	06.04.72	30	49	07.04.56
2)	34	31.12.71	12	36	20.01.70
3)	35	24.09.70	6	46	20.12.59
4)	36	18.06.69	30	40	01.06.65
5)	26	29.08.79	12	31	22.07.74
6)	35	21.05.70	6	46	07.02.59
7)	41	07.05.64	30	36	22.08.71
8)	41	30.10.64	12	28	22.02.77
9)	35	05.08.70	6	43	11.11.62
10)	41	30.05.64	30	35	14.03.70

All involved were female apart from Prover 10

Proving Text Contents

General Features

Energy and temperature fluctuations. Libido.
Left and right sides

Modalities – time, environment

Direction of action of the medicine, and significant locations

Electric lights and switches, and analogies

Burning

Suddenness

Sensations of lightness

Feelings of constriction

'Spreading' or distant effect of the medicine. Coincidences. Dream Links. Telepathic (?) links. 'Journeying.'

Mental and Emotional States

Excitement and exhilaration, uncontrollable or inappropriate giggling. Pace. Emotional roller coaster.

Calm, relaxed, happy and secure, as if there are no time restraints. Calm in situations that are usually stressful. Mentally alert and clear thinking. Fastidious. Able to get on with things and show feelings.

Contrasted with Insecurity, self-conscious and with low confidence. Negativity and tearfulness. Depressed about health. Anxiety. Restlessness. Disorganized, unable to carry out tasks, clumsiness, bad writing and spelling errors. Forgetfulness, repetition of words. Difficulties concentrating. Irritability and wanting to be alone.

'My fault.' Judgments. Reconciliation within families.

Return of old symptoms. The need to sort out unresolved issues. Clearing out junk: 'yucky things'.

Teenage resonances

Claustrophobia

Body Parts and Functions

Head/Headaches/Vertigo/Light-headedness

Eyes + vision/nose + smells

Face

Mouth/Tongue/Teeth

Food and drink. Appetite and thirst. Effects of alcohol.

Stomach, nausea and feelings of intoxication. Abdomen and bowel movements.

Urine and bladder

Female

Throat/cough/breathing

Skin (and respiration – Prover 6)

Heart

Back, neck and shoulders

Extremities – limbs

Sleep
Dreams

Provers' Reviews (at the time and later on)
Supervisors' Reports during the Proving (and other parallel experiences)

Proving Text

You can make your own way through these records, either in the sequence of features or by using a Prover's number to pick out that person's particular experience, as it shows up in the different sections.

You will notice that parts of the text show up more than once. For example – Headaches at 2 p.m. will appear in the headache as well as the time modality sections. This is so that each headed section is complete in itself.

A = New symptoms, B = Familiar symptoms, C = Old symptoms returning.

General Features

Energy and temperature fluctuations. Libido.

1) *Seven days before the proving:* Feeling tired. Achy all over. Limbs feel heavy. Felt slightly nauseous. Appetite less than normal. Felt better about 7 p.m.

Two days before: Lots of energy. I feel more 'alive'. Giggly. Appetite normal now.

The day before: In the morning woke very awake, and energetic. This is very unlike me. Still high energy. I feel in great spirits; I feel I could do anything. Had irritable spell between 2–4 p.m. Snappy, especially towards family. Had to meet a friend, but felt worse from having to converse.

Felt better again in the evening.

Day 1. *The day the proving began.* 10.20 a.m. Hot flushes. Heat radiated from inside, lasting from a few seconds to a minute.(B) 12.30 p.m. Still hot flushes, waves of heat, all over but especially on my face. Face also very itchy.(B) 12.45 p.m. Took second (and final tablet). 12.50 p.m. Felt slightly light-headed, almost drunk feeling, straightaway.(A) Good spirits. Very giggly. Laughing at inappropriate moments e.g. when my husband was speaking about his work over lunch, I could not resist the urge to laugh!(A) 12.55 p.m. Eyes feel noticeably wide and big.(A) I wondered if it was a hallucinogenic remedy? 1 p.m. Again I have increased energy.(A) 2.15 p.m. Felt slightly headachy, for half an hour.(C) My energy slumped and I felt a bit tired. 5 p.m. Energy back again.(A) Loads of energy, abnormally so. I feel in good spirits.(A) Still have the hot flushes. Very cold feet, > warmth.(B)

Very warm all over. It feels lovely.(A) (Usually I am a very cold person.) Lots of energy, and mentally very calm.(A) No light-headedness or giggling today. I think, 'This is quite good fun.' My mind is not quite right: I have to think longer about things.

2 p.m. Heat in face again, twice. Waves of nausea and slight

dizziness.(A) Felt sick straight after lunch.(A) Still felt very warm, not a fever, just hot and a bit sweaty, especially in my armpits.(A) (I'm not usually a sweaty person at all.) I even went out on school run with just a cardigan and no coat. (A) 5.30 p.m. I had lots of energy all day again, quite steady, even with the nausea. 8.30 p.m. Still very warm all over.(A) (Day 2)

12 noon onwards. Lots of energy again.(A) Later: I've had loads of energy. I could keep going, but I've got to stop now. Night time: Went to bed – not tired at first. Read two pages of book and suddenly, like switching off a light, felt very tired.(A) My feet felt icy cold, > covering them with two blankets as well as wearing socks.(C) At night time, every night since taking the tablets, my feet get really cold. Within seconds they warm up once I am in bed – again like a light switch. Generally I'm cold all over, but since the proving began I'm warm, just a nice temperature. My feet have been cold, but just at night. No hot flushes today (Day 3).

Eyes: wide awake feeling again: and full of energy all morning.(A) I feel the best I've felt in a long time. I could do anything. *Supervisor's observation (they met up that day): Despite this aliveness she is sitting quite still with her hands clasped around her knees.*

2.20 p.m. No physical energy. Mentally want to get on with things, but physically can't.(C) Burnt out. Crave chocolate again.(C) Thirsty for water.(C) I have felt cold all day. Feet especially cold. 5.30 p.m. I found it was a real effort to think about household chores, for example cooking the dinner. I felt I just couldn't be bothered; I didn't feel I had the mental or physical energy to do it.(C) Although once I got started this improved. I had fluctuations of hot and cold.(B) (Day 4)

7.15 a.m. Felt I couldn't get out of bed. Feeling so tired physically and mentally.(A) 4.45 p.m. I'm a bit tired, haven't got as much energy. I'm not sure if the proving's effects are wearing off. Temperature: more warm than cold today. Feet have been fine so far. 8 p.m. Sweating once again – sweaty armpits (Day 5).

8 a.m. Felt really tired when I woke; I couldn't get out of bed, and

then all of a sudden my eyes felt really wide awake, even though they felt tired when I was in bed.(A) Again it's like flicking a switch. 3 p.m. Craving for a chocolate bar. Normally if I have sugar, within half an hour I'm tired, but I wasn't. It didn't affect me. 7 p.m. Temperature: not as cold, feeling a bit warmer than usual. Sweaty again, slightly, armpits and feet only (Day 6).

8 a.m. It was an effort to get up: it took a good ten minutes for my eyes to feel properly awake. I couldn't get up when the alarm went off – normally I'm straight up when the alarm goes off. I kept dropping back to sleep. 11.30 a.m. Feet cold today. 8 p.m. Sweatiness: none today (Day 7).

7 a.m. This morning when the alarm went off, I kept turning it off. I couldn't get up at all, I was really tired; I just wanted to go back to sleep.(A) 2 p.m. Had sweaty armpits (never normally sweaty) although I generally felt cold (Day 8).

7.30 a.m. Awoke feeling very awake. My eyes felt wide-awake.(A)

8 a.m. Very hungry. (Unusual for that time of day.) 8.30 a.m. Lots of energy. (Also unusual for that time of day.) 2 p.m. Feet cold.

9.50 p.m. My feet felt icy cold again, as they did throughout the afternoon. Around about the same time my face, especially my cheeks, felt hot and flushed again. Almost like being sunburnt – that kind of heat sensation (Day 9).

7.15 a.m. The alarm went off and I literally jumped out of bed. I sprang up and felt really wide-awake (including eyes).(A) 8 a.m. Again, and unusually, I felt hungry for breakfast. 10 a.m. I just want to get on and do something. My eyes feel wide-awake.(A) I wonder if I have picked up some energy from the proving co-ordinator. (I saw him two days ago.) 12–1 p.m. Loads of energy again.(A) 2 p.m. I had a hot flush in my face. I looked at it and it was quite red and at the same time I felt sweaty in the armpit area.(A) 6 p.m. Feet: icy cold again.(B) 8 p.m. My face felt really hot and flushed again.(A) 9.20 p.m. I had my warmest socks on my feet, but my feet felt as cold as ice – they were not cold to touch, except my toes.(B) I've been very chatty today, with quite a lot of energy.(A) (Day 10)

7.30 a.m. I jumped out of bed, my eyes feeling wide awake but my body felt tired.(A) 8 a.m. Feeling irritable generally. 8.30 a.m. Still feeling irritable because the housework needs doing again. My face looked tired.(A)

11 a.m. My right hand is really cold when using the computer keyboard.(A) Just the one hand, and one cold area. I am right-handed. This lasted approx half an hour. 5 p.m. I had lots of energy and felt like going for a walk; but I couldn't be bothered, or to do the housework etc. – I have an aversion to it at the moment.(C) 6.30 p.m. Throbbing toothache; two more Paracetamol.(C) 7.15 p.m. I felt hot in the face with the toothache, but otherwise my normal temperature. Feet normal, not icy cold (Day 11).

I woke up at 3 a.m. and had real problems getting back to sleep again. I kept clock-watching until about 5 a.m. I felt really wide-awake and could have got up.(A) 7.15 a.m. My eyes are very awake although my body is a bit tired and heavy.(A) 8 a.m. onwards. Lots of energy.(A) 9.30 a.m. Face felt hot and flushed.(A) 8 p.m. Feet icy cold again.(C) I was OK earlier, much better. 8.50 p.m. I still had hot face flushes intermittently (Day 12).

8 a.m. I felt really wide awake but very cold. I felt cold for most of the day.(B) (Day 14)

7 p.m. I had very cold feet today. They were literally icy cold, as if I had no socks on. I used a hot-water bottle to warm them up but it still took a good few minutes to warm up.(C) 8 p.m. I had a very cold body; I had to put on my dressing gown in bed, and have a hot-water bottle, but felt I had a cold coming (probably from getting a bit of a chill that day).(B) I felt very cold all day, but was outside much of the time.(C) (Day 15)

Midnight I went to bed, really cold, with a hot-water bottle.(C) (Day 16)

8 p.m. Very tired, especially eyes (Day 17).

Temperature: I have felt comfortable all day (Day 21).

Morning. I have had a temperature and frequent stools this morning, but my daughter has a bug too. With the flu-like virus, I felt my limbs, especially my legs, were achy, heavy. I had a bit of nausea and loss of appetite. My body heat has gone up today (could be the temperature). I've been warm all day. The cold hands and feet have stopped. I had a slight temperature, but nothing major. I was very, very tired. I didn't have any striking symptoms, but just generally felt horrible (Day 22).

Temperature? I'd say I'm a bit warmer than normal (Day 26).

I felt improved, but tired and lethargic and generally quite depressed.(C) Could still be post-viral (Day 27).

I was in almost a hot flush, babbling to the proving co-ordinator today. I told him half my life history (Day 29).

3.30 p.m. Tired. I could have nodded off. 5 p.m. More awake now, but feeling low (Day 30).

Temperature? A bit of both. Real hot and cold spells. More cold flushes – the cold starts in my hands, then a shiver goes all through me and my whole body feels cold. My feet have not been cold recently though. I had to stand by a radiator or put on an extra layer of clothing. I get that if I haven't eaten.(C) So I'm > eating (Day 34).

I felt I had no energy, was tired. Once I started the housework though, felt I could not stop and was being very fastidious (Day 36).

Felt fine all day (Day 40).

3) I've had two very mild hot flushes since taking the last tablet (Day 1).

I had a hot flush after taking the 6th tablet. The flushes have all been very mild and rise from the stomach upwards over the back of my head. I don't normally experience hot flushes. The onset was sudden, but the effect was not dramatic. There was a slight rise in body temperature, ascending to and affecting the area between breasts and face, and head. I was not aware of any observable rednesses or flushing of the skin, although the sensation was of being flushed. I was warm each time for about an hour. Whilst I was having the flush I felt emotionally calmer than I would have expected, and did not feel at all anxious about the flush. Afterwards

I felt quite normal (Day 2).

Got a sudden stomach-ache in the upper abdomen, in the centre just below my ribs, < pressure, < doubled-up, > stretching out. I also had a slight hot flush as the tummy pains started (Day 6).

Review: Since the proving began I have been sneezing two or three times a day, very mild sneezes that are actually quite pleasant! Also my libido has been a bit higher this week, but I'm wondering if that is just related to my menstrual cycle (Day 8).

Libido still higher than normal (Day 9).

4) *Six days before the proving:* Woke up approx 7.30 a.m. feeling physically exhausted. Lower back ache, period started last night. Libido is much higher. (It was very low over past few months.)

Five days before the proving: Awoke at 7.30 a.m. by my daughter, felt very irritable and tired. Went back to sleep, felt disorientated and muggy-headed on waking from a dream.

Dream: I was in a supervision class at college. My supervisor told me I needed to take *Phosphorus 200*. I took it, then I felt myself falling off my chair, a sinking sensation, I thought I'd fainted. I was aware of people around me, yet unable to move or open my eyes. I thought this must be the *Phosphorus* burned out state. It felt very real.

At around 2.20 p.m. Still feeling muggy-headed and tired despite having a normal night's sleep last night. I had to sleep for about three quarters of an hour.

Boyfriend came to see me this evening. Libido still high, but felt a bit detached from him (Day 1).

I got up around 11.45 a.m. to do housework, feeling dull-headed and tired (Day 4).

Tired again in the morning (Day 5).

I had some time to myself this morning and ended up sleeping for three more hours after waking up, when I only meant to have a catnap. I woke up approx 2 p.m. feeling muggy-headed (Day 9).

5) *Seven days before the proving:* I felt very 'alive', my body felt as if right into my stomach there was a tingling/moving sensation. I was very aware of my feet in my shoes and not being flat!

6) *During the week before the proving begins (remedies in the house at this stage)*: Loads of energy during this week.

Very tired in the evening (Day 4).

Very tired in the evening again (Day 5).

Generally I feel warmer in my body. *(It is January.)* (Day 6)

(Days 7 and 8) Feeling very tired in the evening. *(This is unusual for me.)*

7) I notice that other family members feel weary and rather tired – 'a bit flat'. My daughter speaks of feeling the way I look: 'tired and lethargic' (Day 1).

My daughter says she feels very tired, weepy and seems very lethargic (Day 4).

Awoke feeling parched and dehydrated with mouth dry. Drank two glasses of water. Unusual for me. Body feels limp and weary, > for drinking.(B) (Day 9)

8) 5 p.m. Very tired, lethargic want to lie down, but didn't. I haven't got time. Cleared the kitchen, energy started to flow again (Day 1).

Woke feeling very cold, despite the weather being very mild. I was OK once I got moving (Day 2).

Mentally/emotionally brighter but tired after sitting in at clinic all day. Felt shattered when got home. Went to feed horse; felt re-energized and lifted.

Supervisor's report: When I saw her today she seemed calmer than when I've seen her before. She looked well in herself. (Day 8)

Woke up feeling tired and still a little low. Went back to bed at 7 a.m. until 9.30 a.m. Felt better after. Started decisive action. Felt better for it (Day 17).

Chilly – had to have warm shower for ten minutes to get

warm.(C)

Slept quite well, woke 6 a.m. Went to do horse, felt OK (Day 19).

Came back home 7 a.m. Spent time lying on floor stroking the cat. Got stuff organized for college, and daughter to go to friends. Made breakfast for family. Feeling chilly (Day 22).

Evening: Felt very cold (Day 23).

Morning: Pins and needles in left arm despite not laying on it.

Evening: Cramp in both feet. Feet felt cold but when wrapped in duvet they cramped. Had to put feet in sink in hot water to relax the muscles (Day 24).

5.20 a.m. Woke up, came over very hot: I thought I was going to be sick. No period, so thought, 'Morning sickness – oh great!' Had diarrhoea instead, black liquid (Day 29).

9) *Four days before the proving*: 10 p.m. I had a sense of my spine concertina-ing down, slumped, no inner strength.

Period began. 9 a.m. Very grumpy and irritable, want my own space to get on with things. I feel trapped. Later that morning I felt great when I was able to do some lengths of swimming. 5 p.m. I feel stressed about getting everything done in the house so that I can work in the evening (Day 9).

I feel a lot lighter and happier today, with a clear head for studies. Decided to go for a swim, which was great. I felt very energized, breathing well despite not having swum more than twenty lengths for a long time, and was able to swim fifty lengths easily (Day 11).

This has been a good day, I feel brighter and lighter with more energy (Day 12).

11 a.m. to 1 p.m. Very sleepy, I'm finding it very difficult to study. 2.30 p.m. When swimming I felt physically very clear and fluid, with no aching in my shoulders/neck (Day 13).

I woke grumpy and tired, wanting my own space before having to deal with children. Snappy with them through breakfast. I feel like a terrible mother and feel exhausted (Day 14).

10) Very tired around 3 p.m. Possibly normal for me, but I felt it more so than usual. I slept for about one and a half hours (Day 1).

Felt physically and emotionally fine all day but very tired in the afternoon and slept on the train both into work and on the way back (Day 5).

Felt very tired in the afternoon (around 2–3 p.m.) and didn't get much done until about 4.30 p.m. (Day 9)

Broken night – woken in early hours by shouting in the street. Woke very tired in the morning. Productive day despite physical tiredness and pleased with my creativity (Day 13).

Rubrics

The rubrics for each section are presented, as is customary, with a key word first, then the rest of it as if back to front!

Examples:

Fear, falling of, walking when = fear of falling when walking.

Body, general, unattractive feels = Feels generally unattractive.

Water, drinking, as if one glass of seemed many = when she had drunk just one glass of water, she felt like she had drunk lots more than that!

Remember that they are compact, pithy, verbal signposts to help homoeopaths find a particular remedy. It's a Nineteenth Century equivalent to an Internet word search engine.

The Rubrics used and page numbers are as in Robin Murphy's Homeopathic Medical Repertory, 2003.

NR = New Rubric. These are needed to reflect new states and symptoms that have not appeared before in repertories. They represent many of the striking features of the remedy. They have been devised by myself and two of the provers, now homoeopaths.

Rubrics
Energy and Temperature Fluctuations
High Energy then Burnt Out
Libido

Chills

Beginning, in hand 294

Chilliness, body, night 295

Chilliness, body, perspiration, with 295

Chilliness, heat, alternating with NR

Chilliness, waking, on 296

Generals

Cold, body temperature 756

Cold, body temperature, low vital heat 756

Heat, alternating with chills 763

Heat, flushes of 763

Heat, flushes of, emotions from NR

Heat, flushes of, exertion from least 763

Heat, calmness, with NR

Heat, flushes of, perspiration, with 764

Heat, flushes of, pain, stomach with NR

Heat, flushes of, upwards 764

Heat, flushes of, upwards, from stomach to back of head NR

Heat, flushes of, waking, on NR

Warmth, desire for 801

Warmth, desire for warm clothing 801

Head

Heat, sensation 881

Heat, sensation, rising up, chest, from 883

Heat, sensation, occiput 884

Heat, sensation, occiput, flashes of 884

Vertigo

Intoxicated, as if 1882

Eyes

Open, eyelids, sensation as if wide 550

Enlargement, sensation 540

Enlargement, sensation, morning, on waking 540

Face

Heat 583

Heat, burning 584

Heat, cheeks 584

Heat, flashes 585

Heat, flashes, cold feet, with NR

Heat, flashes, itching, with NR

Heat, flashes, sunburn like NR

Heat, sudden 586

Heat, sensation of 585

Heat, toothache, with 586

Shoulders

Perspiration, axilla 631

Hands

Coldness, hands 828

Coldness, hands, right 828

Feet

Coldness, feet 608

Coldness, evening 608

Coldness, warm, become suddenly, after getting into bed NR

Coldness, hot, face, with 609

Coldness, icy, cold 609

Perspiration 626

Stomach

Nausea 1748

Nausea, vertigo, with 1755

Nausea, vertigo, during 1755

Food

Appetite, general, increased, hunger 725

Appetite, general, increased, hunger, waking, on 726

Chocolate, desires 732

Generals

Contradictory, and alternating states 757

Energized NR

Energized, exertion, by NR

Energized, exertion, mind, body exhausted with NR

Energy, lots of, anything feels possible NR

Energy, alternated, switch like NR

Energy, increased NR

Energy, decreased NR

Energy, decreased, no inner strength NR

Energy, high, waking, on NR

Energy, Kundalini, internal circulation, raising of NR

Energy, switches on, light switch, like NR

Female

Sexual, desire, increased 684

Generals

Weakness, Diarrhoea, from 804

Weakness sensation, rest, desire to NR

Weakness sensation, eating after 804

Weakness sensation, exertion amel. 805

Weariness, aching, with NR

Weariness, sensation 811

Weariness, sensation, evening 811

Weariness, waking, on 812

Mind

Exhaustion, mental 1323

Exhaustion, mental. Burnt out. NR

Exhaustion, mental. Burnt out, after a period of high energy. NR

Exhaustion, mental, waking, on 1324

Confidence, lacking, no self-esteem 1290

Alert, mentally 1265

Fastidious 1326

Fastidious, with desire to clear clutter NR

Housework, aversion to NR
Intoxication, sensation, as if 1356
Laughing 1363
Laughing, desire to 1363
Lively 1366
Positiveness 1381
Tranquillity 1416
Tranquillity, with lots of energy NR
Sleep
Sleepiness 1704
Sleepiness, sudden 1710
Sleepiness, sudden, like switching off a light NR
Waking, energy, with lots of, immediately NR
Waking, sudden 1717
Waking, sudden, as if flicking a switch NR

Left and right sides

As yet (August 2011) we have not seen a dominant side in the cases. However, the bringing together, connecting up aspect of the remedy may be reflected in one-sided symptoms. The rubrics are derived from only two provers' detailed symptoms and are included for completeness.

1) *Left side (mostly)* 8.30 p.m. Tickling in upper nose, as if I was going to sneeze, but didn't. It lasted for about five minutes. Then suddenly my left nostril started running clear 'water.' No sneezing.(A) 9.15 p.m. Had an itch on the left side of my head, and when I scratched it, it hurt like a burning sore. It remained sore and painful for a few minutes even after I stopped scratching it and even though there was nothing there.(A) The whole of the top of my head felt sore to touch, like it would if I'd brushed my hair too hard.(A) 11 p.m. I had a pain in my head, on the top of my head on the left side – quite an intense pain. I wondered if it could be related to my neck (referred pain).(A) (Day 6)

9.40 p.m. Severe itch on base of left foot, right in the centre.(A) This lasted for about one minute (Day 8).

10.50 p.m. Itchy inside left nostril, for a couple of minutes.(A) (Day 9)

1.45 p.m. I had a really itchy left eye again. (Nothing to see, not red; it just felt a bit sore.) Lasted for ten minutes.(B) (Day 10)

8.30 p.m. Very tired eyes, and I had a headache over my left eye area.(C) Didn't have it when I woke up (Day 13).

10 a.m. Itchy left eye, which was slightly sore, when rubbed for about five minutes, and slightly bloodshot (Day 17).

8 p.m. My arms and legs just ached and I had darting pains in all my limbs on the outside areas. (Not hands/feet.) I had exactly the same kind of pains in my arms and legs. It could have been referred pain from my back from sitting in a bad chair doing my homework. It lasted most of the evening, on and off (Day 18).

On waking I still had the pain in my left leg on waking (the same as the darting pain yesterday), but it wore off quickly. I'm very tired (but was up late). I was still feeling anxious/aware of heart flutterings. They've all stopped now I've finished my homework. 1 p.m. I started to get a headache, the one I get with my period. It was worse for moving around.(C) I did take two Nurofen (usually helped by *Belladonna 200*). 4.30 p.m. I still had the headache, with pain around the left eye area as usual. I was tired and irritable. I felt frustrated with everything – it felt like I was not getting anywhere.(C) (Day 19)

10.15 a.m. Itchy left eye again.(A) 2 p.m. I suddenly had a headache (left-sided) coming on again, but it only lasted about ten minutes. I often get a headache at the end of a period.(C) 7.30 p.m. I had that itch on my foot again, but the right foot this time.(A) (Day 20)

7.30 a.m. I had a pain in my right knee, on the left inner side, < bending knees, going up and down stairs. It lasted for an hour and then just went.(A) (Day 21)

9) I woke with a sore left eye; it feels as if I may be developing a sty on the lower lid. It feels as if there's an infection at the base of the eyelash (Day 3).

The sty has gone, and on my left forearm I have a spot that's slightly itchy and raised. It feels as if it is an infected pore. When I squeezed it clear pus came out. Actually feels like a hard lump under the skin. It's been coming up for two days (Day 6).

Rubrics
Left and right sides

Generals

Sides, left 787

Eyes

Itching, left NR

Feet

Itching, soles of, left NR

Itching, soles of, right NR

Head

Itching, scalp, left NR

Itching, scalp, left, painful NR

Headaches

Extending to, head pain, eyes, left 924

Forehead, extending to eyes, left NR

Forehead, extending to eyes, left, above 928

Left-sided headaches 936

Sharp, pain, vertex, left NR

Vertex, left NR

Knees

Pain, right, inner side NR

Pain, right, inner side, stairs agg. NR

Legs

Pain, walking, left leg NR

Nose

Discharge, watery, left 1507

Itching, nostril, left 1513

Modalities – time, environment
Time of day < 2–5 pm

1) *The day before the proving:* Still high energy. I feel in great spirits; I feel I could do anything. Had irritable spell between 2–4 p.m. Snappy, especially towards family. Had to meet a friend, but felt worse from having to converse. Felt better again in the evening.

First day: 1 p.m. Again I have increased energy.(A) 2.15 p.m. Felt slightly headachy, for half an hour.(C) My energy slumped and I felt a bit tired. 4 p.m. Tearful, all of a sudden, about a situation at my daughter's school. (Return of old symptom, which had cleared with a constitutional remedy in previous months.) Forgetful, for the second time today – went to my mother's house to collect some photos and left without them.(A) 5 p.m. Energy back again.(A) Loads of energy, abnormally so. I feel in good spirits.(A)

2 p.m. Heat in face again, twice. Waves of nausea and slight dizziness.(A) Felt sick straight after lunch.(A) Still felt very warm, not a fever, just hot and a bit sweaty, especially in my armpits. (I'm not usually a sweaty person at all.) I even went out on school run with just a cardigan and no coat.(A) Still nauseous throughout the afternoon, > sips of cold Diet Coke and < water.(A) I'm not sure if the nausea is caused by the remedy. My husband has an upset tummy, but hasn't felt sick. 5.30 p.m. I had lots of energy all day, quite steady, even with the nausea (Day 2).

Eyes: wide awake feeling again: and full of energy all morning.(A) I feel the best I've felt in a long time. I could do anything. 2.20 p.m. No physical energy. Mentally want to get on with things, but physically can't.(C) Burnt out. 5.30 p.m. I found it was a real effort to think about household chores, for example cooking the dinner. I felt I just couldn't be bothered; I didn't feel I had the mental or physical energy to do it.(C) Although once I got started this improved. 8 p.m. Generally I feel fine this evening, with no anxiety; just my eyes are tired and I'm generally tired.(B) (Day 4)

2 p.m. Felt suddenly slightly irritable.(B) My nose just suddenly

ran. Dripping from my left nostril like water. It came out of nowhere. Just an isolated event.(A) Suddenly felt very tired (Day 7).

Felt sad, low and sorry for myself most of the afternoon (Day 8).

2 p.m. My writing is terrible again this afternoon – I could barely read it (Day 9).

2 p.m. I was very tired. I could have gone to sleep.(B) 3 p.m. More awake, but I could nod off if I sat down.(B) 3.15 p.m. I felt almost withdrawn, worse for talking, for approx half an hour. I felt I'd be better for fresh air. I don't normally feel better for it, although I do like being out in the air.(A) (Day 17)

2 p.m. I suddenly had a headache (left-sided) coming on again, but it only lasted about ten minutes. I often get a headache at the end of a period (Day 20).

2) I felt nauseous from around 3 p.m. until after my dinner, four hours later. I'd had a spoonful of an oil supplement, which I do most days, and it kept repeating on me. I could taste it in my throat, which made me feel sick. I had no appetite and felt worse for the thought of food. Although I don't find the taste of the oil pleasant, it hasn't had this effect on me before (Day 3).

2 p.m. I had a piercing, throbbing, radiating pain on my left upper arm. It lasted approx five minutes (Day 14).

After lunch I had a feeling of extreme tiredness and irritability. I had cycled a few miles with my daughter on the back in the morning, which usually leaves me invigorated, but it left me feeling drained. I had no patience with my daughter for the rest of the day and found her hard to cope with – everything felt like a battle. The feeling remained for the rest of the day (Day 25).

4) *Eight days before the proving:* 1.50 p.m. Felt very dizzy after walking in rain, had to sit down on a chair when coming inside. Felt a bit spaced out.

Felt really dizzy approx 1.45 p.m. – 3 p.m. I felt sensitive to everyone's moods around me. As I walked down the street I imagined that some people were literally barging through my aura. I felt very dizzy at one stage in a large high street shop, a bit breathless approx 2.30 p.m. I thought I was going to pass out and kept knocking things off shelves as I turned around, with a slight spinning sensation in my head (Day 3).

5) I have realized that I ate meat (chicken) for the third time in two days (which I rarely do) and then had a really painful stomach-ache where I was bent double, from about 2 p.m. to 5 p.m. Then it passed (Day 3).

6) Heartburn rising to throat. *(Aggravation of a familiar symptom.)* (Day 1)

Raging heartburn, rising and felt in the throat, < swallowing (Day 3).

No heartburn (Day 4).

Heartburn, burning sensation rising up to the throat, < belching (Day 10).

Heartburn rising again. *(Consistently < 2 p.m.)* (Day 12)

10) Very tired around 3 p.m. Possibly normal for me, but I felt it more so than usual. I slept for about one and a half hours (Day 1).

Very sleepy around 3 p.m. again. This is not unusual for me at this time of year (I find the cold and dark difficult to tolerate) but this seems more extreme than usual (Day 3).

Felt physically and emotionally fine all day but very tired in the afternoon and slept on the train both into work and on the way back (Day 5).

Felt very tired in the afternoon (around 2–3 p.m.) and didn't get much done until about 4.30 p.m. (Day 9).

Sleepy again after lunch (Day 10).

Rubrics
Modalities
1/Time Of Day

Face

Heat, afternoon, 2 p.m. 584

Generals

Afternoon, agg. 750

Energized, amel., morning NR

Energy, decreased, agg 2 to 5 p.m. NR

Energy, increased, 5 p.m., from NR

Mind

Depression, afternoon 1308

Exhaustion, afternoon, 2 p.m. 1324

Irritable, afternoon, 2 to 4 p.m. NR

Weary, of life, afternoon 1418

Sleep

Sleepiness, afternoon, agg 2 till 4 p.m. 1704

Stomach

Nausea, afternoon 1748

Vertigo

Afternoon, agg 2 p.m. NR

2/Environment – > Fresh air > walking

1) 3.15 p.m. I felt almost withdrawn, worse for talking, for approx half an hour. I felt I'd be better for fresh air. I don't normally feel better for it, although I do like being out in the air.(A) (Day 17)

3) *(The 'grounding'? benefits of walking.)* I had to admit to feeling quite confused. I'm having to concentrate a lot harder on things I would normally find quite easy or would just say or do. I had to keep my mind really focussed on what I was trying to say. Also when a friend gave me directions to the café I was meeting her in yesterday, I found it really hard to grasp. I do feel confused. Concentrating was difficult in town today. I tried some boots on in a shoe shop and when the assistant asked if I needed help, I found it really hard to explain what I was doing or what I wanted. Aware that I was confused, I was trying to hide it; I didn't want people to notice that I was not 'quite right.' Once I realized that it may have been the proving tablet making me feel that way I was OK with it. I felt a bit lost – almost a childlike feeling, like a child trying to behave like an adult.

I walked around for a long time this afternoon and feel better and less confused tonight at home. Normal again, I think (Day 3).

I felt very nauseous on the train to London this morning. It came on about 8.30 a.m. and carried on until about 9 a.m. It gradually got worse while I was sitting still on the train but cleared and went completely when I got off the train and walked in the fresh air (Day 11).

5) My train journey home was seriously delayed and I became hugely claustrophobic and needing to get off the train. Obviously I didn't, but have never had such a problem with being stuck on a train before. I found the central heating unbearable and craved fresh air (Day 16).

I have been at home with my son who is unwell and again found the heating unbearable (Day 17).

Rubrics
Fresh Air

Environment – Fresh Air

Air, gen, indoor air, agg. 517

Air, gen, open air, outside amel. 517

Air, gen, open air, outside, desire for 518

Warm, warm, room, agg. 525

Mind

Confusion, walking, amel. 1293

Fear, claustrophobia, closed places, trains of 1328

Confusion, mental, walking, air, in open, amel. 1293

Walking, amel. 1417

One further modality – Throat constriction, > drinking water.

(See Prover 7's entry in Constriction section. Page 107.)

Direction of action of the medicine, and significant locations

1) I can almost feel the remedy working downwards through the body (Day 34).

3) I've had two very mild hot flushes since taking the last tablet (Day 1).

I had a hot flush after taking the 6th tablet. The flushes have all been very mild and rise from the stomach upwards over the back of my head. I don't normally experience hot flushes. The onset was sudden, but the effect was not dramatic. There was a slight rise in body temperature, ascending to and affecting the area between breasts and face, and head. I was not aware of any observable rednesses or flushing of the skin, although the sensation was of being flushed. I was warm each time for about an hour. Whilst I was having the flush I felt emotionally calmer than I would have expected, and did not feel at all anxious about the flush. Afterwards I felt quite normal (Day 2).

Got a sudden stomach-ache in the upper abdomen, in the centre just below my ribs, < pressure, < doubled-up, > stretching out. (I also had a slight hot flush as the tummy pains started.) Pains – twisting inside, gripping, quite sharp and a little bit nauseous. Intense for a couple of minutes, then easing off, and just slightly achy and nauseous after that. It comes in waves. The duration was from about 4.15 p.m. to 6.15 p.m. I also felt nauseous and had a rise in temperature with a feverish feeling, accompanying the pain. I felt panicky about the pains. I was worried something serious was wrong but this panic didn't last (Day 6).

(All her symptoms and the solar plexus location, as described in this section, are highly characteristic of the remedy. Ed.)

I've noticed two spots under the skin – one above each eyebrow, an unusual place for me to get spots. (The spots themselves are normal for me.) *(Later on, when reading through the co-ordinator's proving diary, he describes a pink spot at the 'third eye' point, a similar area to my unusual spot.)* (Day 7)

9) *Four days before the proving*: 9 p.m. I get a sense of hilarity about this remedy. Overwhelming laughter, bubbling up from my throat, irresistible need to laugh. I see this as the potential for this remedy. 10 p.m. I had a sense of my spine concertina-ing down, slumped, no inner strength.

Day 1 7.30 a.m. Took first tablet. I was very struck by the undertaking of what this may involve. I felt my mood sink. I was able to lie for half an hour and in this relaxed state. I suddenly felt the impact of the remedy. It was as if a light went through me from the top of my head down. I don't know if this is the impact of this remedy in particular or how remedies in general take effect on our systems.

I get a sense that this remedy affects the heart and sacral and crown chakras. The words amethyst and quartz come to mind, but I do not know about them for their possible relevance. I have a sense of calmness, love, and serenity (Day 11).

I'm stuck in old patterns and can't move on. I want to clear this state of stress and anxiety; I've had enough of it now. In the evening I did a latihan (spiritual practice) to try and break through this, clear the darkness. My latihan concerned my heart, about joy and love, the potential of how I could be in my heart. I'm aware of the lower heart with feelings of anger and frustration and my upper heart with a sense of lightness and love. There is a disconnection and I need to find a bridge (Day 14).

10) Persistent asthmatic cough most of the day, triggered by very cold air cycling to the station in the morning. It feels like a return of the chest infection treated homoeopathically prior to the proving. Maybe it is caused by my emotional state regarding my mother.

My sense of the proving is that it is bringing up old issues; so could it be bringing up old (physical) symptoms too? (Day 9)

Rubrics
Direction of Medicine/ Significant Locations

Back

Spine, inner strength, sinks down NR

Female

Sexual, desire increased 685

Generals

Energy, inner strength, sinks down NR

Heat, flushes of, upwards 764

Heat, flushes of, calmness with NR

Heat, sensations, rising up, chest, from NR

Sensations, direction, downward NR

Electric lights and switches, and analogies

1) When I went to bed, I felt wide-awake, as if my brain was over-stimulated. Then, all of a sudden, it was like a switch and I went tired, and soon went to sleep (Day 2).

I was standing in the kitchen and a light bulb flashed, a bit like lightning. It was like a lightning strike between three bulbs. The light bulbs didn't blow (Day 4).

Three light bulbs blew this morning when my daughter put the lights on (Day 5).

8 a.m. Felt really tired when I woke; I couldn't get out if bed, and then all of a sudden my eyes felt really wide awake, even though

they felt tired when I was in bed.(A) Again it's like flicking a switch. *Later on:* Lights keep flickering in different rooms (Day 6).

I put the light in the bathroom on, and the light flickered.(A) (Day 7)

No electrical things happening (Day 10).

9 p.m. The bathroom light has flickered a couple of times.(A) (Day 19)

Some of the lights went by themselves sometime through the morning. It was a fuse (Day 26).

The bathroom light still keeps flickering, and all of them went out in the kitchen yesterday (Day 31).

9) Feeling very low, but aware it's almost like flicking a switch and that I can be positive and happy. I keep having flashback memories to when I used to be anorexic, remembering exactly what I allowed myself to eat. Struggling to keep balanced as my husband has had enough of this (Day 29).

Rubrics
Electric Lights/ Switches

Environment

Light bulbs, flickering NR

Light bulbs, blow, suddenly NR

Mind

Depression, happiness, alternating, like a switch NR

Sleep

Sleepiness, sudden, like a switch NR

Sleep, Waking, sudden, like a switch NR

Burning

1) About five times this week, mainly in the daytime, I've smelled a burning smell. I didn't think much of it at the time. Always a burning smell, but different burning smells – sometimes it's like rubber burning. For example, I leant over to kiss my daughter and I thought I could smell burning.

9.15 p.m. Had an itch on the left side of my head, and when I scratched it, it hurt like a burning sore (Day 6).

Burning smells: none (Day 7).

No electrical things happening or burning smells (Day 10).

9 p.m. I smelt a burning smell when sitting in the lounge. I got up to look around but there was nothing. It lasted a few seconds. The bathroom light has flickered a couple of times.(A) (Day 19)

Rubrics
Burning

Nose

Smells, burning, something 1523

(Compare my accounts of burning things (Ed.) Page 48 and Case 7 Page 349.)

Suddenness

1) 12.45 p.m. Took second and final tablet.

12.50 p.m. Felt slightly light-headed, almost drunk feeling, straightaway.(A)

4 p.m. Tearful, all of a sudden, about a situation at my daughter's school (Day 1).

3.30 p.m. I felt suddenly fastidious so had the urge to keep tidying and cleaning,(A) to the point where I had to empty all the bins in the house, something that was normally done on a set day. I spent two hours doing my daughter's bedroom, and then began cleaning round the bathroom sink with a toothbrush. Usually I'd let it wait. *That night:* when I went to bed, I felt wide-awake, as if my brain was over-stimulated. Then, all of a sudden, it was like a switch and I felt tired, and soon went to sleep (Day 2).

10 a.m. I feel a lot more tired, all of a sudden, and slightly irritable. 8.45 p.m. Three times within the space of an hour I had a

sudden quick sharp pain in my right abdomen, perhaps the ovary area.(B) It came on just like a switch. (I have an ovarian cyst but on the left side.) Feelings of anxiety (B) throughout the evening, as if fight or flight reflex. Went to bed – not tired at first. Read two pages of book and suddenly, like switching off a light, felt very tired.(A) My feet felt icy cold, > covering them with two blankets as well as wearing socks.(C) At night time, every night since taking the tablets, my feet get really cold. Within seconds they warm up once I am in bed – again like a light switch. I'm normally cold all over, but since the proving began I'm warm, just a nice temperature. My feet have been cold, but just at night.

Perhaps less forgetful? But then I suddenly couldn't remember if I had phoned my mother or not; I'm still getting my words jumbled, but my head feels clearer about everything. I feel like I can achieve anything (Day 3).

7.45 p.m. A constant high pitched sound in my left ear, it lasted for about half a minute.(A) It was very irritating and annoying. I was standing in the kitchen and a light bulb flashed, a bit like lightening. It was like a lightening strike between three bulbs. The light bulbs didn't blow.

11 p.m. Period-like pains. (My period isn't due for two weeks.) In lower abdomen and an achy lower back, > lying down and > passing wind.(B) It came on suddenly and lasted until I went to sleep (Day 4).

Three light bulbs blew this morning when my daughter put the lights on (Day 5).

8 a.m. Felt really tired when I woke; I couldn't get out of bed, and then all of a sudden my eyes felt really wide awake, even though they felt tired when I was in bed.(A) Again it's like flicking a switch. 8.30 p.m. Tickling in upper nose, as if I was going to sneeze, but didn't. It lasted for about five minutes. Then suddenly my left nostril started running clear 'water.' No sneezing.(A) (Day 6)

2 p.m. Felt suddenly slightly irritable.(B) My nose just suddenly ran. Dripping from my left nostril like water. It came out of

nowhere. Just an isolated event.(A) Suddenly felt very tired.(A) 10.35 p.m. I suddenly had a craving for tandoori chicken or Indian food of some kind.(A) (Day 7)

6 p.m. Itchy shins, it drove me mad. It came on so suddenly. It was like a burning itch (Day 8).

9.20 a.m. I suddenly had real cramping tummy pains – I thought I was going to have diarrhoea but didn't. They were like burning pains. I got goose bumps and felt slightly nauseous.(C) (Day 12)

1 p.m. I had a couple of palpitations, and my period started today. But it was unusual. I have been tired and irritable, but my mood was better instantly, rather than in a few days of period starting as it normally is (Day 17).

2 p.m. I suddenly had a headache (left-sided) coming on again, but it only lasted about ten minutes. I often get a headache at the end of a period (Day 20).

Afternoon: I had an itchy tummy (like I'd been bitten). It was under the rib cage, centrally. It just stopped suddenly – it had been intermittent during the afternoon. There was nothing to see.(A) All of a sudden the period came back on today but had gone again when I got home from college (Day 21).

The bathroom light still keeps flickering, and all of them went out in the kitchen yesterday (Day 31).

3) I had a hot flush after taking the 6th tablet. The flushes have all been very mild and rise from the stomach upwards over the back of my head. I don't normally experience hot flushes. The onset was sudden, but the effect was not dramatic. I was warm each time for about an hour. Whilst I was having the flush I felt emotionally calmer than I would have expected, and did not feel at all anxious about the flush. Afterwards I felt quite normal (Day 2).

Got a sudden stomach-ache in the upper abdomen, in the centre just below my ribs, < pressure, < doubled-up, > stretching out. (I also had a slight hot flush as the tummy pains started.) Pains – twisting inside, gripping, quite sharp and a little bit nauseous. Intense for a couple of minutes, then easing off, and just slightly achy and nauseous after that. It comes in waves. The duration was from about 4.15 p.m. to 6.15 p.m. I also felt nauseous and had a rise in temperature with a feverish feeling, accompanying the pain. I felt panicky about the pains. I was worried something serious was wrong but this panic didn't last (Day 6). (This is a return of old symptoms.)

(See also her review Page 250 and its description of the sudden change after hearing a radio programme.)

8) *College group meeting day.* Felt a little low at college, mind going over prior day. I guess it is normal to feel a little sad at ousting a family member. Sad because they were not there to support me, never had been and always had their own agenda. By the time we got to the proving group session I felt totally OK about it. Cried when telling of my symptoms in class because it feels like I have got postnatal depression all over again. Relived it at that moment. OK after. Diet – very bad today. Trapped wind this afternoon; > farting. Hubby had made tea when got home which was great. He is very supportive of me at college now. Played with daughter and had fun. 8 p.m. Suddenly very tired. Daughter won't go to bed, but dealt with it without getting cross with her. Went to bed early myself as very tired (Day 22).

9) 7.30 a.m. Took first tablet. I was very struck by the undertaking of what this may involve. I felt my mood sink. I was able to lie for half an hour and in this relaxed state. I suddenly felt the impact of the remedy. It was as if a light went through me from the top of my head down. I don't know if this is the impact of this remedy in particular or how remedies in general take effect on our systems (Day 1).

7.30 a.m. Left eye suddenly bleary, opaque white discharge in the corner of the eye. Not itchy, slightly red (Day 7).

Feeling very low, but aware it's almost like flicking a switch and that I can be positive and happy (Day 29).

Rubrics
Suddenness

Environment

Light bulbs, blow NR

Feet

Coldness, feet, warm, sudden, like a switch NR

Female

Pain, uterus, sudden NR

Menses, stops and starts, sudden NR

Generals

Heat, flushes of, sudden NR

Headaches

Sudden pains NR

Hearing

Noises, shrill sound, sudden NR

Mind

Crying, sudden NR

Depression, alternating with happiness, sudden NR

Exhaustion, sudden NR

Suddenness, behaviour in NR

Suddenness, emotions NR

Suddenness, physical ailments NR

Nose

Coryza, watery discharge, sudden NR

Skin

Itching, sudden NR

Itching, stops suddenly NR

Stomach

Cramping, sudden NR

Sleep

Waking, sudden, like a switch NR

Other miscellaneous symptoms

To Do With Cancer

1) 8.30 a.m. Funny ache in right breast/chest area – like a muscular nagging ache.(C) I thought, irrationally, that it was breast cancer. I had the same thought some years ago. That night I had a vivid dream: I used to have a phobia of cancer. I was at a hospital or a huge doctor's surgery and I was told that I had been diagnosed with cancer of the teardrops! Bizarre.(A) (Day 2)

Popping, Tapping Sensations

1) 7.30 p.m. I had a 'popping, tapping' sensation under my right ribcage.(A) It lasted for about half a minute. Then, two hours later, the same sensation, this time on my left side at the back. (Supervisor's experience: *I had similar sensations shortly before and after my prover's second lot!)* (Day 3)

Rubrics

Generals

Tapping sensation NR

Popping sensation NR

Broody

1) 11.30 a.m. I felt really wide-awake.(A) Felt in good spirits – happy.(A) I'm feeling broody; I keep noticing babies.(B) I do go through bouts of this, but haven't for six to eight months. I found myself weighing up the positives and negatives about having another baby and even talking about it with my husband (Day 7).

Cigarettes

1) One thing I have noticed in the last few days, because I smoke, I haven't fancied a cigarette and when I do I get a horrible taste afterwards.(A) I imagine it is like a sulphur taste (Day 12).

Sensitivity

4) I felt sensitive to everyone's moods around me. As I walked down the street I imagined that some people were literally barging through my aura (Day 3).

I felt extremely sensitive to people's moods. I feel as though I can tell what people are feeling inside. Strangers appear to be talking to me a lot on the street and in the park (Day 6).

Rubrics
Sensitivity

Generals

Sensitive, energy field of others, to NR

Mind

Awareness, heightened 1281

Impressionable 1350

Sensitive 1393

Sensitive, mental impressions, to 1394

Sensitive, external impressions, to 1394

Sensitive, moods of others, to the 1394

Sensitive, sensual impressions, to 1395

Fingers Crossed

4) I've not remembered to note it before but over the past couple of weeks I've fallen asleep with my fingers crossed together, joining my hands, usually above my head. It felt relaxing to stretch the fingers while crossed or linked as well. This has happened about four or five times (Day 11).

Soul-Body Alignment

9) 7.30 a.m. Took first tablet. I was very struck by the undertaking of what this may involve. I felt my mood sink. I was able to lie for half an hour and in this relaxed state, I suddenly felt the impact of the remedy. It was as if a light went through me from the top of my head down. I don't know if this is the impact of this remedy in particular or how remedies in general take effect on our systems (Day 1).

8.30 p.m. During latihan (a spiritual exercise) I felt as if my soul was completely within my body, determining every movement which was graceful, and holding me upright, so I was unaware of the physical weight of my body (Day 3).

Kookaburras and Kingfishers

9) Woke with a dream: 1. I saw two birds in a niche in the wall. They were soft, grey, black and white with long beaks. I didn't know what they were at first and then suddenly realized they were kookaburras. They were sitting together, looking down on myself and others (Day 38).

I searched on the Internet to find out what the kookaburra bird symbolizes. On Australian Bird Essences site: *'Giving expression to all parts of the self, saying what needs to be said. Unblocks the throat chakra, ease congestion from stuffing your feelings.'*

Kingfisher/Kookaburra's Wisdom Includes:

- *Connection to peaceful seas*
- *Happiness and love*
- *Peace*

- *Indifference to surroundings*
- *Clear vision through emotional waters*
- *Ability to dive (focus) into emotional waters and catch one's dreams. (Further references to Kingfishers – Supervisor of Prover 8, and my account. Ed. Pages 284 and 18.)*

Dangers and vulnerability

10) Cycling to and from work I had unusual feelings of vulnerability. More aware of the inherent danger than normal, as if I could see myself from a remote viewpoint. I realize this has been happening quite a lot recently. Maybe part of a general change of perception (Day 13).

Rubrics

Mind

Sensitive, sensual impressions, to 1395
Awareness, heightened 1281
Fear, danger, of impending 1328,
Vulnerable, feels 1417

Sensations of lightness

7) Went swimming and felt a real sense of lightness in the water. On reflection this was akin to lightness in the head that I had felt yesterday.(A) (Day 2)

9) 8.30 p.m. During latihan (a spiritual exercise) I felt as if my soul was completely within my body, determining every movement which was graceful, and holding me upright, so I was unaware of the physical weight of my body (Day 3).

Rubrics
Sensations: Lightness

General

Lightness, sensation 767

Delusions

Floating in air 367

Body, general, lighter than air 362

Feelings of constriction

(See also claustrophobia section, Page 169.)

7) Dose 1. Throat dry > drinking water.(B) 7.40 p.m. Unusual feeling in throat; not a sore throat but more a constriction, as if the throat was closing up, > drinking water.(A) I felt a bit panicky; this feeling subsided after a while (Day 1).

7.30 a.m. Dose 4. Throat constriction still present.(A) Feel really thirsty and a little dehydrated with it, > drinking water.(B) (Day 2)

As a result of the proving discussion I realized that I have suffered from sore, restricted throat sensation intermittently during the last month, > drinking water (Day 22).

Throat constricted, > drinking water; also feeling wobbly emotionally (Day 25).

Anxious about intended meeting so rang a friend for emotional support and felt she was not able to give it. Feeling rather angry with my friend as if this has thrown into relief my issues over friendship. Is this an old issue which has never been confronted? Almost feel that this is the last straw if she does not come to the meeting. Feel rather angry and irritable and feel that this mood has descended since the college weekend.(B) (Day 26)

I dreaded the meeting this afternoon. However, my friend came and was very supportive. She seems to have responded to the plea for support. The meeting was difficult and potentially very conflictual, and I was worried beforehand that I was angry and might explode, but I managed to release this anger in a measured and assertive way.(B) On reflection, I feel as if a weight has been lifted from my shoulders (Day 27).

Still very dry mouth (Day 32).

No further report of the sensation of constriction in her throat after Day 24. Ed.

Rubrics
Constriction

Generals

Constriction, sensation, internal 757

Throat

Constriction, throat, external 1818

Constriction, throat, external, water, drinking amel. NR

'Spreading' or distant effect of the medicine. Coincidences. Dream links. Telepathic (?) links. 'Journeying'.

Supervisors' experiences (Pages 261 to 291) reflect the group dynamic of provings. The wide spreading impact is particularly characteristic of this remedy.

1) 7.30 p.m. I had a 'popping, tapping' sensation under my right ribcage.(A) It lasted for about half a minute. Then, two hours later, the same sensation, this time on my left side at the back. (Day 3)

(Supervisor's experience: *I had similar sensations shortly before and after my prover's second lot!)*

Perhaps less forgetful? but then I suddenly couldn't remember if I had phoned my mother or no. *(Parallel effects) – My husband ran a bath then forgot to have it.*

2.15 p.m. Couldn't remember a friend's phone number whom I call regularly, and the same thing had happened to her that morning apparently.(A) *Later that day*: a couple of times I noticed that my eldest daughter was about to speak and then forgot what she was about to say. She never did remember it.(A) (Day 4)

10 a.m. I just want to get on and do something. My eyes feel wide-

awake.(A) I wonder if I have picked up some energy from the proving co-ordinator. (I saw him two days ago.) *Supervisor's comments: We've both noticed we can't get our homework done. We've got lots of notes on separate pieces of paper, but just can't get on with it. We feel disorganized.(A) Early on in my conversation with my prover on the phone I couldn't stop giggling, despite her telling me fairly serious symptoms. It just welled up from nowhere when she started to speak – I'm doing it again now even though I'm off of the phone. Uncontrollable giggling. She was giggly too, but less than me.* (Day 10)

My daughter complained of an itchy left foot, in the arch underneath (Day 14).

2) *This prover had many 'coincidental' experiences.*

Six days before the proving. When Stuart, the proving co-ordinator was talking, I was thinking of *Lycopodium* (as an example of a remedy to note as having previously benefited from) and then he said it.

Four days before the proving. As I was strapping my daughter into the car seat, I realized I felt hungry and decided I would get an oat cake from my bag to eat after I'd strapped her in. She immediately said, 'Mummy, can I have an oat cake?'

Also: I borrowed a catalogue from a neighbour (also a student in my class) three months ago and had finally made arrangements with her to order something. As we were meeting this evening, she was to bring with her a list of items she wanted me to order for her along with my order. When we met, she had the new catalogue with her that had arrived in the post that morning, meaning that the products would have changed. The timing of this seemed a coincidence, since I'd had the catalogue for so long.

Having dreamt of chocolate money last night, my daughter offered me pretend chocolate money half an hour after I got up (Day 1).

My partner was telling me about a compass he had that might help me with a college assignment, but he had no idea where it was.

Several hours later in the day he saw a tin in the spare room, wondered what was in it and there was the compass! (Day 5)

During breakfast, my partner told me the name of the road where his brother's workshop is. That triggered my memory of a dream I'd had the night before, where I was his brother and I was ordering something by phone to be delivered to the workshop. I have the address as Unit 23… (can't remember the rest). This wasn't the real address, but strange I should have dreamt that and then it be mentioned (we don't see much of him either).

Later: My partner, daughter and I were on our way to the supermarket. As we passed the health food shop, I thought about getting some ice cream from there. Then my partner said, 'Shall we pop in there on the way home?' and our daughter asked, 'Why does ice cream melt?' My partner subsequently told me that he had thought of buying ice cream on the way home, otherwise it would melt. All three of us were tuned into the same thought, even though my daughter doesn't know that we intended to get ice cream or even where we buy it (Day 8).

During dinner, my partner told me that the main ingredient he'd used to flavour the curry was tamarind. He then went on to say that it tasted quite strongly of citrus and if you didn't know it was tamarind, you could easily think it contained lots of lemon or lime juice. Later on, watching a cookery program, the chef said this recipe usually contained tamarind, but as he didn't have any, he was substituting with lemons (Day 11).

Whilst pouring cornflakes for myself and my daughter, I noticed we were running low and thought I might buy Rice Puffs if we ran out before the next purchase from the food co-op scheme I'm involved in. We haven't had Rice Puffs for about six months (since being in the co-op). When we sat down to eat, my daughter said, 'Mummy, do Rice Puffs have eyes?' and then 'Can we have Rice Puffs?'

Whilst talking to a friend on the phone, my daughter was climbing all over me, making a lot of noise and generally making a nuisance of herself. I apologized to my friend who said she understands. She said, 'You wouldn't believe the things my kids ask me for when I'm on the phone. They know I'll say yes just so they'll leave me alone.' When my supervisor came for her weekly visit, I told her I'd had a difficult day with my daughter and I mentioned her behaviour when I was on the phone. She said almost exactly the same about kids asking for things they know you would normally say no to because they know you're distracted and will say yes (Day 13).

One of my classmates from college rang to discuss some homework. She also told me that she'd been having ideas about what the remedy might be and said that grasshopper kept coming into her head. Then she suddenly exclaimed that as she'd said 'grasshopper', one had appeared on TV!!

At lunchtime, my partner asked if I remember the lions of Longleat from the 1970s, a popular destination for children to go on visits. I had never heard of it before. When my daughter came back with her grandparents four hours later, her grandfather told us as soon as they got in the door that they had just been telling her about the lions of Longleat on the drive home (Day 14).

When speaking to my supervisor in the evening, I mentioned that my partner and I had just scoffed a whole box of Maltesers. Half an hour later, I got a message from her saying that her partner had just come back from the shops with a box of Maltesers! (Day 16)

Whilst visiting a friend, she mentioned a mutual friend and asked if she was still in Spain (where she'd been for several months). I said as far as I knew she was. An hour and a half later, as I drove into the car park at home, I saw the mutual friend, having no idea that she was back (Day 17).

I slept heavily and can only remember one snippet of a dream. I was talking to some people from college and said my/our experience was mainly related to coincidences. They said theirs was mainly about sarcasm! (Day 18)

3) *Four days before the proving:* I dreamed that I was talking to the detective sergeant who is investigating the robbery that I walked in on at my ex-partner's house. In the dream he sat me next to the criminal who they'd caught. I knew it was him, and confirmed this to the detective (but it didn't look like the burglar I saw in real life). I remember feeling worried that this guy had seen me identify him to the police.

Three days before the proving: Today I got an unexpected phone call from the police requesting I do a photo fit on the man I saw in the burglary. (This is real life not a dream!) I thought it coincidental that I had dreamed about that the night before.

I didn't think to write this down, but when my supervisor asked if I had felt nauseous at all, I thought, 'How did she know?' I said that I had but that it was so mild and fleeting that I had disregarded it. The reason she asked was that she had been experiencing nausea! (Day 7)

In part of this dream a girl who works for me told me very accusatorily that I was going to get a £2,000 pay rise, as 'you're all managers.' (Day 17) *In mid March 6 weeks after this dream, we had our pay review and I had a letter through saying I was to be given a pay rise of £2,000. I had no idea that I would be given this sum and was not expecting to be given quite as much.*

4) I felt sensitive to everyone's moods around me. As I walked down the street I imagined that some people were literally barging through my aura (Day 3).

I felt very sick this morning, I think I have a stomach bug, very bad diarrhoea, watery, lots of it approx 8.30 a.m. My daughter woke me in the early hours and threw up everywhere, also has diarrhoea. I felt as if I wanted to be sick but couldn't. Felt very weak, very pale in the face, but felt better after more sleep (Day 4).

Stomach bug appears to be a lot better and I haven't suffered as much as my daughter and mother did with it (no vomiting and less long lasting). (Day 5)

I felt extremely sensitive to people's moods. I feel as though I can tell what people are feeling inside. Strangers appear to be talking to me a lot on the street and in the park (Day 6).

5) I have had an un-restful night. I had a very vivid dream. A face of a man appeared in a window and it gave me such a fright, I woke up with a start. That is all I can remember. I then went back to sleep much more deeply for an hour before the alarm went off (Day 4). *Review:* Does the man represent Stuart, the proving co-ordinator?

I've had a dream that I had just had a baby. Myself and my sister were choosing a name for the baby. That's all I remember (Day 21). *My sister told me she was pregnant a week after this dream.*

(Compare Prover 1 feeling broody. Page 200.)

6) Days 1–3 Slept very well – like a log.

Very restless sleep, after speaking to co-ordinator (Day 20).

Restless sleep again (Day 21).

Very restless night. I did not get to sleep until very late; I was still awake at 5 a.m. I feel this was the effect on me of the energy of the proving group at college today (Day 22).

7) I notice that other family members feel weary and rather tired – 'a bit flat'. My daughter speaks of feeling the way I look: 'tired and lethargic' (Day 2).

My daughter says she feels very tired, weepy and seems very lethargic (Day 4).

My son is at home sick. He says he has this feeling that he will be unwell. Lo and behold by the late afternoon he is pale, white and can hardly stand up. On reflection this was almost a clairvoyant feeling by him (Day 6).

My son has had 'delusions that people were in his bedroom'. This is very rare – he never has nightmares or talks of bad dreams (Day 9).

8) *Retrospective entry after twelve week scan in hospital (March 27th).* As a result of my scan at twelve weeks, I discovered that I was carrying twins, which died at nine weeks and two days (March 7th). I wasn't aware of this as no spotting occurred until 25th and only on 25th. Scan showed two embryos and no foetal heartbeat in either. Termed as incomplete miscarriage. Subsequently didn't miscarry naturally; had to have D&C to abort foetuses (Day 53).

From her supervisor's diary – I saw two large bits in my period that looked like a tiny miscarriage, which is odd for the third/fourth day of my period (Day 51).

This is one of many examples of provers and supervisors having similar experiences. Ed.

9) 7 a.m. I'm very tired, just want to be left alone. Everything's too chaotic; I can't keep on top of it all. 9 a.m. Chatting to a friend, she said she couldn't understand why she was feeling so angry at the moment. She was aware she needed to 'let go of something', something had to give. This made me realize that another close friend of mine had been feeling similar yesterday. She knows I'm doing the proving and wondered if she's been affected. She feels unusually stressed and is getting into struggles with her toddler (Day 7).

5.15 p.m. My sister has just given birth to a baby boy! I'd just been remembering the sensation of my babies' bodies as they came out. My dad called five minutes later to give me the news (Day 9).

When I saw a close friend this morning she described a dream that she had after we had met up last week. She also told me that she hadn't been aware of her dreams for a long time, but was aware that with me doing the proving, this is the second time she had had a very clear dream (Day 12).

Telepathic things keep taking place: I heard my advisor's voice in my head only to find a phone message later, which would have been at the same time. Another time picked up the phone to dial the number of a close friend when it rang and it was her (Day 31).

10) *(Effect of proving on someone else?)* My friend who has been working for me told me he had had a dream with me in it; we were working together and had seen a tsunami coming but had escaped it together, despite the building we were in and all those around it being demolished. I do not ever remember him telling me about a dream before. (I have known him for more than fifteen years). (Day 11)

Cycling to and from work I had unusual feelings of vulnerability. More aware of the inherent danger than normal, as if I could see myself from a remote viewpoint. I realize this has been happening quite a lot recently. Maybe part of a general change of perception (Day 13).

Rubrics
Spreading Effects etc

Mind

Danger, aware of NR

Synchronicity and coincidences, frequently noticed NR

General

'Astral' travelling, heightens potential for NR

Thoughts and prayers make an impact, heightened awareness, that NR

Interconnectedness of everything, heightens awareness of the NR

Reactions to remedy, wide-spreading NR

Mental and Emotional States

Contents

Excitement and exhilaration. Uncontrollable or inappropriate giggling.

Pace. Emotional roller coaster.

Calm, relaxed, happy and secure, as if there are no time restraints. Calm in situations that are usually stressful. Mentally alert and clear thinking. Fastidious. Able to get on with things and show feelings.

contrasted with

Insecurity, self-conscious and with low confidence. Negativity and tearfulness. Depressed about health. Anxiety. Restlessness. Disorganized, unable to carry out tasks, clumsiness, bad writing and spelling errors. Forgetfulness, repetition of words. Difficulties concentrating. Irritability and wanting to be alone.

'My fault'. Judgments. Reconciliation within family.

Return of old symptoms. The need to sort out unresolved issues. Clearing out junk: 'yucky things'.

Teenage resonances

Claustrophobia

Excitement and exhilaration, uncontrollable or inappropriate giggling.

1) *Two days before the proving:* Lots of energy. I feel more 'alive'. Giggly.

Day the proving began: 12.45 p.m. Took second and final tablet. 12.50 p.m. Felt slightly light-headed, almost drunk feeling, straightaway.(A) Good spirits. Very giggly. Laughing at inappropriate moments e.g. when my husband was speaking about his work over lunch, I could not resist the urge to laugh!(A)

4.45 p.m. I'm a bit tired, haven't got as much energy. I'm not sure if the proving's effects are wearing off. No giggling (unfortunately!) (Day 5).

I've been very chatty today, with quite a lot of energy.(A) Twice today I have laughed at something when perhaps I would normally just smile.(A)

Supervisor's evening report: Early on, in my conversation with my prover on the phone, I couldn't stop giggling, despite her telling me fairly serious symptoms. It just welled up from nowhere when she started to speak – I'm doing it again now even though I'm off of the phone. Uncontrollable giggling. She was giggly too, but less than me. (Day 10)

Supervisor's observations at college: lots of people had had their hair cut. One minute people seemed 'jolly', then the next they turned and seemed a bit low and tired. (Day 20)

I was in almost a hot flush, babbling to the proving co-ordinator today. I told him half my life history.(A) (Day 29)

5) *Seven days before the proving: in the group at college.*

This usually very chatty/vocal group now seems very quiet; slight apprehension and nervous giggles. Now feel we are each alone and unsure.

I felt very 'alive', my body felt as if right into my stomach there was a tingling/moving sensation. I was very aware of my feet in my shoes and not being flat!

6) *Seven days before the proving:* I felt great excitement and silliness. I felt as if I wanted to do something really exhilarating.

Six days before: Excited. Supervisor and year group giggly with lots of laughter.

Five days before: Bubbly feeling, really excited.

Four days before: While at work, watching the sea, I felt as though I wanted to go windsurfing. I don't know how! Still very excited. I have been achieving a lot during the last few days, as though I am on a mission?

Three days before: Very happy, bubbly and feeling excited; about what? I don't know. I seem to be whizzing around at work and at home. I feel like a runaway train, I just can't stop.

Two days before: Still feeling very excited, but my body and energy levels are beginning to flag. Feeling much better with more energy after evening meal.

One day before: Feeling more excitement. I feel as though I need exciting challenges; I just want to play practical jokes on people. I took my son to football training and felt as though I could play as well.

Looking back at the whole week before the proving begins: Loads of energy during this week.

Still feeling a little excited (Day 3).

Still feeling happy, things are not getting me down (Day 4).

Silly mood. Annoyed husband, poking him when he was trying to sleep! (Day 20)

Still in a silly mood, wanting to run around and 'wag my tail' and go crazy (Day 21).

Feeling excited again; felt in the throat area. It is like that roller-coaster feeling I had before the proving began. This time it seemed to affect my breathing. *(Has asthmatic tendency, which alternates with her skin symptoms.)* (Day 24)

Excitement calming down now, not running around so much (Day 25).

9) *Four days before the proving:* 9 p.m. I get a sense of hilarity about this remedy. Overwhelming laughter, bubbling up from my throat, irresistible need to laugh. I see this as the potential for this remedy. 10 p.m. I had a sense of my spine concertina-ing down, slumped, no inner strength.

Rubrics
Exhilaration – Elation

Mind

Cheerful feelings, happy 1285

High-spirited 1345

Elated, state of mind 1319

Excitement, excitable 1321

Excitement, excitable, alternating with sadness 1321

Exhilaration 1324

Mind, excitement, desire for 1322

Mind, excitement, throat area, felt in NR

Exhilaration, alternating with sadness 1324

Playful 1381

Laughing 1363
Laughing, serious, matters, over 1363
Laughing involuntarily 1364
Laughing, silly 1364
Mind, foolish behaviour 1337
Talking, excessive 1409
All these possibly alternating with feeling alone and insecure.

Some states for which we haven't made rubrics –

Loads of energy, but it's like he is riding a bike with no brakes on.

'Delusion' – feels like he is on a roller coaster. Can't switch mind off.

Calm, relaxed, happy and secure, as if there are no time restraints. Calm in situations that are usually stressful. Mentally alert and clear thinking. Fastidious. Able to get on with things and show feelings.

contrasted with

Insecurity and low confidence. Self-conscious. Negativity and tearfulness. Depressed about health. Anxiety. Restlessness. Disorganized, unable to carry out tasks, clumsiness, bad writing and spelling errors. Forgetfulness, repetition of words. Difficulties concentrating. Irritability and wanting to be alone.

This section, with its long individual contributions, can be read as a focal centre of the proving experiences (Ed.)

1) *The day before:* Still high energy. I feel in great spirits; I feel I could do anything. Had irritable spell between 2–4 p.m. Snappy, especially towards family. Had to meet a friend, but felt worse from having to converse.

Felt better again in the evening.

Day 1. 8.30 a.m. Slight pain in groin area and needed to pee twice in half an hour. It felt like my UTI had come back.(C) It lasted for about half an hour, I passed a small quantity of urine, then just suddenly the pain stopped; this was then followed by a couple of minutes of flatulence.(B) Mentally throughout this I felt relaxed and calm.(A) 4 p.m. Tearful, all of a sudden, about a situation at my daughter's school. (Return of old symptom, which had cleared with a constitutional remedy in previous months.) Forgetful, for the second time today – went to my mother's house to collect some photos and left without them.(A) 5 p.m. Energy back again.(A) Loads of energy, abnormally so. I feel in good spirits.(A)

9 a.m. Lots of energy, and mentally very calm.(A) No light-headedness or giggling today. I think, 'This is quite good fun.' My mind is not quite right: I have to think longer about things. I noticed today that my writing skills appear very messy; I seem to have lost full control of the pen. Usually I am neat. My supervisor noticed that in the emails that I sent her I was missing out letters: e.g. Jdy instead of Judy. 12 midday. Forgetful – forgot to call back a close friend. 5.30 p.m. I had lots of energy all day again, quite steady, even with the nausea. I felt suddenly fastidious so had the urge to keep tidying and cleaning, to the point where I had to empty all the bins in the house, something that was normally done on a set day. I spent two hours doing my daughter's bedroom, and then began cleaning round the bathroom sink with a toothbrush. Usually I'd let it wait. 9 p.m. Forgetful – couldn't remember if I had made a phone call yet or not. Even when I made the phone call could not be certain at first.(A) (Day 2)

Calmer than usual before a school run. I took it all in my stride.(A) 10 a.m. I feel a lot more tired, all of a sudden, and slightly irritable.(C) There is so much that I wanted to do, and I felt I was completely on my own to do it. I almost resented my husband for sitting at his computer while I was running around. I feel I want to get on with homework but I can't because of my circumstances: home educating my daughter.

A few moments throughout the afternoon when I thought, 'How can I cope with everything I've got to do, it's not fair.'(C) (It reminded me of a *Sepia* state.) But then I just couldn't stop: I've been cleaning everything. I just *had* to do it – for example I had to do my kitchen windows. Normally I would fit it in whenever.

Generally I have felt happy this afternoon.(B) I've had loads of energy. I could keep going, but I've got to stop now. Perhaps less forgetful? But then I suddenly couldn't remember if I had phoned my mother or no. I'm still getting my words jumbled, but my head feels clearer about everything. I feel like I can achieve anything. *(Parallel effects)* My husband ran a bath then forgot to have it (Day 3).

My mum told me that in the morning on the phone I had been repeating myself. I hadn't noticed.(A) 2.15 p.m. Couldn't remember a friend's phone number whom I call regularly, and the same thing had happened to her that morning apparently.(A)

2.20 p.m. No physical energy. Mentally want to get on with things, but physically can't.(C) Burnt out. *(Parallel effects)* A couple of times I noticed that my eldest daughter was about to speak and then forgot what she was about to say. She never did remember it.(A) 5.30 p.m. I found it was a real effort to think about household chores, for example cooking the dinner. I felt I just couldn't be bothered; I didn't feel I had the mental or physical energy to do it.(C) Although once I got started this improved. Cleaning has died down but I'm still keeping on top of things – e.g. I had to do the washing up straight after the meal; normally I would let the food go down first. Irritability spells. Got irritable very quickly, especially if my daughters or husband appeared to be making a mess. It has been a bit like PMT symptoms: I snapped when my daughter interrupted me talking to my husband. He said I had been very irritable today. This made me even more irritable: I didn't think I had been. Writing seems to be neater now (Day 4).

7.15 p.m. Felt I couldn't get out of bed. Feeling so tired physically and mentally.(A) 4.45 p.m. I'm a bit tired, haven't got as much energy. I'm not sure if the proving's effects are wearing off. No giggling (unfortunately!) No forgetfulness, nor in family either (Day 5).

9.30 a.m. I keep repeating myself still. 3.30 p.m. Felt the house was untidy again so I had to tidy it up.(B) 7 p.m. Strong PMT feeling. Irritable. The girls had their dressing up things out; then they went out with their dad and everything was left out and not in its place and I had to tidy it away. This annoyed me but I felt I had to do it (Day 6).

11.30 a.m. I felt really wide-awake.(A) Felt in good spirits – happy.(A) 2 p.m. Felt suddenly slightly irritable.(B) 7 p.m. Still have to be clearing things away.(B) As soon as we got home from the day out I had to put everything away, e.g. empty all the picnic bag etc., before sorting out and bathing the children. I felt it just had to be done immediately. Forgetful still (Day 7).

11.30 a.m. Felt irritable. Felt I just wanted to be on my own (B) and get on with my homework but again couldn't because I am home educating. 3 p.m. Irritable. I feel that I have to cope with everything.(B) I got so irritable that I ended up having a massive row with my husband. I never shout normally. I think that this remedy has brought up everything to do with the school/home-educating business again. Now I can't do my college homework when I want to. Uncontrollable crying. I wanted to be on my own afterwards to sulk, but did feel generally better for letting it out. (*Nitric acid* had previously helped me in this kind of thing.) Felt sad, low and sorry for myself most of the afternoon (Day 8).

10 a.m. A bit 'fastidious' again: I just had to do things. Not as much this way as I was last week; I could have waited but I felt better if I did them.(A) Felt I wanted to be alone today.(C) 2 p.m. My writing is terrible again this afternoon – I could barely read it. 11 p.m. Felt like doing homework, so did so until midnight.(B) Went to bed, felt restless, tossing and turning. Didn't sleep until about 1.00 a.m.(A) (Day 9)

11 a.m. My supervisor noticed that I was getting words wrong: I said hast instead of fast heartbeat. *Supervisor's comments: We've both noticed we can't get our homework done. We've got lots of notes on separate pieces of paper, but just can't get on with it. We feel disorganized.* (Day 10)

7.30 a.m. I jumped out of bed, my eyes feeling wide awake but my body felt tired.(A) 8 a.m. Feeling irritable generally. 8.30 a.m. Still feeling irritable because the housework needs doing again. My face looked tired.(A) 9 a.m. I've got toothache again, and would take something if I could. My teeth have been sensitive since starting the proving.(A) 11 a.m. I'm disorganized. I can't concentrate on my homework. I can't seem to give it full attention although I want to. 6.30 a.m. My writing is still very messy. I haven't got any control over the pen.(A) (Day 11)

I have been feeling calm generally today (Day 12).

Throughout the day, I was generally feeling calm – strange, as I was at a funeral.(A) (Day 15)

9.30 a.m. I felt really irritable and wanted to be on my own.(C) 11 a.m. Very hungry, still very irritable and wanted to be alone (could be PMT).(C) 3 p.m. I still wanted to be on my own (Day 16).

Daytime: No real symptoms to report, just feelings of my homework being a real struggle. I can't focus 100%.(A) I have a lack of confidence in doing the homework. *(Supervisor: I too have had great trouble getting my homework finished this month. I just couldn't seem to finish it however much I worked on it.)*

I did homework until 12.30 a.m. By then I was overtired so when I eventually went to bed I was very restless. My mind was spinning. I had thoughts of not feeling happy and confident with my homework. I couldn't switch my mind off; it was racing with thoughts about the remedy *Mercury*. I had to lay down and do relaxation techniques to calm myself down. I had a couple of palpitations and then started getting anxious: worried in case I have something wrong with my heart. I was very aware of my heart beating, aware of palpitations. It took a good hour to get to sleep (Day 18).

6 p.m. onwards. I felt I want to be cuddled, by my daughter or husband. I felt soothed by it. It was almost a craving for a cuddle.(B) 9 p.m. I keep misplacing my proving book.(A) (Day 19)

College weekend: I felt wide-awake in the morning, but flustered and clumsy throughout the day at college: I broke a bottle, spilt tea and tripped down the stairs.(A) *Supervisor's comment: everyone seemed to be clumsy at college. T fell over someone's bag, and said she's not usually clumsy. Lots of people dropped papers on the floor on Sunday. Lecturers forgot things too.* (Day 20)

I have noticed I keep forgetting lots of things, losing my train of thought.(A) I've been feeling sorry for myself.(A) (Day 22)

Days 23–25. These were really bad days. I felt poorly, low and depressed. I wanted to have homoeopathic remedies or get some St John's Wort, but didn't.(C) In the mornings, getting out of bed was really difficult – I had to drag myself out.

I woke up a lot better this morning. I feel more myself now, but I'm un-motivated. I just left the washing up. The place is like a bombsite.(C) (Day 26)

I felt improved, but tired and lethargic and generally quite depressed.(C) Could still be post-viral (Day 27).

I feel lots better but not quite 100% (Day 28).

About midday: I felt like I couldn't cope with things at home, thinking, looking around, 'I don't know where to start.'(C) (Day 29)

We were playing Snakes and Ladders. My husband said I was getting everything jumbled but I'd not noticed. I got things back to front. A strange concoction – I felt calm in myself, yet depressed. I felt I had all the time in the world, a laid-back feeling. I was almost floating around, almost in a dream. *(Supervisor's comment: unusual for her, she usually rushes around.)* I went shopping and was forgetful – I left my card behind (Day 31).

I woke up irritable, but managed to get organized quite quickly.(B) (Day 34)

I felt I had no energy, was tired. Once I started the housework, though, felt I could not stop and was being very fastidious (Day 36).

Felt fine all day (Day 40).

At college – the day we found out what the proving substance was: Overwhelmed. Calm. Mind not clear. I had wondered if the remedy was yellow or connected to the colour yellow in some way (Day 48). *(See also Prover 8's supervisor's text about the remedy Yellow. Page 285.)*

2) Day 1 9.30 a.m. I was feeling a bit tired and grumpy as I took the remedy. 1 p.m. I felt very irritable, this lasted about two hours. I took the second dose at 5.30 p.m. 6 p.m. I felt very irritable again. Felt crowded by my daughter who kept leaning on me and climbing on me. Lasted till bedtime.

I felt very wound up by my daughter all day. She was being very bossy and demanding, which ground me down (Day 4).

I felt very tired and lethargic all day despite getting a much-needed lie-in. I just wanted to lie on the sofa and watch TV on my own all day (Day 16).

After lunch I had a feeling of extreme tiredness and irritability. I had cycled a few miles with my daughter on the back in the morning, which usually leaves me invigorated, but it left me feeling drained. I had no patience with my daughter for the rest of the day and found her hard to cope with – everything felt like a battle. The feeling remained for the rest of the day (Day 25).

I had an overwhelming feeling of negativity and tiredness all day. My daughter was at her grandparents'. I had a row with my partner. I spoke my mind on an issue that I knew he wouldn't like, but I didn't care how it made him feel, I just said it. He was upset, but I felt numb and could barely react.

I went and met my supervisor to discuss the proving. I told her how I felt and realized I have felt like this once before. This was in December, starting about three weeks before Christmas (which I usually really enjoy) and up to New Year's Eve when I had a really good dance and felt better after that. During December my homoeopath prescribed *Sepia,* which helped my period a bit. I told my supervisor I thought I needed it again. When I got home I apologized for being so negative and I explained I couldn't shake off this feeling (Day 26).

My supervisor rang me and said my negative feelings could be to do with the proving. I agreed it sounded similar to some experiences others had shared at college. I decided not to take *Sepia,* although I remain uncertain as the feelings are just like those I had in December before the proving commenced and even before the advance notice lecture at college the month before starting the proving (Day 27).

I didn't feel quite so negative today, but still not right (Day 28).

I felt more energetic and positive during the day. In the evening I went to a pub then a party. Although I had a nice time, I was a bit flat and didn't enjoy dancing as much as usual. Everything was such an effort (Day 29).

3) I was in town and only had one hour spare and had to get a lot done. Normally, I would get into a real flap about this and get stressed but today I didn't. I wandered round feeling calm and measured. I felt like my heart rate should be rising and I should be panicking but I wasn't (Day 1).

The 'grounding' benefits of walking. I had to admit to feeling quite confused. I'm having to concentrate a lot harder on things I would normally find quite easy or would just say or do. I had to keep my mind really focussed on what I was trying to say. Also when a friend gave me directions to the café I was meeting her in yesterday, I found it really hard to grasp. I do feel confused. Concentrating was difficult in town today. I tried some boots on in a shoe shop and when the assistant asked if I needed help, I found it really hard to explain what I was doing or what I wanted. Aware that I was confused, I was trying to hide it; I didn't want people to notice that I was not 'quite right'. Once I realized that it may have been the proving tablet making me feel that way I was OK with it. I felt a bit lost – almost a childlike feeling, like a child trying to behave like an adult. I walked around for a long time this afternoon and feel better and less confused tonight at home. Normal again, I think (Day 3).

I got confused and lost trying to find a clinic this morning. I work in the town and know the area quite well so it was odd that I just couldn't work it out (Day 4).

I feel very bright and in a good mood today. It's the first time in a few days, but I think that's normal due to my period. I feel more together, more 'me' (Day 10).

I keep getting this urge to clean the house and clear my desk at work and put my cupboards together (still in cardboard boxes since they were delivered a few weeks ago); and to unpack my remaining boxes from moving in a couple of months ago (Day 15).

In my dream I fed my friend's cat but dropped cornflakes and milk in its bowl. I was quickly trying to repair the damage by scooping them out with a spoon (Day 20). *I'm being clumsy in my dream.*

I completely forgot to go to a college tutorial this week (Day 30).

During this week I forgot to buy my dad's birthday card – I've never forgotten him before, and what's even worse is that he was coming to see me on his birthday yesterday. I knew he was coming and I knew I should buy a card, yet still forgot. I forgot my good friend's birthday card also earlier this week. This really isn't like me at all. I tend to make a point of remembering close friends' and family's birthday cards (Day 36).

Reflecting on forgetting my dad's and friend's birthday cards and the tutorial, I realized that: 1. this is not like me; 2. when I realized I'd forgotten, I just shrugged to myself and thought 'Oh well.' I didn't care (Day 43). *This is really strange. I normally really worry about things like that and feel tremendously guilty.*

This week my apathetic attitude has continued. I feel I have reached a point where I can't worry about things that I would normally worry and get stressed about. I'm behind with lots of college work, which would really normally bother me, but I'm just not bothered by this. It's a nice liberating feeling in a way. I really can't remember ever not being bothered by this sort of thing (Day 50).

4) *Eight days before the proving:* 1.50 p.m. Felt very dizzy after walking in rain, had to sit down on a chair when coming inside. Felt a bit spaced out. I nearly left my favourite jumper behind when leaving college.

Six days before the proving: I forgot that someone was coming around to buy some baby equipment I had advertised in the local paper. I was also shocked to realize that I'd left my proving supervisor's notes behind at college. I was convinced I had, but found them at a later date.

Day 1 *Clarity of thought and calmness.* After taking second remedy, I felt like I was a bit out of my body, spaced out, but also focussed. My daughter was very demanding of my attention, whilst I had other pressures to think about such as work for college, finances and paperwork stacking up. I was feeling frustrated and ended up shouting at her, almost wanting to hit her. About ten minutes later I was full of remorse and took her to the park, tried to be cheerful, but still felt irritable.

I forgot to take remedy at lunchtime. I also sent an email with notes on my dreams and symptoms to someone else by mistake. She had the same first name as my proving supervisor (Day 2).

I've been awake since 5 a.m. It's now approximately 6.40 a.m. and though I'm physically tired, my eyelids feel heavy. I feel as though I want to get on with some work, while my daughter is still asleep (very unusual for me at this time of day). Felt really dizzy approx 1.45 p.m. – 3 p.m. I felt sensitive to everyone's moods around me. As I walked down the street I imagined that some people were literally barging through my aura. I felt very dizzy at one stage in a large high street shop, a bit breathless approx 2.30 p.m. I thought I was going to pass out and kept knocking things off shelves as I turned around, with a slight spinning sensation in my head. I stopped taking the remedies today as I feel I have come out in symptoms, the main one being dizziness and a spaced-out feeling. I found myself venting feelings of anger about my daughter's father to his parents; this was to do with maintenance for child support. I informed them I would take him to court if he doesn't get his act together. Fairly unusual for me to vent my feelings like this but felt better for it (Day 3).

Still clumsy, knocking things over, spilling drinks etc. throughout the day (Day 5).

Still forgetful with appointments, and buying essential items like toilet roll etc. Also forgetting to write in my proving notebook (Day 9).

Feeling very content, calm and able to get on with things (Day 12).).

Confusion of words in writing and speaking. I forgot to mention that over the past couple of weeks I've been getting my words muddled up. I've been speaking sentences with words in the wrong order. I've also been typing words with the letters jumbled (Day 19).

5) *Seven days before the proving in the group at college:* All female group – a feeling of nurturing; looking out for one another. Relaxed, comfortable feeling. This usually very chatty/vocal group now seems very quiet, slight apprehension and nervous giggles. Now feel we are each alone and unsure.

Two days before the proving: These past few days I have had a real sinking feeling in my stomach. A kind of anxiety. I've felt clumsy in my words and actions. Most strongly I feel very self-conscious with low confidence. Today I felt so embarrassed by the way I have been behaving towards friends and colleagues. I feel I'm acting silly and dumbing down, unable to think before I speak. This has gone on since the college weekend. The only time I can recall feeling as self-conscious as I'm feeling now is when I was in my teens.

The day before the proving: My mood lifts in the afternoon; I finally sense I'm coming out of this period of clumsiness and low confidence.

Day 1 *in the evening*. Feeling slightly nauseous. I have come off the phone from my supervisor feeling angry. I did not feel supported, I cannot discuss my feelings/symptoms with anyone else and am wondering why I'm doing this proving at a time when my stomach hurts, I've got a cold sore and my supervisor doesn't seem to take this as seriously as me. Humph!

Later review. I felt alone all the way through the proving. It is an issue for me, because I'm alone with my son and dealing with life. Why do I have to end up with a supervisor whose English isn't very good when I'm the one who most needs support in the group? Unsupported and alone – familiar feelings. No matter who I was paired with, I'd have had that feeling anyway – it's very familiar. I'd been working too hard before taking the remedy, cold sore, run down...

My mood is upbeat and relaxed. I feel my confidence crisis has gone (Day 2).

My mood seems as usual. My general feeling is that of a return of old ailments, but nothing wildly new! (Day 3)

Another night of waking and vivid dreams. I feel tired and un-refreshed. I dreamed I was at a huge ball and my body started to swell. I swelled up like a balloon and a doctor was called. I urged myself to sort out my stomach problems.

Physically I have not noticed anything, apart from still being slightly clumsy.

I feel very emotional, weepy. My general mood is one of worries rearing their head and needing my attention (Day 5).

Again this evening I feel tired and my mood is low (Day 6).

My mood is more upbeat (Day 7).

Again bad night's sleep. Emotionally I feel really well. I definitely feel I have been through 'old stuff' in the last week (e.g. family relationship problems) as well as the feeling of clumsiness and insecurity, but now feel I've come out the other side. I'm feeling very calm and secure. I've noticed I'm taking real pride in my home, cleaning and decorating, but mainly sorting out old junk and clutter (Day 8).

Review: Emotionally – going through old stuff. Clumsy. Insecurity. Desire to clear clutter and sorting out old junk. Still enjoying this feeling of calm. Have even decided to leave my monthly weekend job, so that my weekends are more free.

Generally my mood feels un-relaxed again. However, there have been family changes, and I have been given notice on my house/home, so this current feeling of anxiety about the future may be natural. I do not feel I'm 'going with the flow' well though. My mood is one of anxiety (Day 13).

I have been staying with friends and, though happy to see them, feel very depressed about my surroundings and desperate to go home, which is very unlike me, as I enjoy moving around (Day 15).

My mood is full of anxiety; I'm worrying about the future (Day 18).

After work I feel very tired and get a bit tearful. I am short-tempered with my son – not able to cope with his noise. I feel I need rest and am anxious about work tomorrow. Period finished (Day 19).

My mood is calmer and I do not feel tearful today and my mood is fine towards my son. Reflecting on how I felt yesterday when I was tearful, I felt very alone with coping with my job, change of home and problems my son is having at his new school. I felt there was not much to look forward to. If I did take a remedy now, it would be *Sepia*, my mood is one of drudgery – all work and no play! (Day 20)

I feel emotionally/mentally that I have definitely come through a change. Looking back over the pages, I felt very confused and clumsy. My writing is full of spelling mistakes, and I felt as if I was revisiting old anxieties. This feeling has passed now and I feel mentally alert again (Day 21).

Alone/emotional roller coaster: I seemed to have totally disconnected from the proving for the last week. I found the whole experience such an emotional roller coaster and felt as if I was going through the experience alone – not really being able to talk with anybody, that I wanted to disconnect a bit, simply to protect myself. I'm feeling concerned about how much work I have to do. Also, all my positive resolve and clearing out which occurred during the proving seems to have gone (Day 31).

I am feeling full of anxiety about where my future is going to be, e.g. new home. I don't feel as if I'm going with the flow at all. I do feel better for having spoken with Stuart. I think my feeling of being alone was creeping back (Day 32).

I realized when typing yesterday, also, how my spelling is still completely muddled. I still feel calm again, and looked after a child who was being difficult, yet I did not get stressed (Day 33).

Having recently spent time with relatives, I'm back to that feeling of insecurity and low confidence. Due to having been given notice to move, I'm full of anxiety and, at times like that, my stomach and digestion can be problematic (Day 34).

I am feeling very 'blue'. I can't seem to shake off my anxiety about moving house. I feel the proving and even my college work is the furthest thing from my mind. I have had to move many times before, yet this time I feel very uncertain and not hopeful about the future. I am eating a lot of things that are not good for me and give me stomach-ache, bread, croissants, chocolate and coffee. I am also going to bed late. My mood is not one of 'taking care' of myself. I can't shake this 'doubting' and lack of confidence (Day 35).

My mood has been more relaxed and I feel more hopeful about the future. Less anxiety. I have been very calm. I do not feel this proving has affected my relationship with my son. That side of things remains fine and peaceful (Day 36).

Showing feelings more. My mood is happy at work, but as soon as I'm on my own I feel anxious again. I always used to be like that, happy at work but since the remedy I've been more willing and able to show my feelings at work. Really proud about that. People expect me to be fun. I generally feel responsible for others and their feelings. Reflecting on my general mood the past month, I feel slightly vulnerable and fragile. I think I'm coming out of that 'state' but feel disconnected and rejected by my family, which is shaking my confidence (Day 39).

I found it hard to go to bed until quite late, 1 a.m. yesterday evening. My mind seems to be racing and I was tearful about family issues. I feel fragile. This morning my son and I had a row; I remained fairly calm throughout but just felt exhausted by him and his needs. At work I am able to switch off and have a lot of fun and laughs – so my mood is up and down I suppose. Finally this evening I have had some clarity about our house move plans and feel much calmer (Day 40).

My mind is still slow (Day 41).

I'm still muddling up words and spellings. I keep daydreaming instead of concentrating. I have spent the whole day rowing with my son. I feel sad and exhausted. My confidence as a mother is low tonight (Day 42).

I have spent the day scrubbing my house. I feel much calmer now! I have hardly been smoking cigarettes these last two days (Day 43).

My mood is very calm today (Day 44).

I've realized I'm sleeping better at night again. My mood is relaxed (Day 45).

Family/awaited change: I had a horrible phone call from my mum and got very upset – very tearful. I feel I need to really distance myself from my family. It think it's taken me a while to come to this much-needed conclusion. Last time I felt it was when I was fifteen and then left home – and was happy again! (Day 46).

My mood is fine and calm (Day 47).

Feel very happy and calm. I have also been giving up smoking and finding that not too stressful at all (Day 48).

At college together, I feel relaxed and hopeful. The group seems relaxed but dopey! I feel those in our group who were very confident are more confused and questioning things, and those who lacked confidence seem surer (Day 49).

Review: Now I feel the proving has completely changed my relationship with my son – much more detached and healthier. He feels somehow less of a responsibility for me.

7) Clumsy, constantly dropping, knocking or tripping up, noticeably at college. This is rare because generally I am none of these.(A) Generally felt that the mood at college was irritable and angry and that people seemed to be at a low ebb. Felt that this mood transferred itself to me by the end of the day. Period lessening – but still ongoing. *(See Prover 7 in Female section. Page 202.)* (Day 22)

Anxious about intended meeting so rang a friend for emotional support and felt she was not able to give it. Feeling rather angry with my friend as if this has thrown into relief my issues over friendship. Is this an old issue, which has never been confronted? Almost feel that this is the last straw if she does not come to the meeting. Feel rather angry and irritable and feel that this mood has descended since the college weekend.(B) (Day 26)

I slept better last night – no waking at 4 a.m. I woke at about 6 a.m. This was the first morning in ages that I did not have to rush to get up; but I could not settle.(A) So I got up. I tried to have a leisurely breakfast, but it didn't work. My mood is very irritable and I am short-tempered with everyone in the family. I had an argument with my husband about family 'priorities'. Atmosphere is heavy and not one of resolution. Funny taste in mouth, like 'fusty'. Taste buds seem shot. Not hungry for anything (Day 29).

Feel a little more settled than yesterday, but conscious of mood swings. Generally far less irritable than yesterday. *Later on:* Much more restless by the end of the evening. Lots of children in the house on sleepover, even this did not lift spirits. Normally would have enjoyed this.(B) (Day 30)

8) *(This section for this prover combines with her description of dealing with unresolved issues, and gives a thorough text of her overall experience. Ed.)*

5 p.m. Very tired, lethargic; want to lie down, but didn't. I haven't got time. Cleared the kitchen, energy started to flow again (Day 1).

Mind: Irritable in spurts, short fused. Overall I realize that I express now and don't suppress. Difficult to suppress, except around my mother who does the 'poor me' routine (Day 3).

Mind: Irritable like PMT. Irritable with husband and daughter. Shouting at my daughter then feeling remorseful. Shirty with husband but kept it in. I knew I was crabby though. Suppressing my anger, resorting to eating chocolate instead. *(A reminder of the postnatal depression that I had two years ago.)* (Day 4)

More emotional crap. Angry outbursts getting worse, especially at my child. Shouting so loud throat is sore. Depressed. Want to stay alone, curl up and sleep. Can't be bothered to do anything, least of all take daughter to music club.

It's almost like I've got full blown post-natal depression again, as I had two years ago after my daughter was born. I was shouting at my daughter in a way that I wouldn't normally and that overall I felt bloody, wildly irritable. A lot of mental and emotional feelings. 'Christ, what is happening here?' Definitely a return of old symptoms. I'm expressing so much more, rather than suppressing my feelings; yesterday, I felt so angry. I felt like I wanted to smash an empty bottle of wine against the wall and wanted to walk out of my home. I didn't. I ate some Maltesers and had a cup of tea instead. It's like a flash in minutes – some stupid little thing will trigger it. I feel more relaxed when I am down with my horse. My stress levels are really high if I have a lot to do in a short space of time. Cleared old clothes from cupboard, maternity wear, cot sheets and blankets. Felt no point to keeping them, obviously not going to get pregnant (Day 5).

Very depressed 8.30 a.m. Curled up went to sleep on bed. Don't want to be bothered to do anything. Cried. Woke feeling better but couldn't be bothered to do anything. *(Similar to postnatal depression of two years ago.)* Decided to clear out some clutter from the house. Took loads of stuff to charity shops and tip. Took a friend and her son and visited beach and café. Walked along the front. Felt so much better. On the way home kids screaming, felt very irritable and shouted. Very short fused. Child behaviour driving me crazy. Angry with the constant whingeing and screaming. Shouting again. Remorseful after (Day 6).

Last night: Interrupted sleep. Husband had emotional crisis at 1 a.m. Just got off to sleep about 2.30 a.m. Broken again. Slept very deeply till 6 a.m. Very difficult coming to, to get up when alarm went off. Felt tired through lack of sleep. Irritable, short fused.

Had lovely relaxing afternoon at stables with my child. On the way home, she screamed to get out of her chair. This tipped me over the edge and I really screamed and shouted back at her. I unleashed everything at her. Her distress made me do it more. I didn't want to know her, just wanted to be far away from her, to be alone. She became distressed, so I picked her up and felt bad about my behaviour. That night I lay in bed and thought about her distressed face and sobbed and sobbed about how nasty I was to her (Day 7).

Mentally/emotionally brighter but tired after sitting in at clinic all day. Felt shattered when got home. Went to feed horse; felt re-energized and lifted (Day 8).

Supervisor's report: When I saw her today she seemed calmer than when I've seen her before. She looked well in herself.

Mid morning: feeling irritable and impatient especially with husband's driving. Incident at stables made me very angry but didn't see the person responsible for initiating the anger to let it go, so the anger festered. I am just going to cut her dead from now on. (C) *Irritable, like in my time of postnatal depression.*

Angry again when I returned to stables in evening. Calmer when I left there, but still got the anger because I can't confront the issue.(C) *I'm generally like this.* Noticed: irritability > after stool (Day 9).

6 p.m. Felt very depressed, apathetic, didn't go for my weigh in at slim club – I couldn't deal with the disappointment of having gained. (I don't know if I had or not, just couldn't deal with it if I had.) (C) 10.30 p.m. Very down, cried, fed up with having to struggle financially all the time. Felt better after (Day 10).

Irritable, developing to outbursts of anger (Day 12).

Woke OK, but irritable mid morning (Day 13).

Irritable throughout the day with daughter because of her constant whining and tantrums. On-edge feeling. Depressed. Violent outbursts, throwing things, desire to smash things up; then I break down in tears. 'Can't take any more.' Need to escape; > crying (Day 14).

Woke OK, then irritable mid morning when daughter wouldn't

behave. Daughter irritating me a great deal with whingeing, screaming and tantrums. Depressed, feel very low, apathetic. Can't be bothered to do anything; > after shower (Day 15).

Morning: Feeling much brighter and energetic, got a huge amount done. No anger, irritability.

Afternoon: Met confrontation with one source of anger. Expressed my feelings and stood my ground. Angry afterwards because of the accusations, injustice and lies thrown at me. Realization of person's true nature. (Coming round from numb.)

Upset over injustice. Decided to take decisive action and remove myself (and horse) from the cause.

Evening: Still upset and feeling low. Reliving the words spoken and analysing it. Realization their story doesn't add up and I was being victimized (Day 16).

Woke up feeling tired and still a little low. Went back to bed at 7 a.m. until 9.30 a.m. Felt better after. Started decisive action. Felt better for it (Day 17).

Evening: Morale very low. Mother pissed me off. I so need to confront this issue. Feeling like I will but need to remove the anger first. She has let me down on childcare for this college weekend with two days' notice when she knew about it over ten days ago (Day 19).

Got very angry with daughter when she persistently tried to scribble in my repertory despite being told three times not to. Hit table, tea bounced off it all over laminate floor – lost the plot, got very angry and shouted at her. She went and stood behind the chair. Felt awful because she was scared of me. Shut down unable to communicate with her or even look at her for half hour. Stuart, the proving co-ordinator, phoned; left message re proving. Listened to the message and broke down and sobbed. Hugged daughter and said I was sorry; > crying, releasing.

Urge to eat chocolate, so ate a big bag of Maltesers, choc raisins and two Freddos. Felt sick! *(Again like my time of postnatal depression.)* One hour later, had to rush to loo, preceded by hot sensation all over. Very watery flatulent stools. Ten minutes later same thing.

Nothing more until 11 p.m. Daughter late to bed and playing up; can't deal with it, getting irritable so walk away. Husband said I was irritable, didn't feel it overly at the time, but was obviously projecting it. Narked with him for going to bed without saying goodnight. Chilly; can't seem to get warm. Sensitive to drafts. (B) 1 p.m. diarrhoea – had to rush to loo, same as earlier. Sensation as if it is coming any minute, > after. Noticed a sensation of bile from stomach last couple of days (Day 20).

Mother is playing the 'poor me' syndrome again. Received a curt email from her. This one broke the camel's back. Liaised with my sister regarding mother's attitude. Received an email from her (my sister), crowing about herself and how she is so wonderful and I am a crap person. Subsequently unleashed anger I have been holding back for thirty years with regard to her, and then cut her out of my life permanently. Don't feel bad about it; it's been long overdue. Felt better – lighter. Spoke to husband and he was 100% supportive.

Night time: reflected – was I right to do that? I knew it would upset my mother but she is the next one I have to deal with. Realized that mother controls family members through emotion by emotional blackmail – her 'poor me' dramas (Day 21).

College group meeting: Slept quite well, woke 6 a.m., went to do horse, felt OK. Came back home 7 a.m. Spent time lying on floor stroking the cat. Got stuff organized for college, and daughter to go to friends. Made breakfast for family. Feeling chilly. Little late leaving but not really stressed. Daughter clingy when dropped off. Her abandonment fear has risen again, I am sure from my distance through emotional outbursts.

Felt a little low at college, mind going over prior day. I guess it is normal to feel a little sad at ousting a family member. Sad because they were not there to support me, never had been and always had their own agenda. By the time we got to the proving group session I felt totally OK about it. Cried when telling of my symptoms in class because it feels like I have got postnatal depression all over again. Relived it at that moment. OK after.

Diet – very bad today. Trapped wind this afternoon; > farting.

Hubby had made tea when got home which was great. He is very supportive of me at college now.

Played with daughter and had fun.

8 p.m. Suddenly very tired. Daughter won't go to bed, but dealt with it without getting cross with her. Went to bed early myself as very tired (Day 22).

Emotionally upset when talking to Dad about recent events. Had his support and that meant a lot. Discovered the depth of my mother's emotional blackmail and that she now knows my feelings on her behaviour. Family member I have cut out passed my email directly to her. Not the way I would have put it to her but nevertheless am glad she knows now. Confirmed I was right to cut out family member and realized the game my mother has been playing for last twenty-six years. Went to bed late as cleared all the ironing!! (Day 24)

Working in London. Felt tired in morning due to late night and early start. Arrived home 8 p.m. – daughter had bath, was so tired could hardly hold my head up so laid on floor with my head on a towel while she washed herself. Was all I could do to finish her off and put her to bed. Went to bed and fell asleep before she did. Slept very deeply (Day 25).

Lethargic today – can't be bothered to go out. Pottered at home instead. Much better with daughter today. Not as many outbursts (Day 26).

Forced myself to take daughter to music club because felt so tired wanted to slob on settee. Irritable with her over stupid minor issue. She cried before she went into the class. First time she has ever done that. Wouldn't leave me (unusual) except to get the instruments. She is stammering a lot in speech (unusual). Felt my irritability was to do with it so felt guilty. Took her to swings and slide to make up for it. She was much better (Day 27).

5.20 a.m. Woke up, came over very hot, had to go to loo because I thought I was going to be sick. No period so thought, 'Morning sickness – oh great!' Had diarrhoea instead, black liquid. One hour later awoke – was sick, yellow liquid. Ate banana and rice cake – went to horse. Felt OK outside in fresh air. Came back felt dreadful again. Was sick again – banana and rice cake mashed. Must be the sickness bug that my friends have had. Exhausted all day, laid on settee but couldn't really sleep as was watching daughter. Later she was sick; gave her a remedy. Laid down on bed with daughter and slept for three hours, woke up, had a drink of water – can't face any other food. Can't face food except melon. Utterly exhausted (Day 29).

Felt much better in morning. Diarrhoea and vomiting stopped, still very tired though. Slight heart palpitations still, but faint, throughout the day. Energy much better than yesterday. Nausea, pit of stomach. Passed parents' house and felt angry at my mother about her 'poor me' attitude towards me.

Evening: Appetite OK while cooking – got to food – appetite gone. Positive pregnancy test (after fifteen months of trying). Hubby stressed about how we'll cope. Felt dejected because of his negative attitude. Very tired 9 p.m. Went to bed (Day 30).

(No further irritability/short fuse/shouting at daughter after diarrhoea and sickness of Day 28. This as physical sequel to emotional clear out of Day 20. Ed.)

Nothing to report all day except very tired in evening (Day 32).

Very tired all day. Wanted to lay down a lot. Couldn't get going. Better afternoon (Day 33).

Dream – about sister getting married. Couldn't be bothered to get ready, so didn't go. No evidence of who she was marrying. She was dressed like Carmen Miranda in blue sequined cloak and wrap type hat!

Good day today. Did lots of baking which I haven't done for years. Took kids to park, had good time (Day 35).

Irritable, especially due to flatulence (Day 36). *(Only reference to irritability since Day 26. Ed.)*

March 4th College weekend: Memory issues today. Sitting in and couldn't get going on the remedies and case taking. Struggling to remember much.

Other symptoms noted after discussion in college: Extreme apathy to the point that my whole body almost ceased. Serious constipation and violent migraine. Unable to function physically. I put this down to my pregnancy but discussing with another two provers they both experienced the apathy as well (Day 43).

Reflections: coming round from numb. Been closed so long, now coming out of it and dreaming a lot more. Feeling of becoming a woman again – motherhood perhaps.

Day 53. *Retrospective entry after twelve week scan in hospital (March 27th).* As a result of my scan at twelve weeks, I discovered that I was carrying twins, which died at nine weeks and two days (March 7th). I wasn't aware of this as no spotting occurred until 25th and only on 25th. Scan showed two embryos and no foetal heartbeat in either. Termed as incomplete miscarriage. Subsequently didn't miscarry naturally; had to have D&C to abort foetuses.

See also her overall review of the time of the proving. Page 259 in proving reviews section.

9) *Seven days before the proving:* Slightly clumsy, keep dropping my pen. Kept getting confused when dealing with numbers – i.e. money change. I also had a very 'clumsy' conversation with someone.

Two days before the proving: I feel that various symptoms mentally and physically have been taking place over the last few days. I don't know whether it's:

1. The effect of the moon – coming up to full moon.

2. It's like PMT – which I normally only get the day before my period begins, but now this is unusual and extreme; every day I've been getting very short with the kids, very little patience.

3. Menstrual cycle appears to have been delayed by two weeks. The last three times I've menstruated just after full moon, whereas I was aware of ovulating two nights ago – sharp pain left ovary.

4. Today I've been very upset about my body. Familiar feelings about my self and appearance.

5. I have a lot of doubt about my ability to take a homoeopathic case tonight.

Are things coming to the surface before the proving?

Day 1 7.30 a.m. Took first tablet. I was very struck by the undertaking of what this may involve. I felt my mood sink. I was able to lie for half an hour and, in this relaxed state, I suddenly felt the impact of the remedy. It was as if a light went through me from the top of my head down. I don't know if this is the impact of this remedy in particular or how remedies in general take effect on our systems.

I've been extremely impatient and had little tolerance for the children today. I want my own space. After taking three doses yesterday, I didn't take any more, because the remedy seems to have taken effect through my dreams. I'd like to blame it for my mood too! (Day 2)

8.15 a.m. I shouted at my eldest son as he was running up the road, for not getting himself together and not thinking for himself (Day 3).

5.30 a.m. I woke again with a significant dream: I was cycling up a very steep hill, finding it difficult, arduous. I thought I knew where I was going because I had to return to somewhere I'd just come from, but got lost.

8 a.m. I shouted and swore at my son this morning, fed up with his predictable behaviour about doing his schoolwork.

I feel very low, tired and like I can't cope with all the continual family stuff. Like in the dream this morning I feel like I've gone back to where I've already come from; I recognize this state from times when I have really struggled with my children and had little support in caring for them. *Sepia* was very helpful at those times (Day 4).

It may be that I'm more rested from a good night's sleep but I feel lighter today and more patient and loving with my children (Day 6).

5.30 a.m. My daughter woke. I was upset and angry that I'm not getting enough sleep. She wanted to get up and wouldn't go back to sleep. 7 a.m. I'm very tired, just want to be left alone. Everything's too chaotic; I can't keep on top of it all. I have a very sore neck < left side. (This soreness lasted several days.) 9 a.m. Chatting to a friend, she said she couldn't understand why she was feeling so angry at the moment. She was aware she needed to 'let go of something', something had to give. This made me realize that another close friend of mine had been feeling similar yesterday. She knows I'm doing the proving and wondered if she's been affected. She feels unusually stressed and is getting into struggles with her toddler (Day 7).

I feel lighter and more refreshed today (Day 8).

Period began. 9 a.m. Very grumpy and irritable, want my own space to get on with things. I feel trapped. Later that morning I felt great when I was able to do some lengths of swimming. 5 p.m. I feel stressed about getting everything done in the house so that I can work in the evening (Day 9).

I still feel agitated about keeping in control over house/family stuff. I felt much better when I managed to get the house cleaned (to a degree!) (Day 10).

I get a sense that this remedy affects the heart and sacral and crown chakras. The words amethyst and quartz come to mind, but I do not know about them for their possible relevance. I have a sense of calmness, love, serenity, clarity.

I feel a lot lighter and happier today, with a clear head for studies. Decided to go for a swim, which was great. I felt very energized, breathing well despite not having swum more than twenty lengths for a long time, and was able to swim fifty lengths easily. I've been able to keep my cool instead of reacting when the kids get wound up. I'm able to stay objective and able to guide the children.

I've been feeling weepy, I want to hear and feel the love of people that I love. I want their reassurance. The wanting to cry has changed from out of frustration to a sense of fragility. This is a familiar feeling at times of extreme difficulty before now, when I didn't know where to get the support and love (Day 11).

8.40 a.m. I flared up at my son again on the way out to school, but calmed down quickly and apologized immediately. I'd been very rough on him, having misread a situation.

Later: This has been a good day, I feel brighter and lighter with more energy (Day 12).

I realize that I keep getting stuck; I know how I want to be as a mother and lover but get stuck and flare up with anger if things aren't going the way I intend or rigidly want them to go. I felt very emotional when my husband was telling me news about a family member who is a young teenager and is being very self-destructive. I feel I could cry easily (Day 13).

I woke grumpy and tired, wanting my own space before having to deal with children. Snappy with them through breakfast. I feel like a terrible mother and feel exhausted. I'm stuck in old patterns and can't move on. I want to clear this state of stress and anxiety; I've had enough of it now. In the evening I did a latihan (spiritual practice) to try and break through this, clear the darkness. My latihan concerned my heart, about joy and love, the potential of how I could be in my heart. I'm aware of the lower heart with feelings of anger and frustration and my upper heart with a sense of lightness and love. There is a disconnection and I need to find a bridge (Day 14).

I woke still tired after a good night's sleep, but determined to make this a good day, I want to break though. I gave myself five minutes to receive how to be for the day, and to have a sense that I could return to if I was struggling in the day. The day got better as it went on. I had been very resentful about going to my mother-in-law's house. I would've loved the day to get on with my work. But the day was lovely, focussed on the children, being together and relaxed (Day 15).

Realized I had left my bag at my mother-in-law's, and had to drive back! Generally a good day, had to fight with myself not to feel buried by children and their needs (Day 16).

From the time I woke I feel positive and bright. I struggled with my two year old – her persistence and determination to get exactly what she wants when she demands it is bewildering. I feel trampled by her, and just want to cry. It takes such a conscious effort to be able to distract her and keep her positive. I wonder if the extremeness is reflecting my own turmoil and shifts. Despite that, generally I feel calmer and clearer (Day 17).

My daughter continues to be really hard to be with, but I'm managing to remain objective (Day 19).

Feel bright and more energized. My daughter is much happier too and not so persistent, more accepting and patient – in fact she's been great all weekend too (Day 24).

I feel depressed, emotional and fragile. I feel that I'm always failing myself. I want to be nurtured and withdraw from practical matters. I feel disgust for myself. Recently I've had a strange movement in my abdomen, which reminds me of the sensation 'something alive in the stomach'. At the time I thought that this must be what *Thuja* has, but at the college weekend I picked up a fourth year project on *Thuja*, I felt led to it. I was also drawn to the sequoia tree in the gardens rather than the oak tree I usually greet (Day 25).

6 a.m. Dream: In a large house, possibly there on holiday; it's spacious, clean, tidy, overlooking fields and a bright open space, with a stream at the bottom of a hill. Beyond I was aware of two volcanoes that were smouldering with lots of smoke. There was also to my left a patch, which appeared to be volcanic mud very close to the house. There were two men present who seemed to be two teachers of homoeopathy of some importance to me. I pointed out the volcanoes, which by now had very little smoke coming from them. What had been dramatic and painful was now only a signal of what had happened before.

Generally I feel really slowed down, calmer and not stressed. There appears to be a link that when I have vivid dreams of some significance, there is some sort of resolution and I am much more relaxed about everything (Day 26).

Feeling very low, but aware it's almost like flicking a switch and that I can be positive and happy. I keep having flashback memories to when I used to be anorexic, remembering exactly what I allowed myself to eat. Struggling to keep balanced as my husband has had enough of this (Day 29).

On waking I managed a few minutes to do an 'angel' meditation before going to the children. I felt able to maintain the calmness and love when dealing with their upsets. We had a lovely day in the park (Day 33).

Very slow mellow day – grey and rainy outside. We all just got on with things indoors. Everything went very well until the children's bedtime when I got impatient and couldn't wait till I could shut the door on everyone and get on with my own stuff (Day 36).

I've been slightly detached all day, very relaxed, almost dreamy. I feel relaxed about my studies, being with the children, with enough time for everyone and everything (Day 39).

10) 7.45 a.m. First dose of remedy. General feeling of well-being and calm, though slightly detached (but not uncaring). Very tired around 3 p.m. Possibly normal for me, but I felt it more so than usual. I slept for about one and a half hours.

Irritated during the day by my wife's negative attitude towards the children and herself. I feel life is good and that her problems are self-inflicted (Day 1).

Still feeling calm and even-tempered all day. Noticed that I was not feeling that I had to compete in the company of male friends where I would normally. Pleased that I have been more even tempered with the children, not shouting or losing my temper (Day 2).

Generally laid-back and calm today. I forgot to bring an important piece of equipment to the studio with me meaning that my whole workday was effectively wasted. I have never forgotten anything that important before. However, I was not all that perturbed by my forgetfulness and still described my day as 'laid-back' (Day 3).

Uneventful day, spoke to a friend involved in a business venture with another close friend that is falling apart. And was able to deal with the situation unusually calmly, not taking on other peoples' responsibilities or condemning either party (Day 4).

Felt physically and emotionally fine all day but very tired in the afternoon and slept on the train both into work and on the way back. Forgot the keys to the studio safe, so was unable to get on with the work planned for the day. This is irritating but not a massive problem, it is surprising though that I would make two such mistakes of forgetfulness in one week. Again I am surprisingly philosophical about this (Day 5).

Woke early because I had to get an early train to London, but felt surprisingly good and well rested. Also very calm considering it was to be a hectic day with people I hadn't worked with before. Remained calm all day and dealt well with client and set builder, both of whom seemed nervous and stressed. In this situation I will usually try to appear calm but in fact let people get under my skin. Today I felt very confident and had a better perspective of the day's importance (not great). So was able to deal with the egos involved well (Day 6).

Slept well and woke feeling rested. Relaxed morning with family.

My younger sister L. is visiting from Canada and is staying at my mother's house (one hour's drive away). My sister and I were close as children but have drifted apart as adults; we are still very loyal to each other though. My relationship with my mother is more troubled and I find spending long in her company difficult. We drive to my mother's house for lunch. I feel distant from L. and fail to close the divide of time and distance. Maybe this is the negative aspect of the emotionally stable feeling I have had recently. I was able to retain a feeling of calm despite mounting irritation towards my mother but just before leaving I was rude to her. Even at this point I am surprisingly self-aware but unable to use this beneficially. I am irritated and have a sense of failing that at this age I can still be so thoroughly upset by my mother. She still manages to make me feel bad about myself. I had thought that I was in a place where I could deal with her, but I couldn't. This kind of thing can affect me for at least a couple of days afterwards.

No physical symptoms (Day 7).

More irritable than of late, I lost my temper with my younger son, aged five (I generally have least patience with him); and also with my oldest child, aged seven, when we were doing his homework. This made me feel cross with myself. I'm still probably wound up from yesterday's difficulty when my mother visited. Had a good talk to my wife about my mother and family. Despite our good relationship it is unusual for me to talk so openly about something like this when it is still so fresh (Day 8).

Felt positive and loving towards my wife and children as if the effects of the weekend have dissipated. (In the past I have carried on feeling bad for up to a fortnight after seeing my mother.) Productive and busy morning at work, felt I dealt with clients particularly well (Day 9).

Snapped at my elder son for not paying attention while doing homework in the morning, but was able to realize that I had overreacted and stop him from being upset. Enjoyed settling debts with tradesmen who have been working for us and felt unusually able in negotiating money – less fear of offending. I feel like I've got on top of things that were needing to be sorted out. Energized. Dull but virtuous day at work again: worked late editing photographic images (Day 10).

A rather distracted afternoon but did good work and dealt with people well. Feeling generally calm and that I have regained my emotional balance from the weekend (Day 11).

Felt calm and focussed today. Productive day at work (Day 12).

Broken night – woken in early hours by shouting in the street. Woke very tired in the morning. Productive day, despite physical tiredness and pleased with my creativity. Cycling to and from work I had unusual feelings of vulnerability. More aware of the inherent danger than normal, as if I could see myself from a remote viewpoint. I realize this has been happening quite a lot recently. Maybe part of a general change of perception (Day 13).

Slept well. Children all exceptionally good this morning. My younger son was rather clingy but I was able to deal with him better than normal (Day 14).

Went swimming with the children in the morning. It can be difficult to control and keep all three happy in these situations but they were all helpful and happy and I felt I was dealing with them better than usual. (More patient and calmer.) My sister and mother visited in the afternoon. I felt relaxed and more determined to deal well with my mother. I did manage to deal with her much better. Things are moving on between us: I feel much more forgiving and accepting. Much happier with how I dealt with her. Communicated better with my sister though irritated by her slipping into a very passive middle-aged lifestyle – controlled by overprotective husband and mother – I remember her as having more spirit and feel disappointed (Day 15).

Rubrics
Calm vs. Irritable

This section is perhaps encapsulated in this image (Prover 9) –

'Lower heart – anger and frustration... Upper heart – lightness and love

There's a disconnection between the two and a need to find a bridge...'

Mind

Contented, feeling 1295

Tranquillity, serenity, calmness 1415

Tranquillity, serenity, calmness. Incomprehensible 1416

Capable, handle anything, feels she can NR

Clear, mind 1287

Impetuous 1350

Quick to act 1382

Anger 1266

Irritability 1357

Irritability, anxiety, with 1357
Irritability, alone, wants to be 1357
Irritability, children, towards, own 1358
Company, aversion to 1287
Company, alone, amel. when 1288
Irritability, family, to her 1358
Irritability, remorse after outbursts NR
Conversation, averse to 1295
Crying, remorse from NR
Concentration, difficult 1289
Concentration, difficult, studying, reading while 1290
Confusion, mental 1290
Confusion, concentrate the mind, on attempting to 1291
Confusion, intoxicated, as if 1292
Confusion, mistakes makes 1292
Memory, forgetful 1370
Memory, forgetful, words while speaking of, word hunting 1371
Memory, weakness of 1371
Memory, weakness of, done, for what he has just 1372
Memory, weakness of, said, for what has 1372
Memory, weakness of, say, for what he was about to 1373
Mistakes, speaking, in 1374
Mistakes, writing in 1375
Awkward, mentally 1281
Awkward, drops things 1281
Anxiety 1270
Anxiety, future, about the 1275
Vulnerable, feeling, with need for protection, or reassurance NR
Apathy 1280
Indifference, apathetic, struggling, unequal, adverse circumstances with 1352
Fear, opinion of others, of 1333

'My fault.' Judgments. Self-doubt. Reconciliation within families. Return of old symptoms. The need to sort out unresolved issues. Clearing out junk: 'yucky things'.

1) I woke up having had the most horrific dream. I dreamt I was in a kitchen and there was a lady a bit like an old neighbour (but it wasn't) and I saw her stabbed to death. I woke up and I thought I hope I didn't do that. I'd watched a program on Jack the Ripper – so perhaps it was a mixture of that and homework (on 'delusions had committed a crime').(A) I felt slightly anxious for most of the day. I even looked it up on the Internet to see what it meant – when there are so many obstacles in your way and you've lost control. When I went back to sleep I had another dream. One of the college teachers was in it, telling me I had to sit all my Materia Medica tests again and do all my homework assignments again (Day 13).

I had another strange dream where I was being chased by somebody. I think it was an ex-boyfriend, and he tried to attack me; so in my defence I climbed on to a climbing frame. He climbed up after me, so I stabbed him with my keys. I felt mortified that I had done that; crying because I thought I'd injured him, but I actually hadn't. I was wide-awake after this.(A) (Day 16)

Early hours. I dreamt that somehow someone had driven into the front and back of my car, where I park for school. I can remember feeling, 'Oh my God, everyone will think it's my fault,' as there was no one around. No cars nearby.(A) (Day 17)

I've been in a bit of a state today because I've still been aware of the odd heart fluttering. My dad's been bad recently – I was really anxious it was to do with his heart. Then I found myself last night wanting to read up all the remedies, looking for a remedy for my dad. As I was reading I felt really negative, thinking I'll never remember all these remedies.(A) (Day 28)

3) Last night I dreamed that I was living with my family in our old house in Worthing. My mum had decided to leave my dad and I was really upset, I felt all the security had been knocked out from under me (Day 3).

My analysis: I think this may be old issues re-surfacing going back to a place where I used to live with my mum and dad. Mum and dad did used to argue badly for a time when we lived in that house but they never split up. We all used to argue and freely express our anger with each other! My family are all pretty close and we know we are a bit dysfunctional but we all love each other. This dream was very unusual as the house in the dream was my actual old house that we all used to live in: our main family home that I grew up in. Normally in my dreams, the location does not reflect reality. This seemed to be a dream about losing that security I feel I have with my family.

Last night I dreamed I had these long artificial nails on and I was trying to fight a witch who was sitting next to me. She looked exactly like me and I scratched her across the face. I woke up very upset (Day 4). *My analysis: Reflecting on this dream, I think this may be an old issue rearing its head that I have not yet been able to deal with. This is about me disliking parts of myself and fighting with myself.*

In my dream last night, I dreamed that I had this crusty and slimy mucus in my mouth which meant I couldn't speak properly… So I started to pull it out of my mouth and I was aware it looked disgusting, so was trying to hide it from others. Anyway this thick white mucus (almost solid, like a solid yogurt) came out of my mouth and the crusty bit on the end looked like the tail of a brown snake (Day 17).

Last night I dreamed that my ex-partner bought a very modern, small, neat, three-bedroom house on the outskirts of everything, in deepest suburbia. I had bought a beautiful but run-down flat in the centre of town. It was full of period features (my building) and some furniture had been left by the previous tenant. When I looked out of my window I could see the previous tenant – a pretty Spanish girl with her boyfriend in a studio flat. The whole side of her studio flat opened up so that you could see everything inside. She was arguing with her boyfriend. I could see he was being a pain. I also found her diary in the flat I bought. It was together with other bits and bobs she had left in a chest of drawers. I can't remember what it said by I did read some of it. I knew she should dump her boyfriend, I could tell he was no good for her. She didn't see that though. I could also sense that she was somehow restricted by staying with him (Day 22).

My analysis: This dream has some parallels to reality. I split up with my ex last February because I felt restricted in that relationship. He stayed in the house we'd bought together on the very outskirts of Brighton in deepest suburbia, while I moved out and bought a new flat which is the top half of a Victorian house and is much nearer town. I'm also friends with a man who I don't think is very good for me and I think I should end our friendship. I think that this dream is symbolic of certain issues in my life that I need to deal with, resolve and move on.

I have to see the friend I'm trying to cut out of my life at work today. I feel more and more angry with him (Day 27).

After discussing the proving at college last weekend the subject of anger came up and I was quite taken aback by this. I have been feeling very angry with this friend since taking the tablets and I didn't note it in my diary but I did acknowledge to myself how angry I suddenly seemed to be with him. He isn't too good for me and doesn't treat me as I'd like him too, but I'd always just accepted the situation and written it off as that's how he is. But I think I just buried the issues. There were a lot of unresolved issues and these seemed to be re-surfacing together with a building anger. It all came to a head on Saturday night when I decided I didn't want him in my life anymore. I was in a complete fury. Then I felt terribly hurt and sad on Sunday at deciding to lose someone I care about. He has been in touch since and I think I probably need to talk through all the problems to get closure (Day 29).

Reading back over the dream where the mucus/snake in my mouth prevents me from speaking, I wonder if this is symbolic of unexpressed anger. When I let the mucus out of my mouth, I am worried that people will see it and it's disgusting. I wonder if this is all wrapped up with concerns that people will not think I'm a 'nice person' if I am expressing anger. Also a woman who works for me is in the dream and I have a lot of pent up anger towards her. She is very negative, tries to do as little as possible at work and takes long breaks and doesn't respect me. I don't think I'm dealing with the situation very well. Also the friend I'm angry with is talked about in the dream. These are two people with whom I have not fully been able to express my anger (Day 30).

I am fuming with a member of staff at work who has been lazy, uncooperative and not working her contracted hours. This has been going on for some time and I have dealt with it, although being someone who dislikes conflict it was very difficult to do. The anger has been bubbling away beneath the surface ever since; especially as the staff member could not see that she has done anything wrong and thinks I am being unfair. Anyway she requested some lieu time off to take back some supposed hours she had worked as overtime. All the anger came to the surface: I had a meeting with her today to clarify things, and assertively raised all the issues. Although she has reacted badly to being told what she can and can't do with the company rules, I feel better in myself for getting it out in the open and actually dealing with it (Day 31).

A colleague of mine put me in a very embarrassing situation at work this week. He decided to work from home. A lady from an external company turned up for a meeting with him. I had to go and tell her he was off sick. We rang and couldn't get hold of him. I asked the lady if she'd come far – she'd flown down from Scotland. I was fuming and embarrassed. Instead of bottling this up, I rang my colleague straight afterwards and told him off. That is not like me!

I'm starting to express my anger. I also told Jim to leave me alone for good. I cried for two days and felt hurt and loss. I had two doses of *Ignatia 30* and felt better after that.

Then I had to see him at work for two or three days this week and we were completely ignoring each other which I thought was stupid so I spoke to him and he was very off with me. Another surge of anger inside me – been thinking about this all day – I eventually called him and said as we had to work together we should get on as colleagues. I'm addressing issues more readily as they come up now and not letting them just fester away underneath. This is happening with things that make me angry in particular. I have more energy and feel less tired. I feel strong and ready to move forward (Day 43).

(See also her review 26/01/08 Page 250.)

4) Dream: About being in East End of London, at a music festival. It was grey and a bit dark. I was on the top deck of a double-decker bus looking down at the streets. I saw the music festival on a big screen and tried to see if I could see myself on the film (I didn't). Then I remember trying to walk home (I used to live in the East End). I got caught up in a wind, which was like a vortex. It spun me around in circles, really fast. I felt dizzy and passed out. I then got up to try and get to a tube station. I was taller than my boyfriend who is 6′ 3″; I think I was wearing very high boots. I had trouble keeping my balance, holding on to stair rails. It felt good being taller than everyone despite this. He disappeared from my dream and then I realized I was on a high unicycle, which spun around, a bit, I managed to get off easily, though I felt a bit panicky that I'd not be able to. I had bought a return ticket at the tube station, was holding my unicycle and going down an escalator. An old lady walked past and said she liked to keep fit by going to the gym, which I said was 'good for her'. I decided I needed to get back out of the tube station to buy something, possibly tobacco, and then found myself in a café amidst some women. I sat down at a spare seat at their table and got the feeling they'd been victims of abuse and were having a refuge meeting. Unable to stop myself, I fell asleep in my chair and woke up realizing I'd lost my daughter (who appeared in the café when I walked in there). I panicked a lot, running to a lift to see if she'd got in there and gone to another floor. I found her on the sofa in the café, tucked behind a big cushion and all right. I was so relieved as I thought she may have been snatched. I left the café and bumped into an ex-boyfriend who was flirting with me. I wanted him to go away (Day 1).

Dreamed about a big manor house I used to live in as a child. There was a wild party going on there and lots of people I didn't know; some people were dressed up in slightly kinky outfits. It was my mum's ex-boyfriend's house and I wondered if he was there (in reality he sold the house years ago). I have dreamed about this house before, having secret corridors and rooms and I went to look for these again. I managed to find a secret passageway by pressing books on a bookshelf (like something I've seen in a film). I entered the corridor, saw some lights on and felt scared and anxious. I turned around and quickly shut the shelves up again. There was a sexual element to the theme of the party, which made me feel uncomfortable (Day 2). *I'm feeling strange as I write this and tearful. I don't know why. I just know I was very unhappy living there as a child. My mum's ex-boyfriend was an alcoholic and they used to fight a lot. I'm wondering whether the private/secret rooms represent something I've repressed in my subconscious; not sure though.*

It seems as though I'm revisiting places in my dreams that I have bad associations with. My dream about the East End of London and sitting with women who I felt had been abused has made me think about the time I was beaten up really badly by an ex-boyfriend when I was living in the East End with him. These are just speculations, and I think possibly I'm analysing things too much. I'm OK within myself; just feel as though something has been stirred up within me.

Cannabis Addiction. I realize I should probably not be smoking cannabis but find I can't help myself. By the time my daughter's asleep it's too tempting; I feel frayed at the edges and don't want to think or worry about anything. It is an addictive feeling, a return of an old symptom. A lot has been stirred within and I've found it hard coping with my feelings and actions (Day 5).

I have a need to feel more in control and have stopped smoking cannabis as I realized it was slowing me down a lot. I no longer feel the need to smoke (Day 11). *This lasted for a few weeks.*

(See also case No 4 – a patient with a long-standing cannabis habit.)

5) I have had an un-restful night. I had a very vivid dream. I remember a part about opening up my flesh with a scalpel (it didn't hurt and there was no blood) and extracting a small hair, which shouldn't have been there, with a pair of tweezers. I felt relief to get the hair out (Day 4). *The small hair represents an impurity, something 'yuck'.*

I feel very emotional, weepy. My general mood is one of worries rearing their head and needing my attention (Day 5).

Emotionally I feel really well. I definitely feel I have been through 'old stuff' in the last week (e.g. family relationship problems) as well as the feeling of clumsiness and insecurity, but now feel I've come out the other side. I'm feeling very calm and secure. I've noticed I'm taking real pride in my home, cleaning and decorating, but mainly sorting out old junk and clutter (Day 8).

Emotionally – going through old stuff. Clumsy. Insecurity. Desire to clear clutter and sorting out old junk.

Still enjoying this feeling of calm. Have even decided to leave my monthly weekend job, so that my weekends are more free. Continued de-cluttering the house (Day 9).

My mood for 'clearing out' is continuing. Going through old boxes, sorting out photos etc. It is a satisfying feeling and I hope it lasts (Day 10).

I'm feeling concerned about how much work I have to do. Also, all my positive resolve and clearing out which occurred during the proving seems to have gone (Day 31).

Teenage resonance. –

Two days before the proving: These past few days I have had a real sinking feeling in my stomach. A kind of anxiety. I've felt clumsy in my words and actions. Most strongly I feel very self-conscious with low confidence. Today I felt so embarrassed by the way I have been behaving towards friends and colleagues. I feel I'm acting 'silly' and 'dumbing down', unable to think before I speak. This has gone on since the college weekend. The only time I can recall feeling as self-conscious as I'm feeling now is when I was in my teens. I have dyed my hair red and thought 'the last time I did that was when I was about thirteen years old.' All through this proving I've had a sensation of 'revisiting' my teens (Day 33).

I do not feel this proving has affected my relationship with my son. That side of things remains fine and peaceful (Day 36).

Family/Things that needed to change.

I had a horrible phone call from my mum and got very upset – very tearful.

I feel I need to really distance myself from my family. I think it's taken me a while to come to this much-needed conclusion. Last time I felt it was when I was fifteen and then left home – and was happy again! (Day 46)

7) Unsettled night – dreams full of anxiety about impending event that I am about to organize. I feel that there may be some conflict ahead. I had a weird feeling during the day that some awful illness will strike at someone in the family and that it will change lives forever. Despite this I still feel very upbeat and positive. I had a good run at the gym – despite my period. *(See Prover 7 in Female section Page 202.)*

Anxious about intended meeting so rang a friend for emotional support and felt she was not able to give it. Feeling rather angry with my friend as if this has thrown into relief my issues over friendship. Is this an old issue which has never been confronted? Almost feel that this is the last straw if she does not come to the meeting. Feel rather angry and irritable and feel that this mood has descended since the college weekend.(B) (Day 21)

I dreaded the meeting this afternoon. However, my friend came and was very supportive. She seems to have responded to the plea for support. The meeting was difficult and potentially very conflictual, and I was worried beforehand that I was angry and might explode, but I managed to release this anger in a measured and assertive way.(B) On reflection, I feel as if a weight has been lifted from my shoulders (Day 27).

Long conversation with my Head of Department. This was a chance to sort out a few things. Seems to have cleared the air. This was a resolution of an ongoing problem which I had been trying to resolve via different means.(C) (Day 38)

9) 5.30 a.m. Dream: I felt imprisoned, possibly in a prison, sitting on the floor with someone standing over about to shoot me. Somehow I broke through the floor to my left and dived through the hole to arrive outside. I felt sullied and had the thought, 'I am no longer the Virgin Queen.' Retrospectively I now see this relates to my first experience of sex, how I lost my virginity against my will.

When I got up I stood on the scales, as I thought I should know where I am at the beginning of this proving (Day 1).

Thinking about my emotions at this time: I'm fed up with my dourness and disappointment in myself. I constantly question whether this mood is anything to do with the proving remedy. I will be glad to find out with other provers what is going on. I want to shift this frustration – things constantly are in the way of what I want to do (Day 11).

I'm stuck in old patterns and can't move on. I want to clear this state of stress and anxiety; I've had enough of it now. In the evening I did a latihan (spiritual practice) to try and break through this, clear the darkness. My latihan concerned my heart, about joy and love, the potential of how I could be in my heart. I'm aware of the lower heart with feelings of anger and frustration and my upper heart with a sense of lightness and love. There is a disconnection and I need to find a bridge (Day 14).

I woke still tired after a good night's sleep, but determined to make this a good day, I want to break though. I gave myself five minutes to receive how to be for the day, and to have a sense that I could return to if I was struggling in the day. The day got better as it went on. I had been very resentful about going to my mother-in-law's house. I would've loved the day to get on with my work. But the day was lovely, focussed on the children, being together and relaxed (Day 15).

At college: I'm responding to the name Ruth being called out. I haven't been called Ruth for fourteen years! My change of name was the beginning of pulling myself out of the difficulties I was experiencing in my early twenties. I'm holding tension in my stomach. Still constipated.

I had a very interesting conversation (last night) with a very close friend of mine about when she couldn't deal with me when we were about twenty/twenty-one, i.e. when I was having anorexia problems. She couldn't deal with my rejection of myself, of food and (what I was surprised about) her (Day 23).

I feel depressed, emotional and fragile. I feel that I'm always failing myself. I want to be nurtured and withdraw from practical matters. I feel disgust for myself. Recently I've had a strange movement in my abdomen, which reminds me of the sensation 'something alive in the stomach'. At the time I thought that this must be what *Thuja* has. At the college weekend I picked up a fourth year project on *Thuja*, I felt led to it. I was also drawn to the sequoia tree in the gardens rather than the oak tree I usually greet (Day 25).

6 a.m. Dream: In a large house, possibly there on holiday, it's spacious, clean, tidy, overlooking fields and bright open space, with a stream at the bottom of a hill. Beyond I was aware of two volcanoes that were smouldering with lots of smoke. There was also to my left a patch, which appeared to be volcanic mud very close to the house. There were two men present who seemed to be two teachers of homoeopathy of some importance to me. I pointed out the volcanoes. By now there was very little smoke coming from them. What had been dramatic and painful was now only a signal of what had happened before.

Generally I feel really slowed down, calmer and not stressed. There appears to be a link that when I have vivid dreams of some significance, there is some sort of resolution and I am much more relaxed about everything (Day 26).

Feeling very low, but aware it's almost like flicking a switch and that I can be positive and happy. I keep having flashback memories to when I used to be anorexic, remembering exactly what I allowed myself to eat. Struggling to keep balanced as my husband has had enough of this (Day 29).

Tired because only got five hours sleep, but went for a swim – desperate for a swim.

Saw photos of myself when I was a teenager, fifteen. I looked awful. I've had strong realizations throughout the day of where some of these patterns come from: memories of feeling different from everyone else, that I was abnormal. Also realizations that other people's perceptions are very different to one's own mindset about oneself. I saw my family today, and chatting to my dad said that I'm revisiting past stuff, of which he was at the time painfully aware but unable to do anything. He told me a way of massaging the forehead whilst accessing these memories and exploring them, but maintaining an objectivity. Then going back further in time to see where these fears come from, still maintaining an objectivity to enable releasing these fears (Day 30).

Feeling better – I like having the kids on holiday. Everyone is pretty mellow and going at a slow pace (Day 31).

Dream: I was with my first boyfriend (true love at fifteen/sixteen!). It was a very sweet, romantic, innocent relationship, which never progressed far physically. We remained friends for years after. I remember very little of the dream, it just seems to be part of the flashbacks that are taking place. Retrospectively I now see this as the oldest flashback, and the beginning of where healing needs to take place (Day 32).

This morning I had a strong impression that I'd just been on a long journey and that I've brought back a piece of information, which has shown me where I've been stuck. Yesterday I walked past a smell that took me back probably twenty years, but I couldn't place what it was (Day 33).

Woke with a dream: 1. I saw two birds in a niche in the wall. They were soft, grey, black and white with long beaks. I didn't know what they were at first and then suddenly realized they were kookaburras. They were sitting together looking down on myself and others. 2. I was on a very steep hillside with other people. There were some craggy rocks and two of the people broke off a rock each. Then coming up the hill, across from another hill, came what appeared to be two park rangers saying that the people couldn't take the rocks away. 'You can't run with those.' My impression is that it is not possible to change our physical body. *(See section on Kingfishers and Kookaburras. Page 286.)*

I've been feeling slightly resentful of the proving over the last couple of days. I'm not quite sure if what's taken place has been necessary and what, if anything, I've learnt from it. It has been very uncomfortable to dig up stuff that I'm very aware of, it's not denied; I just had hoped that over these years I really had moved on.

On another note – my three children have been really infested with parasites over this period. One of my sons caught the worms before the proving began and I don't know when the others got head lice. I've never experienced worms and never had head lice before either (Day 38).

Next day: I've let go of the resentment about the proving because I'm remembering more of what my intentions and reasons for participating were, and of course what provings are about – I agreed to take part in a journey and this has been mine (Day 39).

Day 58 *Synopsis to date:*

I feel that I have brought something to the surface, which has been persisting deep within me. I can now lay it down; it does not need to be part of me any longer. I feel things are resolving. It is parallel to the parasites; they can be cleared, as there is no longer the same detritus to feed from. It has been a deeply healing process and I am still tender from the experience. I frequently feel strong surges of love for my children when I am with them or think about them, I want to cry out of love. This is also more of me available for people who are dear to me.

Day 59. After our advisor/supervisor/prover meeting I feel fantastic. I had been feeling tentative about having to go through all this emotional exploration again but I feel things are settling by witnessing these areas in my life. When I got home my mum had been looking after my daughter, and I kept being surprised at myself by my sense of ease at being with her. Usually, I get irritated by her anxiety over everything and everyone. My daughter was also having a fantastic time with her, whereas a year ago she resented being left with her. Maybe at some level I have forgiven my mum; I am not my mum, I am not really going to turn into my mum, I am myself.

Review after three months: I feel that the distance of time has been important to look at this proving experience and written material objectively. To relive some of the extremely self-destructive period from twenty/twenty-three years old, and the anger and frustration being so surface was very difficult for myself and my family. There is a sense of safety at looking at this, years later and I feel gratitude for understanding something about myself. It is possible to move on from this restrictive thinking, and that I can be expansive in my life. At this point I feel more at ease with myself, more accepting of myself, that I am not different to everyone else, but really quite normal.

Where I have mentioned the lack of internal strength in my spine, I wonder now, whether this could be to do with the Kundalini energy. When I was eighteen/nineteen as part of my healing from two STD's, a healer had to 'replace' my Kundalini, which had been displaced. On days 5 and 48 of the proving I experienced unaided orgasms before waking. I do not remember them being connected to anything particular I was dreaming at the time. I am sure this was part of my development through the proving.

I feel the core energy of this remedy is its potential to bring to the surface unresolved issues that have their roots spread wide in their effect.

25 July 2006 – six months since the proving began: I continue to feel that I have lifted away from a part of myself that was very self-destructive. I am far more accepting of myself than I can ever remember, I feel as if I am growing as a person in self-confidence and that I can grow into my potential capabilities in this lifetime.

10) We drive to my mother's house for lunch. I was able to retain a feeling of calm despite mounting irritation towards my mother but just before leaving I was rude to her. Even at this point I am surprisingly self-aware but unable to use this beneficially. I am irritated and have a sense of failing that at this age I can still be so thoroughly upset by my mother. She still manages to make me feel bad about myself. I had thought that I was in a place where I could deal with her, but I couldn't. This kind of thing can affect me for at least a couple of days afterwards (Day 7).

My sister and mother visited in the afternoon. I felt relaxed and more determined to deal well with my mother. I did manage to deal with her much better. Things are moving on between us: I feel much more forgiving and accepting. Much happier with how I dealt with her. Communicated better with my sister though irritated by her slipping into a very passive middle-aged lifestyle – controlled by overprotective husband and mother – I remember her as having more spirit and feel disappointed (Day 15).

Tired on waking, despite sleeping well. Snapped at wife for being angry with children on leaving the house. Unfocussed and disorganized re work. Behind on work and wasted time. Had to make a trip to London, which could have been avoided if I had been more together. Argument with my wife in the evening for which I apologize after, I am taking my frustration out on her. I have realized that there is too much shouting and anger in the house amongst all of us and feel we must lower the temper (Day 16).

Children lovely this morning and tempers and everyone happy and calm. Very dull day in the studio. I am more unwilling to do dull work recently and more determined to promote myself, to get more interesting jobs. Energy levels low but probably because I am bored and have had to work very late on the computer the last two nights (Day 17).

After this I have stopped taking daily notes as I have the feeling that the immediate effects of the remedy have passed.

Physically I feel perfectly normal as before. Emotionally I feel I have retained a better perspective than before and I am more tolerant and forgiving. I have been able to improve the level of anger in the house and we are working better as parents than before. This is particularly apparent in the behaviour of the two boys, who seem happier and calmer of late. Our two-year-old daughter still has a terrible temper though but maybe this is more a part of her age. I have found myself less judgmental recently (one of my worst character traits) and have been able to enjoy the company of groups of friends amongst whom I had felt uncomfortable and hypocritical recently.

Rubrics
Fault and Judgment
Dislikes himself, or parts of himself

Mind

Blames himself NR

Delusion, wrong, he has done 380

Reproaches himself 1385

Dreams – Crimes, accused wrongly, that he might be NR

Forgiveness – need to forgive himself NR

Clutter, desires to clear NR

'Negative' aspects of himself, has to clear these NR

Personal issues, need to confront and deal with NR

Unresolved issues NR

Family, needs to distance himself from NR

Reconciliation – need for NR

Acceptance of a situation – need for NR

Insecurity, loss of sense of security NR

Protection, and reassurance, need for NR

Critical, censorious 1296

Critical, censorious, disposed to find fault 1296

Critical, censorious, disposed to find fault, and feels bad about this 1296

Anger, absent persons, while thinking of them, at 1266

Anger, about something that has needed to be said NR

Tolerance – need for NR

Will, loss of willpower 1419

Tranquillity, serenity 1415

Anxiety about health. Fears.

1) 8.30 p.m. Funny ache in right breast/chest area – like a muscular nagging ache.(C)

I thought, irrationally, that it was breast cancer. I had the same thought some years ago. Still very warm all over.(A) (Day 2)

I had a vivid dream last night. I used to have a phobia of cancer. I was at a hospital or a huge doctor's surgery and I was told that I had been diagnosed with cancer of the teardrops! Bizarre.(A)

8.45 p.m. Feelings of anxiety(B) throughout the evening, as if fight or flight reflex (Day 3).

8 p.m. Generally I feel fine this evening, with no anxiety; just my eyes are tired and I'm generally tired.(B) (Day 4)

No anxiety (Day 5).

11 a.m. I ran upstairs and had a heart flutter – left-sided. It only lasted a second.(B) *These flutterings started up since I began the proving. Ten years ago I had inhalers for asthma, which caused similar palpitations.* I wasn't short of breath this time, and it didn't frighten me. Later, that night: I felt quite tired in bed. I lay there worrying about my heart. I fear I may have something wrong to have the heart flutterings, although I've had them for many years.(C) (Day 10)

7.15 p.m. I sat thinking about my heart again. I only had one tiny heart flutter today.(C) (Day 11)

I did homework until 12.30 a.m. By then I was overtired so when I eventually went to bed I was very restless. My mind was spinning.

I had thoughts of not feeling happy and confident with my homework. I couldn't switch my mind off; it was racing with thoughts about the remedy *Mercury*. I had to lay down and do relaxation techniques to calm myself down. I had a couple of palpitations and then started getting anxious: worried in case I have something wrong with my heart. I was very aware of my heart beating, aware of palpitations. It took a good hour to get to sleep (Day 18).

I still had the pain in my left leg on waking (the same as the darting pain yesterday), but it wore off quickly. I'm very tired (but was up late). I was still feeling anxious/aware of heart flutterings. They've all stopped now I've finished my homework (Day 19).

I've been in a bit of a state today because I've still been aware of the odd heart fluttering. My dad's been bad recently – I was really anxious it was to do with his heart. Then I found myself last night wanting to read up all the remedies, looking for a remedy for my dad.(A) (Day 28)

7) Throat dry – at time of taking first tablet. After third tablet: unusual feeling in throat – not a sore throat, but more a constriction, as if throat is closing up. Felt a bit panicky, but this feeling soon subsided. (Period almost finished.) (Day 1)

Unsettled night – dreams full of anxiety about impending event that I am about to organize. I feel that there may be some conflict ahead. I had a weird feeling during the day that some awful illness will strike at someone in the family and that it will change lives forever. Despite this I still feel very upbeat and positive. I had a good run at the gym – despite my period. *(See Prover 7 in Female section.)* (Day 21)

Rubrics
Anxiety About Health

Mind

Anxiety, health about 1275

Fear, cancer, of 1327
Anxiety, palpitations with NR
Anxiety, heart condition, about NR

Teenage resonances

3) 8 p.m. Dreadful toe cramps. They go when I apply pressure and hop around on my toes. I haven't had toe cramps for around six months and they haven't been this bad for over a year or more (Day 12). *Return of old symptom first experienced in my late teens.*

5) *Two days before the proving*: These past few days I have had a real sinking feeling in my stomach. A kind of anxiety. I've felt clumsy in my words and actions. Most strongly I feel very self-conscious with low confidence. Today I felt so embarrassed by the way I have been behaving towards friends and colleagues. I feel I'm acting 'silly' and 'dumbing down', unable to think before I speak. This has gone on since the college weekend. The only time I can recall feeling as self-conscious as I'm feeling now is when I was in my teens.

Observation during the proving: Proving relates a lot to early teens (clumsy, low self-confidence).

Later on: I have dyed my hair red and thought, 'the last time I did that was when I was about thirteen years old.' All through this proving I've had a sensation of 'revisiting' my teens (Day 33). *(Other provers died their hair red during the proving. Ed.)*

9) I felt very emotional when my husband was telling me news about a family member who is a young teenager and is being very self-destructive. I feel I could cry easily. Skin – dry patch under my lip, similar to when I was a teenager/early twenties. Often used to get this in very cold winter weather. I keep getting small spots on my face – chin and hairline, which is unusual for me. It is as if I can re-experience various aspects of this period of my life (Day 13).

I had a very interesting conversation (last night) with a very close friend of mine about when she couldn't deal with me when were about twenty/twenty-one, i.e. when I was having anorexia problems. She couldn't deal with my rejection of myself, of food and (what I was surprised about) her (Day 23).

Claustrophobia

5) My train journey home was seriously delayed and I became hugely claustrophobic and needing to get off the train. Obviously I didn't, but have never had such a problem with being stuck on a train before (Day 16).

I have been at home with my son who is unwell and have found the heating unbearable and craved fresh air (Day 17).

7) Awoke feeling a bit claustrophobic, and constricted: hemmed in by all the sickness around me (Day 13).

Rubrics
Claustrophobia

Mind

Fear, phobias, claustrophobia, closed places 1329

Fear, phobias, narrow place, in 1333

Environment

Air, open air, outside, desire for 518

Body Parts and Functions

Contents

Head/Headaches/Vertigo/Light-headedness

Eyes + vision/nose + smells

Face

Mouth, tongue, teeth

Food and drink. Appetite and thirst. Effects of alcohol.

Stomach, nausea and feelings of intoxication. Abdomen, and bowel movements.

Urine and bladder
Female: Menses/feeling broody/libido
Throat/cough/breathing
Skin and respiration
Heart
Back, neck and shoulders
Extremities – Limbs

Head/Headaches/Vertigo/Light-headedness

1) *Her sequence: six days of head symptoms, some of them new to her – a gap of a week – then mostly familiar menstrual headaches.*

Six days before the proving: Urine infection. Peeing frequently. Nausea, headache.

12.45 p.m. Took second and final tablet. 12.50 p.m. Felt slightly light-headed, almost drunk feeling, straightaway. 2.15 p.m. Felt slightly headachy, for half an hour.(C) My energy slumped and I felt a bit tired (Day 1).

No light-headedness or giggling today (Day 2).

1.30 p.m. A dull headache. (B) Muzzy, from my eyes up to the top of my forehead, both sides. It comes and goes. Sometimes it seems to come from my neck. I can't think of anything that makes it better or worse. (It lasted right into the evening.) (Day 4)

9.15 p.m. Had an itch on the left side of my head, and when I scratched it, it hurt like a burning sore. It remained sore and painful for a few minutes even after I stopped scratching it and even though there was nothing there.(A) The whole of the top of my head felt sore to touch, like it would if I'd brushed my hair too hard.(A) 11 p.m. I had a pain in my head – on the top of my head on the left side. Quite an intense pain. I wondered if it could be related to my neck (referred pain).(A) (Day 6)

Gap of a week

8.30 a.m. Very tired eyes, and I had a headache over my left eye area.(C) Didn't have it when I woke up (Day 13).

4 p.m. I have a headache on the left side over my eye again, but I can get it for three or four days before my period (although I haven't had it for two or three months).(C) (Day 14)

Period begins (Day 18).

1 p.m. I started to get a headache, the one I get with my period. It was worse for moving around. (C) I did take two Nurofen (usually helped by *Belladonna 200).* 4.30 p.m. I still had the headache, with pain around the left eye area as usual. I was tired and irritable. I felt frustrated with everything – it felt like I was not getting anywhere.(C) 7 p.m. I'd found that if I used my fingers to put pressure on the eye socket where the headache is, it was better for pressure. Also > cold flannel. The light hurts, with some relief from dimming the light (Day 19).

2 p.m. I suddenly had a headache (left-sided) coming on again, but it only lasted about ten minutes. I often get a headache at the end of a period. The period lasted for about a day and a half. Then it returned the next day.(C) (Day 20)

I had a headache tonight. It continued overnight. It was left-sided, almost like I have pre-menstrually but my period is not due (Day 28).

3) I had a very slight, fleeting tension headache up the back of my head at 7.30 p.m. tonight. This was mild and lasted no more than half an hour (Day 7).

4) *Eight days before the proving:* 1.50 p.m. Felt very dizzy after walking in rain, had to sit down on a chair when coming inside. Felt a bit spaced out.

I had a headache this evening across my forehead and extending to my temples. Dull pain, with sensation of heaviness in my head < tobacco (Day 2).

Felt really dizzy approx 1.45 p.m. – 3 p.m. I felt sensitive to everyone's moods around me. As I walked down the street I imagined that some people were literally barging through my aura.

I felt very dizzy at one stage in a large high street shop, a bit breathless approx 2.30 p.m. I thought I was going to pass out and kept knocking things off shelves as I turned around, with a slight spinning sensation in my head. I stopped taking the remedies today as I feel I have come out in symptoms, the main one being dizziness and a spaced out feeling. Headache across front of forehead extending to temples, dull ache. Heavy-headed sensation and very tired approx 4 to 7 p.m. (Day 3)

Headache 12.40 a.m. < left side extending from left side temple to vertex, and dull pain across forehead. Tired (Day 4).

Still clumsy, knocking things over, spilling drinks etc. throughout the day (Day 5).

Headache, frontal pain extending to vertex and temples, stopping midway across vertex (Day 12).

5) At 10.30 a.m. developed a slight headache, in the back of my head. At 12.45 p.m. took remedy. Headache improved in evening (Day 2).

8 p.m. I feel very tired and sleepy. I still have a slight headache, which seems to have moved forward and is more around the temples (Day 3).

My train journey home was seriously delayed and I became hugely claustrophobic and needing to get off the train. Obviously I didn't, but have never had such a problem with being stuck on a train before. At home I found the central heating unbearable and craved fresh air (Day 16).

I have woken with a sore throat and slight temperature. I've got a lot of mucus and phlegm. My head feels achy and hot (Day 19).

I have a lot of mucus and my head feels hot. My throat is also sore (Day 20).

6) Nausea (I thought I might be sick,) then coughing as it rose up into my throat, then a pounding headache in temples < light (Day 24). *(Sounding wheezy. Supervisor's observation.)*

7) 8.30 a.m. About thirty minutes after taking second dose, I felt a little light-headed and shaky inside.(A) (Day 1)

Went swimming and felt a real sense of lightness in the water. On reflection this was akin to the lightness in the head that I had felt yesterday.(A) (Day 2)

My daughter has headache, aversion to light and tired and a bit irritable (Day 5).

Daughter off sick from school. She has slight headache (Day 13).

I have been at home with my son who is unwell and have found the heating unbearable and craved fresh air (Day 17).

Headache developed during the day and by 3 p.m. I felt that my vision was difficult, and felt very heavy-headed.(B) (Day 23) *(This is during her period. Ed.)*

8) *Seven days before the proving:* Tablets on table beside me – sharp temple pain < left side, sensation as if: someone pressing them, for few minutes. Top of head tingling. Slightly clumsy, keep dropping my pen. Kept getting confused when dealing with numbers – i.e. money change.

Six days before the proving: 10 a.m. I had a very sharp pain in head right side (parietal area – frontal), pain moved as if along a line three or four times and then stopped.

Migraine. Disturbed vision right eye, then pain over eyes then wallop; slept all day.(C) (Day 39)

Other symptoms noted after discussion in college: Extreme apathy to the point that my whole body almost ceased. Serious constipation and violent migraine. Unable to function physically. I put this down to my pregnancy but discussing with another two provers they both experienced the apathy as well (Day 42).

10) Mild headache on and off all day in frontal lobe and slightly sore throat; also a feeling of a lump in my throat (Day 2).

No headaches (Day 4).

Rubrics
Head, Headaches, Vertigo

Head

Heat, sensation 881

Heaviness, sensation 885

Heaviness, sensation, headache from 885

Headaches

Dull pain 922

Forehead 925

Forehead, extending to temples 927

Forehead, extending to vertex 927

Sore, vertex 975

Vertigo

Vertigo 1878

Vertigo, afternoon 1878

Eyes + vision/nose + smells

1) 11 a.m. Had to blow nose. Lots of clear thin catarrh.(B) 1 p.m. Eyes feel noticeably wide and big.(A) I wondered if it was a hallucinogenic remedy? 9 p.m. Had a very itchy left eye, which appeared slightly bloodshot.(A) (Day 1)

12.30 p.m. I felt very catarrhy in the back of my nose. It seemed stuck there.(B) This went away after half an hour (Day 2).

On waking: feel alert, my eyes feel really wide-awake.(A) I'm not usually a morning person at all (Day 3).

8 a.m. Felt really tired when I woke; I couldn't get out if bed, and then all of a sudden my eyes felt really wide awake, even though they felt tired when I was in bed.(A) Again it's like flicking a switch. 8.30 p.m. Tickling in upper nose, as if I was going to sneeze, but didn't. It lasted for about five minutes. Then suddenly my left nostril started running clear 'water'. No sneezing.(A) (Day 6)

My nose just suddenly ran – dripping from my left nostril like water. It came out of nowhere. Just an isolated event.(A) 8.30 p.m.

Very itchy eyes – slightly bloodshot (Day 7).

7.30 p.m. I had a really itchy left eye, again with a slight burning sensation.(A) (Day 8)

11.50 p.m. Itchy inside left nostril, for a couple of minutes.(A) (Day 9)

10 a.m. I just want to get on and do something. My eyes feel wide awake.(A) I wonder if I have picked up some energy from the proving co-ordinator. (I saw him two days ago.) 1.45 p.m. I had a really itchy left eye again. (Nothing to see, not red; it just felt a bit sore.) Lasted for ten minutes.(B) (Day 10)

7.30 a.m. I jumped out of bed, my eyes feeling wide awake but my body felt tired.(A)

3.20 p.m. I had a very itchy left eye for a minute.(A) (Day 11)

7.15 a.m. My eyes are very awake although my body is a bit tired and heavy.(A) (Day 12)

8.30 a.m. Very tired eyes, and I had a headache over my left eye area.(C) Didn't have it when I woke up (Day 13).

6.30 p.m. I had an itchy left eye, sore when rubbed, lasted five minutes.(A) (Day 14)

7.30 a.m. I got up, but my eyes were tired and heavy.(C) The cold symptoms were better (Day 16).

10 a.m. Itchy left eye, which was slightly sore, when rubbed for about five minutes, and slightly bloodshot. 8 p.m. Beginning to feel catarrh, as if a cold is coming on again. Very tired, especially eyes (Day 17).

4.30 p.m. I still had the headache, with pain around the left eye area as usual. 7 p.m. I'd found that if I used my fingers to put pressure on the eye socket where the headache is, it was better for pressure. Also > cold flannel. The light hurts, with some relief from dimming the light. 9 p.m. I smelt a burning smell when sitting in the lounge. I got up to look around but there was nothing. It lasted a few seconds (Day 19).

10.15 a.m. Itchy left eye again.(A) (Day 20)

2) *Six days before the proving.* My left eye was sore and bloodshot in the corner when I awoke. It felt as though it had grit in it. This lasted for an hour, then the discomfort and redness disappeared altogether.

3) *Review: Since the proving began I have been sneezing two or three times a day, very mild sneezes that are actually quite pleasant! Also my libido has been a bit higher this week, but I'm wondering if that is just related to my menstrual cycle* (Day 8).

6) I woke up this morning with a bloodshot right eye, inner canthi. No apparent cause (Day 3).

Eye still bloodshot (Days 4 and 5).

Eye is pink now (Day 6)

Eye going yellow now (Day 7).

8) Dose 1. 6.30 a.m. 8 a.m. Pain in left side of neck on cervical vertebrae nodule of neck extending to under left shoulder blade then disappearing and extending down anterior of left arm to elbow. Continued for half an hour.

Dose 2. 1.10 p.m. Numb sensation down inside of right arm. Tingling on tip of tongue before the remedy dissolved. End of nose numb. Sensation as if coming round from numb as in after anaesthesia at the dentist. Numbness in nose lasted two and a half hours. I became concerned by this numbness in my nose, so I stopped with this second dose. It was an uncomfortable numbness and I was worried that it might extend to other areas of my face (Day 1).

4.30 p.m. Nose feels numb again, not as bad as before but numbish. Lasted about one hour (Day 3).

Right eye painful all day. Felt enlarged compared to left. Neuralgic pain going down right side of face, worse on bone under the eye. << light, touch, OK on hard pressure (Day 23).

Got up to stop alarm clock on phone; when I tried to focus I couldn't see anything for about two seconds then could see and able to focus. Bit frightening until sight came back. Eye better today but still a little sore. Effects faded during the morning (Day 24).

Migraine. Disturbed vision right eye, then pain over eyes then wallop; slept all day (Day 39). (C)

9) I woke with a sore left eye; it feels as if I may be developing a sty on the lower lid. It feels as if there's an infection at the base of the eyelash (Day 3).

The sty has gone, and on my left forearm I have a spot that's slightly itchy and raised. It feels as if it is an infected pore. When I squeezed it clear pus came out. Actually feels like a hard lump under the skin. It's been coming up for two days (Day 6).

7.30 p.m. Left eye suddenly bleary, opaque white discharge in the corner of the eye. Not itchy, slightly red (Day 7).

I realized that I've had a twitch from time to time in my left eyelid, sporadically over several days (Day 51).

10) Attended college discussion of proving and realized through general discussion that I had ignored some symptoms or effects. I remembered that, since the proving began, I have had some difficulty reading a text on the TV screen as if I was unable to focus my eyes. I had my eyes tested recently and they were OK. This did not continue after the proving. (Day 14)

Rubrics

Eyes

Alert, sensation NR

Alert, sensation, suddenly NR

Ecchymosis 540

Enlargement, sensation 540

Heaviness, sensation 543

Itchy 546

Pain, 550

Pain, light 552

Pain, pressure amel. 553

Sore pain 563
Tired, sensation 568
Wide-awake, sensation NR
Vision
Foggy, suddenly NR (original word was bleary)
Nose
Coryza, watery 1502
Coryza, watery, suddenly NR
Obstructed 1517
Smell of burning, something 1523
Sneezing, general 1524

Face

3) I've noticed two spots under the skin – one above each eyebrow, an unusual place for me to get spots. (The spots themselves are normal for me.) *(Later on at college the co-ordinator describes a pink spot at the 'third eye' point, a similar area to my unusual spot.)* (Day 7)

4) Spots on chin since the last two days, not usual, though I do get them occasionally. I put it down to the fact I'd had a late night just before, and drank too much alcohol (Day 1).

8) Dose 1. 6.30 a.m. 8 a.m. Pain in left side of neck on cervical vertebrae nodule of neck extending to under left shoulder blade then disappearing and extending down anterior of left arm to elbow. Continued for half an hour.

Dose 2. 1.10 p.m. Numb sensation down inside of right arm. Tingling on tip of tongue before the remedy dissolved. End of nose numb. Sensation as if coming round from numb as in after anaesthesia at the dentist. Numbness in nose lasted two and a half hours. I became concerned by this numbness in my nose, so I stopped with this second dose. It was an uncomfortable numbness and I was worried that it might extend to other areas of my face. 9 p.m.

Numbness in end of nose returned. Tip of nose cold (Day 1).

Few small spots under nose, probably pre-menstrual. Sometimes get the odd spot (Day 10).

9) Dry patch under my lip, similar to when I was a teenager/early twenties. Often used to get this in very cold winter weather. I keep getting small spots on my face – chin and hairline, which is unusual for me. It is as if I can re-experience various aspects of this period of my life (Day 13).

Right eye painful all day. Felt enlarged compared to left. Neuralgic pain going down right side of face, worse on bone under the eye. << light, touch, OK on hard pressure (Day 23).

10) Spot on left side of upper lip, itchy but nothing visible (Day 14).

Rubrics

Face

Pain, right 590

Pain, eye, below, right NR

Nose

Coldness, tip of 1497

Numbness 1517

Mouth/Tongue/Teeth

1) 9 a.m. I've got toothache again, and would take something if I could. My teeth have been sensitive since starting the proving.(A) 10.30 a.m. Had severe toothache so I took a couple of Paracetamol. It's on the right side, difficult to tell which tooth. I can feel a tiny hole. One of my very back teeth is beginning to recede. I've been getting an almost numb sensation when I grit my teeth together.(A) 6.30 p.m. Throbbing toothache; two more Paracetamol.(C) I felt hot in the face with the toothache, but otherwise my normal temperature (Day 11).

2) Three and a half hours into the proving I had an unpleasant, slightly metallic taste in my mouth, at the front of my tongue, which lasted approx one and a half hours. It went after eating lunch (Day 1).

I had a muscular twinge in my left jaw, moving to the right. It lasted about two minutes. It was a throbbing, stabbing pain (Day 15).

7) Funny taste in mouth like all food is fusty. Taste buds seem really shot.(A) (Day 29)

8) Metallic taste in mouth. Tea tastes horrible and not able to finish it. Reminds me of being pregnant (Day 27).

10) 7 a.m. 4th dose. Slight metallic taste in lower right jaw, where I have a crown (Day 2).

The link with oral toxicity showing up here? Mercury amalgam perhaps. Ed.

Rubrics

Teeth

Numbness of teeth, clenching, when 1800

Pain, teeth, toothaches 1800

Pain, hot face, with NR

Tongue

Taste, bad 1848

Taste, metallic 1851

Taste, musty 1851 (original word was fusty)

Food and drink. Appetite and thirst. Effects of alcohol.

1) *Seven days before the proving:* Feeling tired. Achy all over. Limbs feel heavy. Felt slightly nauseous. Appetite less than normal. Felt better about 7 p.m. 7.30 a.m. Very thirsty for water.(A) Not normally thirsty first thing in the morning. Still nauseous throughout the afternoon, >

sips of cold Diet Coke and < water.(A) The Coke had to be fridge cold. Usually I like to drink water at room temperature. I'm not sure if the nausea is caused by the remedy. My husband has an upset tummy, but hasn't felt sick. 10.30 p.m. Felt I had to eat, very hungry. I craved a sandwich with salad cream and cheese.(A) I would not normally have salad cream (Day 2).

8 a.m. Very thirsty for anything but especially water.(B) (Day 3)

2.20 p.m. No physical energy. Mentally want to get on with things, but physically can't.(C) Burnt out. Crave chocolate again.(C) Thirsty for water.(C) (Day 4)

11 a.m. When shopping my legs felt heavy and very tired.(A) I had a craving for something sweet but especially an apple pastry or cake of some kind.(A) Very thirsty for water.(C) I carry a bottle and drink a cupful at a time, rather than just sips, but only passing normal amounts of urine. Not a very big appetite generally though.(C) 4.45 p.m. Craving for cheese and a yoghurt drink. This is unusual for me in the afternoon (Day 5).

3 p.m. Craving for a chocolate bar. Normally if I have sugar, within half an hour I'm tired, but I wasn't. It didn't affect me. Generally, more appetite today – picking at things between meals.(B) 10.45 p.m. Unusually I craved a glass of Coca Cola – but only had a sip. I could have drunk more of it, but I know it is not good for you, so stopped myself drinking more (Day 6).

8 a.m. Thirsty especially for water. 8 p.m. Slightly nauseous, perhaps trapped wind.(C) Especially before my period, I get it. I craved Coca Cola again; I felt I could drink a big glassful. Nausea was > for drinking Coke.(A) 10.35 p.m. I suddenly had a craving for tandoori chicken or Indian food of some kind.(A) (Day 7)

8 a.m. Had some toast (unusual as never normally can face breakfast as soon as this.) 11 a.m. Craved a packet of cheddar biscuits and a KitKat.(B) This took the sweet craving away. 1 p.m. Craving something sweet again like chocolate (B) but managed to just eat a pear. I am not getting the light-headed/drunk sensation that I used to get when I ate something sweet. This was before I

stopped eating sweet, sugary things about six months ago. 7.30 p.m. I felt really hungry but when the dinner was in front of me I didn't really want it.(A) 9.30 p.m. Craving for chocolate – had a KitKat. (Day 8)

8 a.m. Very hungry. (Unusual for that time of day)

Afternoon: Thirsty for water.(C) 3.20 p.m. Had *huge* sugar craving.(C)

4 p.m. I had the urge to make some biscuits. I actually dipped my finger in the demerara sugar, and I ate I don't know how many biscuits. I couldn't get enough sugar. It made me feel better.(C) 10.50 p.m. Still very thirsty for water.(C) Then I wanted to pee very frequently. Each time after peeing I felt I had to replace the water – I felt really thirsty. Then twenty minutes later the same would happen again (Day 9).

8 a.m. Again, and unusually, I felt hungry for breakfast (Day 10).

8.50 p.m. Very, very thirsty for cold water.(C) I've still got an appetite, but I'm nauseous – strange really.(A) My stomach's been making loads of rumbling sounds. One thing I have noticed in the last few days, because I smoke, I haven't fancied a cigarette and when I do I get a horrible taste afterwards.(A) I imagine it is like a sulphur taste (Day 12).

Not very thirsty today (Day 13).

10 a.m. I was very hungry and craved cheese on toast.(A) 11 a.m. Had a sweet craving. I avoided chocolate – I had a hot cross bun. I've had a big appetite today. (A) (Day 14)

Evening: I craved cherry Coke, sipped some and then had gassy, colicky pains.(A) Throughout the evening I craved chicken korma – and had one at 11.30 p.m.! (A) (Day 16)

4.45 p.m. I craved fruit – quite unlike me. I felt better for it.(A) (Day 17)

I was very hungry, more so in the morning (unlike me). 3.30 p.m. Had a craving for sweets (C) – had about four chocolate biscuits (Day 20).

I was very hungry and thirsty throughout the morning.(B) (Day

21)

I craved cheese and salad cream again.(A) (Day 30)

I had salad cream again.(A) No cravings for Coca Cola (Day 31).

I've been really hungry. I could eat and eat throughout the day.(A) I'm still craving cheese; I even wanted cream cheese and cheese straws.(A) But not wanting Coke or chocolate. I'm craving a lot of vegetables, making vegetable juices, mostly celery and tomato (Day 35).

3) I woke up feeling disproportionately hung-over, considering the amount of alcohol I had. I have a very bad headache and feel very nauseous. I drank two glasses of champagne and five vodka and sodas. This would not normally make me feel this bad (Day 2).

4) *Decreased appetite:* Loss of appetite. I realized I'd only eaten three slices of toast during the day by the evening. Ate tuna and sweet corn with pasta, which tasted like it could be cat food (Day 1).

Increased appetite: Wanting sweet foods, cake, chocolates, crisps, pizza, banoffee pie. I've had cravings for these foods over the past few days (return of old symptom, associated with times of bulimia) (Day 9).

Eating lots of junk food, cakes, pudding with cream, chips, chocolate, crisps. Drinking lots of sweet cold drinks like Ribena and Coca Cola. Appetite may have been increased from smoking cannabis, but it's not usual for me to eat this amount (Day 10).

5) I have realized that I ate meat (chicken) for the third time in two days (which I rarely do) and then had a really painful stomach-ache where I was bent double, from about 2 p.m. to 5 p.m. Then it passed (Day 3).

Another night of waking and vivid dreams. I feel tired and unrefreshed. I dreamed I was at a huge ball and my body started to swell. I swelled up like a balloon and a doctor was called. I urged myself to sort out my stomach problems (Day 5).

I realize I've been craving sweets and chocolate (and eating!) these last few days, which normally only happens before my period (not due for two weeks) (Day 9).

I still have a large appetite, particularly for sweet things (Day 10).

My appetite continues to be huge and feels like my PMT appetite (but it can't be yet). Craving chocolate and bread and sweet things (Day 11).

My appetite shows no sign of decreasing. And I'm still eating lots of sweet things, chocolate, biscuits, hot chocolate etc. (Day 13).

I have started my period about ten days early this evening. All day I was very tired, but at least my craving for chocolate can now be explained. I have never had an early period before; I am always very regular. My period is heavy. In the evening I was full of wind, my stomach very bloated. This was painful – a sharp pain (Day 14).

I've been eating unhealthily and going to bed late (Day 31).

Woke with excruciating stomach cramp. Feels very much like trapped wind (Day 32).

I have had a bad night's sleep due to stomach cramps. I am windy this morning but still have a slight stomach-ache and constipation (Day 33).

I have also been craving and eating chocolate again, yesterday and today, my period is not yet due, so it isn't my usual PMT cravings (Day 34).

Review: Stomach – digestion, worse from anxiety.

I am feeling very 'blue'. I can't seem to shake off my anxiety about moving house. I feel the proving and even my college work is the furthest thing from my mind. I have had to move many times before, yet this time I feel very uncertain and not hopeful about the future.

I am eating a lot of things that are not good for me and give me stomach-ache, bread, croissants, chocolate and coffee. I am also going to bed late. My mood is not one of 'taking care' of myself. I can't shake this 'doubting' and lack of confidence. I am still bloated and only half go to the toilet, but remain slightly constipated (Day 35).

I have slept better. My mood has been more relaxed and I feel more hopeful about the future. Less anxiety. I have been very calm (Day 36).

Review: My stomach was not crampy today – but in the evening again I am full of wind, which does not alleviate. I was not constipated today. I am still eating unhealthily and craving all that is bad for my stomach – pizza and chocolate!

Having gone for a meal yesterday evening and drank too much wine, I have had vomiting and diarrhoea all night, with cold sweats. I felt so hot I had to quickly take my clothes off – but the sweat felt cold. I became so desperate to stop the vomiting that I took *Arsenicum 30C* thinking it may be food poisoning. I then tried *Nux vomica 30* an hour later and another an hour after that. I have had no more diarrhoea, but still feel very queasy.

This evening my appetite is returning, I have eaten porridge, rye crackers and crisps. I feel very sleepy despite having slept a lot today (Day 38).

Still feeling slightly queasy from Tuesday's sickness, but well enough to go to work. All day I have been craving chicken again and looking forward to being able to go and buy some (Day 39).

I'm eating lots of chocolate, I think it may be PMT (Day 42).

I have a huge appetite today (Day 43).

I cannot stop eating, my period is due.

As the proving seems to have come to an end for me – I feel that I am going to have to start some healing treatment for my stomach (Day 44).

I have got my period today, normal cycle time. I'm eating lots of chocolate and cheese on toast (Day 46).

I have a huge appetite and eat every hour (Day 47).

I am eating lots, particularly bread and chocolate (Day 48).

7) Throat dry – at time of taking first tablet. After third tablet: unusual feeling in throat – not a sore throat, but more a constriction, as if throat is closing up. Felt a bit panicky, but this feeling soon subsided. Period almost finished today (Day 1).

7.30 a.m. Dose 4. Throat constriction still present.(A) Feel really thirsty and a little dehydrated with it.(B) (Day 2)

I have been drinking a lot of water. Feel thirsty a lot.(A) (Day 3)

Awoke feeling parched and dehydrated with mouth dry. Drank two glasses of water. Unusual for me. *Later:* Body feels limp and weary, > for drinking.(B) (Day 9)

Very thirsty, trying to increase water consumption and feel better for it.(B) (Day 10)

Woke up at night, dry and thirsty.(B) (Day 16)

Dryness continues (Day 24).

Still rather thirsty (Day 37).

8) Irritable like PMT. Irritable with husband and daughter. Shouting at my daughter then feeling remorseful. Shirty with husband but kept it in. I knew I was crabby though. Suppressing my anger, resorting to eating chocolate instead. *(A reminder of the postnatal depression that I had two years ago.)* (Day 4)

I'm expressing so much more, rather than suppressing my feelings; yesterday, I felt so angry. I felt like I wanted to smash an empty bottle of wine against the wall and wanted to walk out of my home. I didn't. I ate some Maltesers and had a cup of tea instead (Day 5).

9) *Her previous history of bulimia/anorexia (and associated issues) resolved substantially during this proving. (See her synopsis, Page 260.)*

10) Big appetite all day (Day 2).

7.30 a.m. Woke feeling very thirsty (Day 3). *Later review: This was unusual at the time, though has become the norm now five weeks on.*

Not particularly thirsty today (Day 4).

Rubrics

Food

Appetite, increased, hunger 725

Appetite, increased, hunger, afternoon 725
Cheese, desires 732
Cold, drinks, water, desires 733
Fruit, desires 737
Meat, desires 739
Spicy, food, desires 743
Sugar, desires 743
Sweets, general, desires 743
Thirst, general 744
Alcohol, general, aggravates, easily intoxicated 724

General

Weariness, water, drinking amel. NR

Stomach, nausea and feelings of intoxication. Abdomen and bowel movements.

1) *Seven days before the proving:* Feeling tired. Achy all over. Limbs feel heavy. Felt slightly nauseous. Appetite less than normal. Felt better about 7 p.m.

8.30 a.m. Slight pain in groin area and needed to pee twice in half an hour. It felt like my UTI had come back.(C) It lasted for about half an hour, I passed a small quantity of urine, then just suddenly the pain stopped; this was then followed by a couple of minutes of flatulence.(B) (Day 1)

2 p.m. Heat in face again, twice. Waves of nausea and slight dizziness.(A) Felt sick straight after lunch.(A) Still felt very warm, not a fever, just hot and a bit sweaty, especially in my armpits. (I'm not usually a sweaty person at all.) I even went out on school run with just a cardigan and no coat.

Still nauseous throughout the afternoon, > sips of cold Diet Coke and < water.(A) The Coke had to be fridge cold. Usually I like to drink water at room temperature. I'm not sure if the nausea is caused by the remedy. My husband has an upset tummy, but hasn't felt sick (Day 2).

11 p.m. Period-like pains. (My period isn't due for two weeks.) In lower abdomen and an achy lower back, > lying down and > passing wind.(B) It came on suddenly and lasted until I went to sleep. Slight nausea after this pain began, for a few minutes. I thought it might be a urine infection (Day 4).

9 p.m. Lots of belching and flatulence.(A) This lasted for most of the evening. Also slightly nauseous.(B) (Day 5)

8.30 a.m. Lots of belching and some flatulence.(B) 2 p.m. I felt slightly nauseous for a couple of minutes. 8 p.m. Slightly nauseous, perhaps trapped wind.(C) Especially before my period I get it. I craved Coca Cola again; I felt I could drink a big glassful. Nausea was > for drinking Coke.(A) 9.30 p.m. Felt slightly nauseous again > belching. Acid, sicky belching.(A) 10.35 p.m. I suddenly had a craving for tandoori chicken or Indian food of some kind.(A) 10.40 p.m. In bed my stomach was making loud rumbling noises.(B) (Day 7)

7.45 a.m. As soon as I got up had to go and open my bowels.(A) 8 a.m. Had some toast (unusual as never normally can face breakfast as soon as this.) 8.45 a.m. After breakfast I had to open my bowels again, quite loose.(A) (Day 8)

3.20 p.m. I started to make more biscuits, but felt a bit sick, like morning sickness. I think it was trapped wind.(B) (Day 10)

9.20 a.m. I suddenly had real cramping tummy pains – I thought I was going to have diarrhoea but didn't. They were like burning pains. I got goose bumps and felt slightly nauseous.(C) 9.30 a.m. Face felt hot and flushed.(A) 10 a.m. I have felt a bit nauseous today. My daughter has too, so it could be something going around. 2.30 p.m. I had cramping pains again, but not as bad.(C) 7 p.m. Stomach started to feel better.(C) 8.50 p.m. Very, very thirsty for cold water.(C) I've still got an appetite, but I'm nauseous – strange really.(A) My stomach's been making loads of rumbling sounds (Day 12).

I've had loads of flatulence the last few days. (Husband commented on this.)(A) (Day 16)

I had a spell of nausea early evening.(C) (Day 19)

5 p.m. I had colicky pains in my stomach, from holding on to flatulence.(C) This lasted about half an hour (Day 20).

3.15 a.m. Awoke feeling very nauseous. Was actually sick. Felt better afterwards. *Later:* Slight loss of appetite and a bit nauseous (Day 41).

2) I felt nauseous from around 3 p.m. until after my dinner, four hours later. I'd had a spoonful of an oil supplement, which I do most days, and it kept repeating on me. I could taste it in my throat, which made me feel sick. I had no appetite and felt worse for the thought of food. Although I don't find the taste of the oil pleasant, it hasn't had this effect on me before (Day 3).

3) Got a sudden stomach-ache in the upper abdomen, in the centre just below my ribs, < pressure, < doubled-up, > stretching out. (I also had a slight hot flush as the tummy pains started.) Pains – twisting inside, gripping, quite sharp and a little bit nauseous. Intense for a couple of minutes, then easing off, and just slightly achy and nauseous after that. It comes in waves. The duration was from about 4.15 p.m. to 6.15 p.m. I also felt nauseous and had a rise in temperature with a feverish feeling, accompanying the pain. I felt panicky about the pains. I was worried something serious was wrong but this panic didn't last (Day 6). *This is a return of old symptoms.*

I experienced a very mild and fleeting nausea sensation today (Day 7). *(See also her entry Day 6 in Coincidences section.)*

I felt very nauseous on the train to London this morning. It came on about 8.30 a.m. and carried on until about 9 a.m. It gradually got worse while I was sitting still on the train but cleared and went completely when I got off the train and walked in the fresh air (Day 11).

I had a very fleeting feeling of nausea around 8 a.m. in the car on the way to work (Day 12).

I had nausea on the train again this morning from 8.45 to around 9 a.m. I had a funny taste in my mouth along with it (Day 18).

4) *Eight days before the proving:* Awoke around 3–3.15 a.m. Felt slightly nauseous. Not sure whether to attribute this to the fact I'd had a few drinks last night celebrating a friend's birthday. Still awake at 4.40 a.m. Acid feels like it's rising in my chest. *Context:* Dwelling on new relationship, unable to sleep. Not sure what I want out of this relationship (with someone I met a week ago on New Year's Eve.) 8.25 a.m. Diarrhoea. Watery, with bits – grey/brown colour water.

I felt very sick this morning, I think I have a stomach bug, very bad diarrhoea, watery, lots of it approx 8.30 a.m. My daughter woke me in the early hours and threw up everywhere, also has diarrhoea. I felt as if I wanted to be sick but couldn't. Felt very weak, very pale in the face, but felt better after more sleep (Day 4).

Stomach bug appears to be a lot better and I haven't suffered as much as my daughter and mother did with it (no vomiting and less long lasting). (Day 5)

My stomach is bloated; I look about five months pregnant, < approx 9 a.m. after getting up around 8.10 a.m. Still bloated throughout day and into the night. Symptoms of IBS appear to be returning with stomach cramps, < lower abdomen; and slight flatulence. Heavy sensation around lower abdomen. Cutting, stabbing pains intensifying from dull pains, lasting approx five minutes at a time. Approx every one and a half hours (since around 9 a.m.) (Day 11).

Stomach has gone down, still a bit protruded, but I weighed myself to find I've put on half a stone.

I felt better after some exercise and a sauna/steam. Stomach is still a bit tender around lower abdomen and across it. It feels a little inflamed (Day 12).

5) *Day before the proving begins:* Today I have stomach-ache and am constipated. I feel tired.

3 p.m. Took remedy, went to the toilet within twenty minutes of taking remedy having been constipated before (Day 1).

I have realized that I ate meat (chicken) for the third time in two days (which I rarely do) and then had a really painful stomach-ache where I was bent double, from about 2 p.m. to 5 p.m. Then it passed. I am constipated today, but have no stomach-ache (Day 3).

My period is still heavy, which is normal for me. My mood is impatient and slightly irritable and I feel very sleepy – also normal during periods. In the evening I was full of wind, my stomach very bloated. This was painful and felt like a sharp pain (Day 15).

Woke with excruciating stomach cramp. Feels very much like trapped wind.

I am feeling full of anxiety about where my future is going to be, e.g. new home. I don't feel as if I'm going with the flow at all. I am slightly constipated and have a feeling of 'fullness' (Day 32).

I have had a bad night's sleep due to stomach cramps. I am windy this morning but still have a slight stomach-ache and constipation (Day 33).

Bad night's sleep – kept waking and needing a pee. Slightly less constipated. Through being at work, it has reminded me that my flatulence is not a problem in the daytime, but appears more in the evenings.

Woke with excruciating stomach cramp, again like trapped wind.

Due to having been given notice to move, I'm full of anxiety, and at times like that my stomach and digestion can be problematic (Day 34).

*Review: Stomach, digestion – worse anxiety.*I am feeling very 'blue'. I can't seem to shake off my anxiety about moving house. I feel the proving and even my college work is the furthest thing from my mind. I have had to move many times before, yet this time I feel very uncertain and not hopeful about the future. I am eating a lot of things that are not good for me and give me stomach-ache, bread, croissants, chocolate and coffee. I am also going to bed late. My mood is not one of 'taking care' of myself. I can't shake this 'doubting' and lack of confidence. I am still bloated and only half go to the toilet, but remain slightly constipated (Day 35).

My mood has been more relaxed and I feel more hopeful about the future. Less anxiety. I have been very calm. My stomach was not crampy today – but in the evening again I am full of wind, which does not alleviate. I was not constipated today. I am still eating unhealthily and craving all that is bad for my stomach – pizza and chocolate! (Day 36)

I have no stomach-ache or constipation today (Day 37).

Having gone for a meal yesterday evening and drank too much wine, I have had vomiting and diarrhoea all night, with cold sweats. I felt so hot I had to quickly take my clothes off – but the sweat felt cold. I became so desperate to stop the vomiting that I took *Arsenicum 30* thinking it may be food poisoning. I then tried *Nux vomica 30* an hour later and another *Nux vomica 30* another hour later. I have had no more diarrhoea, but still feel very queasy (Day 38).

I have spent the whole day rowing with my son. I feel sad and exhausted. My confidence as a mother is low tonight. I am still constipated and windy (Day 42).

My mood is very calm today. I cannot stop eating, my period is due. I have not been constipated today. As the proving seems to have come to an end for me – I feel that I am going to have to start some healing treatment for my stomach (Day 44).

I've realized I'm sleeping better at night again. I am still constipated and have wind (Day 45).

I have got my period today, normal cycle time. I'm eating lots of chocolate and cheese on toast. I'm no longer constipated (Day 46).

6) *Stomach.* Heartburn rising to throat. *(Aggravation of a familiar symptom.)* (Day 1)

Raging heartburn, rising and felt in the throat, < swallowing (Day 3).

No heartburn (Day 4).

Heartburn, burning sensation rising up to the throat, < belching (Day 10).

Heartburn rising again. (Consistently < 2 p.m.) (Day 12)

No further heartburn (Day 13).

Nausea and feelings of intoxication. I had a few sips of an alcoholic drink. Later, when I lay down, the room was spinning. I could not focus and felt sick. It was < laying on my back. I had to lay on my front with my head hanging over the edge of the bed facing the floor. I kept trying to be sick but all I produced was phlegm (Day 1).

Morning: I slept well, and my stomach feels fine today after last night.

Evening: Feeling a bit nauseous, as if I might be sick (Day 2).

Nausea (I thought I might be sick,) then coughing as it rose up into my throat, then a pounding headache in temples < light (Day 24). *Sounding wheezy. (Supervisor's observation.)*

Abdomen and sides. Cramping pain below umbilicus, with flatulence, < movement, > sitting still (Day 1).

Evening: Sharp pain under ribs, left side (Day 29).

Evening: Pain under my ribs again (Day 37).

Bowel movements: Diarrhoea, after stomach-ache and abdominal wind (Day 1).

7) Daughter says she has 'gurgling, nausea in her stomach as if it was churning.' This is accompanied by mild diarrhoea (Day 14).

My stomach is gurgling and I feel a little nauseous all day. It seems like a milder version of what my daughter has had (Day 17).

All ailments from yesterday are gone – nausea and gurgling stomach (Day 18).

Her period began the next day. *(See Prover 7 in Female section. Page 202)*

I have been experiencing nausea on and off again. Period has now finished (Day 23).

I still feel the constriction in my throat and nausea too; and still feeling emotionally unsettled, as I did during my period. It is unusual for this to carry on after my period has ended.(A) (Day 25)

8) Foul smelling flatulence. Stomach slightly distended; clothes feel tight (Day 3).

Very flatulent, foul smelling, metallic. Not ameliorated when passed, just makes way for the next one. Stools a tad watery. Nothing in diet that could really account for it.(B) (Day 4)

Really bad wind today. It never seemed to stop. It didn't feel any better when I had let some of it out. Stools a bit watery today, 'splattery'. I forced it out to get rid of it (Day 5).

Flatulence < night (Day 7).

Flatulence < evening (Day 8).

Mid morning: feeling irritable and impatient especially with husband's driving. Incident at stables made me very angry but didn't see the person responsible for initiating the anger to let it go, so the anger festered. I am just going to cut her dead from now on.(C) (Postnatal depression.)

Angry again when I returned to stables in evening. Calmer when I left there, but still got the anger because I can't confront the issue. Irritability > after stool (Day 9).

10 p.m. Pain in lower abdomen for five minutes, then had to rush to loo. Went two more times before it stopped (Day 19).

Urge to eat chocolate, so ate a big bag of Maltesers, choc raisins and two Freddos. Felt sick!(C) (Postnatal depression.) One hour later, had to rush to loo, preceded by hot sensation all over. Very watery, flatulent stools. Ten minutes later, same thing. Nothing more until 11 p.m. Husband said I was irritable, didn't feel it overly at the time, but was obviously projecting it. Narked with him for going to bed without saying goodnight. Chilly, can't seem to get warm. Sensitive to drafts.(B) 11 p.m. Diarrhoea – had to rush to loo, same as earlier. Sensation as if it is coming any minute, > after. Noticed a sensation of bile from stomach last couple of days (Day 20).

Diet – very bad today. Trapped wind this afternoon; > farting (Day 22).

Nausea feeling in pit of stomach – ate banana. Nausea >. Occurred to me I could be pregnant as had same feeling before and period still not arrived. (38 days since last period.) (C) Horrendous trapped wind in stomach; had to undo jeans. Unable to fart due to environment. Wind was going up rather than down to point that developed pain in back under right shoulder blade. Felt trapped over diaphragm. Wanted to burp but it wouldn't come up (Day 25). *(Familiar symptom of about ten years ago.)*

Ate out – bad indigestion about half hour later (Day 26).

5.20 a.m. Woke up, came over very hot, had to go to loo because I thought I was going to be sick. No period so thought, 'Morning sickness – oh great!' Had diarrhoea instead, black liquid. One hour later awoke – was sick, yellow liquid. Ate banana and rice cake – went to horse. Felt OK outside in fresh air. Came back felt dreadful again. Was sick again – banana and rice cake mashed. Must be the sickness bug that my friends have had. Exhausted all day, laid on settee but couldn't really sleep as was watching daughter. Later she was sick. Laid down on bed with daughter and slept for three hours, woke up, had a drink of water – can't face any other food. Can't face food except melon. Realize I am pregnant. Utterly exhausted (Day 29).

Felt much better in morning. Diarrhoea and vomiting stopped, still very tired though. Nausea, pit of stomach (Day 30).

Constipated (related to pregnancy). (Day 33)

Constipated again (Day 35).

Sluggish digestion. Seriously foul smelling flatulence after stool. Irritable, especially due to flatulence (Day 36).

Other symptoms noted after discussion in college: Extreme apathy to the point that my whole body almost ceased. Serious constipation and violent migraine. Unable to function physically. I put this down to my pregnancy but discussing with another two provers they both experienced the apathy as well (Day 43).

9) Period began. 9 a.m. Very grumpy and irritable, want my own space to get on with things. I feel trapped. 8 p.m. Stomach pains have started, it feels uncomfortable, not severe, just as if slightly constipated, but the constipation seems to be affecting my stomach

(Day 9).

8 p.m. Aching in my abdomen again, feels slightly bruised, as if constipated. This is the same as Day 9. Period has finished (Day 13).

Had slight stomach pains on and off today, feels like small intestine (Day 14).

I'm constipated today which is unusual for me unless just before my period (Day 15).

I'm holding tension in my stomach. Still constipated (Day 22).

Bowels have cleared (Day 23).

Stomach – feels slightly crampy since 7.30 a.m. (Day 24).

I've started taking a liquid aloe vera supplement, as my stomach still feels bruised and crampy. I had assumed it was because I've been keeping the gastritis away that my daughter was very poorly with. She was the only one who got ill, but then she was the only one who took a chemist medication, whereas the boys and I took herbal tinctures. I want to tend to our digestive systems. The boys keep getting little pimples on their cheeks, so I'll boost us all with some probiotics (Day 55).

The aloe vera seems to have done the job; my stomach feels normal again (Day 57).

10) Bowels – looser than normal (and for the following two days as it turns out,) but I have been doing a general de-tox (Day 1).

Urine and bladder

1) *Six days before:* Urine infection. Peeing frequently. Nausea, headache. Took *Cantharis 30.*

Five days before: Feeling slightly better. Still peeing lots. Took another *Cantharis 30.*

Four days before: Mostly better, feeling glum though. Sleepy in afternoon about 3 p.m. Took another *Cantharis 30.*

Because of her urine infection, to which she is susceptible, I suggested she waited to start the proving. She started two days after the rest of the group. As far as I can judge it, her symptoms 'of the proving' can be seen clearly enough despite the returning of her familiar urinary symptoms. Ed.

10–11 a.m. Frequent urination (Day 10).

1 p.m. I went to pee and I had a pain in the urethra tube – before and after.(C) 2 p.m. I started peeing frequently, literally every twenty minutes. It was like when I have a urine infection – very little urine passed and slightly cloudy looking. With this my face was hot and my body cold. I was peeing throughout the afternoon. I had pain during and after, in the groin area each time(C). (Day 14)

I feel lots better but not quite 100%. I awoke in the morning with left side uterine discomfort and I was peeing all day. I thought I'd got another urine infection.(B) I drank loads of water all day.(C) 10.30 p.m. I had real cystitis symptoms. My uterus felt really full and distended. I had the urge to pee but couldn't – it took me about an hour before I eventually went.(B) (Day 28)

I woke up with backache, which eased every time I spent a penny. I was going frequently. I drank loads and it went.(B) (Day 31)

I had a very bad backache in the morning, better after urinating, so it was a urine infection. I was peeing lots – wanting to go frequently. I had the sensation of needing to go but nothing would come out. This was throughout the day. I had to wake at night to pee (Day 32).

I still had slight signs of a urinary infection. My urine had a muddy smell.(C) I felt in a better mood (Day 33). *I phoned Stuart and we decided to bear with it.*

The urine infection was better. 1 p.m. I had a slight pain in the left, lower abdomen, the area where the ovaries are. I was not peeing so much and it was a normal colour – it had been cloudy.(C) I can almost feel the remedy working downwards through the body (Day 34).

There was no sign of a urine infection (Day 35).

7) *Normal state of urine: pale, yellow, no strong odours. The fact that, since the proving began, it is now different and colourless may well be of signif-*

icance. Note also that there was a significant change in diet over these weeks with a big increase in fluid consumption.

Passed urine that was clear. A conversation with supervisor jogged my memory on this. It is a rarity for me to have urine that is completely clear.(A) I have been drinking a lot of water. Feel thirsty a lot (Day 3).

Urine is clear (Day 5).

Urine seems constantly to be clear (Day 6).

Noticed that my urine is again clear. This now seems to be a regular occurrence. I am very thirsty (Day 15).

Days 16 and 19: Urine is still clear.

Urine clear but with a strange smell, a bit acrid (Day 32).

Urine still pale (Day 41).

Rubrics

Intestines

Flatus 1060

Flatus, evening 1061

Flatus, night 1061

Stomach

Belching 1723

Nausea 1748

Nausea, Coca Cola, drinking, amel. NR

Nausea, eating, after 1750

Nausea. water, after 1750

Nausea, faint-like 1751

Nausea, vertigo, with NR

Vomiting, morning 1777

Appetite

Diminished 725

Loss of, food, at thought of NR

Vertigo

Nausea, with 1884

Abdomen

Cramping, pains 11
Distension 16
Sharp, pains 54
Rectum
Constipation 1596
Diarrhoea 1601
Diarrhoea, morning 1605
Diarrhoea, waking, with urging 1605
Urging, sudden 1624
Urine
Colourless 1869
Pale 1872
Yellow 1877

Female
Menses/feeling broody/libido

1) Irritability spells.(B) Got irritable very quickly, especially if my daughters or husband appeared to be making a mess. It has been a bit like PMT symptoms: I snapped when my daughter interrupted me talking to my husband. He said I had been very irritable today. This made me even more irritable: I didn't think I had been. 8 p.m. Generally I feel fine this evening, with no anxiety; just my eyes are tired and I'm generally tired.(B) 11 p.m. Period-like pains. (My period isn't due for two weeks.) In lower abdomen and an achy lower back, > lying down and > passing wind.(B) It came on suddenly and lasted until I went to sleep. Slight nausea after this pain began, for a few minutes. I thought it might be a urine infection (Day 4).

7.30 a.m. My hair has gone really dry, drier than usual. It feels almost brittle, as if it could break. The skin on my legs, especially the shins, is dry – almost flaky.(A) Still had pain in lower abdomen, around my left ovary area, travelling around to my back also.(C) Not long after this slightly nauseous again, like last night (Day 5).

9 a.m. Had a few period-like pains again only lasting a couple of minutes.(C) In my lower abdomen area and a couple in my back. (There were no more later in the day.) 7 p.m. Strong PMT feeling. Irritable. The girls had their dressing up things out; then they went out with their dad and everything was left out and not in its place and I had to tidy it away. This annoyed me but I felt I had to do it (Day 6).

11.30 a.m. I felt really wide-awake.(A) Felt in good spirits – happy.(A) I'm feeling broody; I keep noticing babies.(B) I do go through bouts of this, but haven't for six to eight months. I found myself weighing up the positives and negatives about having another baby and even talking about it with my husband. 8 p.m. Slightly nauseous perhaps trapped wind.(C) Especially before my period, I get it (Day 7).

4 p.m. I have a headache on the left side over my eye, but I can get it for three or four days before my period (although I haven't had it for two or three months).(C) (Day 13)

Period begins (Day 18). *All familiar symptoms, not apparently modified by the proving. Ed.*

1 p.m. I started to get a headache, the one I get with my period. It was worse for moving around.(C) I did take two Nurofen (usually helped by *Belladonna 200)*. 4.30 p.m. I still had the headache, with pain around the left eye area as usual. I was tired and irritable. I felt frustrated with everything – it felt like I was not getting anywhere.(C) 7 p.m. I'd found that if I used my fingers to put pressure on the eye socket where the headache is, it was better for pressure. Also > cold flannel. The light hurts, with some relief from dimming the light (Day 19).

2 p.m. I suddenly had a headache (left-sided) coming on again, but it only lasted about ten minutes. I often get a headache at the end of a period. The period lasted for about a day and a half. Then it returned the next day.(C) (Day 20)

10.30 p.m. I had a headache tonight. It continued overnight. It was left-sided, almost like I have pre-menstrually but my period is not due (Day 28).

3) *Review:* Since the proving began I have been sneezing two or three times a day, very mild sneezes that are actually quite pleasant! Also my libido has been a bit higher this week, but I'm wondering if that is just related to my menstrual cycle (Day 8).

My period started six days ago, almost a week early. I didn't have the usual tearful emotional state with it but today, after it has finished, I feel sad, tearful and sorry for myself. I should have got my period today and these feelings would normally reflect that (Day 30).

5) I realize I've been craving sweets and chocolate (and eating!) these last few days, which normally only happens before my period (not due for two weeks). (Day 9)

I still have a large appetite, particularly for sweet things (Day 10).

My appetite continues to be huge and feels like my PMT appetite (but it can't be yet). Craving chocolate and bread and sweet things (Day 11).

My appetite shows no sign of decreasing. And I'm still eating lots of sweet things, chocolate, biscuits, hot chocolate etc. (Day 13).

I have started my period about ten days early this evening. All day I was very tired, but at least my craving for chocolate can now be explained. I have never had an early period before, I am always very regular. My period is heavy (Day 14).

My period is still heavy, which is normal for me (Day 15).

I woke up having had dreams all about cleaning. I felt I immediately wanted to go home and clean my home (even though I did before we left!) (Day 16).

My period is lighter today (Day 17).

My period is light today and seems almost finished (Day 18).

Period finished (Day 19).

I feel emotionally/mentally that I have definitely come through a change (Day 21).

I have also been craving and eating chocolate again, yesterday and today, my period is not yet due, so it isn't my usual PMT cravings (Day 34).

I'm eating lots of chocolate, I think it may be PMT (Day 42).

I have got my period today, normal cycle time. I'm eating lots of chocolate and cheese on toast (Day 46).

I have a huge appetite and eat every hour. My period is quite heavy (Day 47).

6) *This prover is on the contraceptive pill.*

- Period started early (Day 11).
- is very heavy (gushing.) Dark red (Day 12).
- returning to normal: medium flow (Day 13).
- now very light in colour, but three days longer than usual (Day 16).
- starts again (two weeks after previous one). Lasted four days (Day 25)
- started again (three and a half weeks). (Day 48)

7) My skin is extremely dry on my hands, faintly cracking, like a map with lines over hands, they are very feint. Still very dry and I am drinking lots.(B) (Day 16)

Dry hands still – put lots of cream on. I woke up in the night with a dry mouth, and thirsty again. My stomach is gurgling and I feel a little nauseous all day (Day 17).

All ailments from yesterday are gone – nausea and gurgling stomach. Hands are still dry. Despite putting on moisturizer and drinking lots.(B) (Day 18)

Period begins today. *(Timing unaffected as yet by the proving. Ed.)* Feeling generally well and upbeat. Positive.(C) (Day 19)

Period very profuse, literally streaming out – bright red (Day 20).

Unsettled night – dreams full of anxiety about impending event that I am about to organize. I feel that there may be some conflict ahead. I had a weird feeling during the day that some awful illness will strike at someone in the family and that it will change lives forever. Despite this I still feel very upbeat and positive. I had a good run at the gym – despite my period (Day 21).

I have been experiencing nausea on and off again. Period has now finished (Day 23).

I still feel the constriction in my throat and nausea too; and still feeling emotionally unsettled, as I did during my period. It is unusual for this to carry on after my period has ended.(A) (Day 25)

Period has arrived but with little pain.(A) The onset of the period was very early, only twelve days from the end of the last one. It is extremely rare for me to be irregular.(A) Also blood was scanty and dark. This too is unusual. In good spirits (Day 36).

Period continues – still dark and scanty (Day 37).

Period ends (Day 40).

8) Few small spots under nose, probably pre-menstrual. Sometimes get the odd spot (Day 10).

Menstruation now seven days late, not bothered and not doing a pregnancy test until it's over two weeks. Don't want to get hopes up and be disappointed again (Day 21).

Nausea feeling in pit of stomach – ate banana. Nausea >. Occurred to me I could be pregnant as had same feeling before and period still not arrived (38 days since last period). (Day 25)

Still no menses; I am wondering if I am pregnant. Will test after forty-three days, as that was longest time between periods. Metallic taste in mouth. Tea tastes horrible and not able to finish it.(C) (Day 27)

5.20 a.m. Woke up, came over very hot, had to go to loo because I thought I was going to be sick. No period so thought, 'Morning sickness – oh great!' Had diarrhoea instead, black liquid. One hour later awoke – was sick, yellow liquid. Ate banana and rice cake – went to horse. Felt OK outside in fresh air. Came back felt dreadful again. Was sick again – banana and rice cake mashed. Must be the sickness bug that my friends have had. Exhausted all day, laid on settee but couldn't really sleep as was watching daughter. Later she was sick. Laid down on bed with daughter and slept for three hours, woke up, had a drink of water – can't face any other food. Can't face food except melon. Utterly exhausted (Day 29).

Positive pregnancy test (after 15 months of trying). Hubby stressed about how we'll cope (Day 30).

College weekend. Reflections: coming round from numb. Been closed so long, now coming out of it and dreaming a lot more. Feeling of becoming a woman again – motherhood perhaps (Day 43).

Retrospective entry after twelve week scan in hospital (March 27th). As a result of my scan at twelve weeks, I discovered that I was carrying twins, which died at nine weeks and two days (March 7th). I wasn't aware of this as no spotting occurred until 25th and only on 25th. Scan showed two embryos and no foetal heartbeat in either. Termed as incomplete miscarriage. Subsequently didn't miscarry naturally; had to have D&C to abort foetuses (Day 53).

From her supervisor's diary around this time: I saw two large bits in my period that looked like a tiny miscarriage, which is odd for the third/fourth day of my period (Day 51).

9) *Two days before the proving:* I feel that various symptoms mentally and physically have been taking place over the last few days. I don't know whether it's:

1. The effect of the moon – coming up to full moon.

2. It's like PMT – which I normally only get the day before my period begins, but now this is unusual and extreme, every day I've been getting very short with the kids, very little patience.

3. Menstrual cycle appears to have been delayed by two weeks. The last three times I've menstruated just after full moon, whereas I was aware of ovulating two nights ago – sharp pain left ovary.

4. Today I've been very upset about my body. Familiar feelings about my self and appearance.

5. I have a lot of doubt about my ability to take a homoeopathic case tonight.

Are things coming to the surface before the proving?

Period began. 9 a.m. Very grumpy and irritable, want my own space to get on with things. I feel trapped. Later that morning I felt great when I was able to do some lengths of swimming. 5 p.m. I feel stressed about getting everything done in the house so that I can work in the evening. 8 p.m. Stomach pains have started, it feels uncomfortable, not severe, just as if slightly constipated, but the constipation seems to be affecting my stomach (Day 9).

8 p.m. Aching in my abdomen again, feels slightly bruised, as if constipated. Period has finished. Very easy and light (Day 13).

I may be ovulating from my right ovary today, which is unusual, as I tend to be aware of ovulating from the left (Day 38).

My period began – the moon is waxing so I wonder if I'm getting back in sync with the moon. My last two periods have been six weeks apart, which I assume is the effect of the proving, as they have recently been around the time of the full moon (Day 50).

Rubrics

Female

Menses, bright red 665

Menses, dark 666

Menses, frequent, too early, too soon 666

Menses, late 668

Menses, scanty 672

Menses, profuse 674

Throat/cough/breathing

1) 7 p.m. Feels like a lump in the throat on swallowing and my glands are tender and sore.(C) Slight sore throat (Day 6).

6.45 p.m. I had a sore throat again, especially glands on the right side; it lasted for about half an hour.(C) Just sore; not a lump sensation today (Day 7).

Throughout the afternoon I had a dry irritating cough, with a sensation as if cold air had got on to my chest, making me cough.(B) Throat feels dry – croaky voice, from coughing.(B) Nothing comes up. Face feels flushed with this coughing.(A) Slightly catarrhy also (Day 9).

1.30 a.m. I woke up with a very sore throat and blocked nose. I managed to get back to sleep quite quickly.(C) (Day 16)

2) I had a feeling like a lump or a small ball in my throat. It wasn't sore, just a sensation. It felt stronger on swallowing anything. The only time I have had this before has been when I have felt nauseous or have vomited (Day 3).

3) Mild cough this evening. A bit of mucus in my throat, tickling dry cough (Day 5).

Slight, dry cough (Day 11).

I've got a tickly cough, which sometimes sounds like a bark, which seems to be worse during the day. It is mild and uncomfortable but not debilitating (Day 12).

The dry, tickling occasional 'bark' cough returned again this evening around 7 p.m. and until I went to bed (Day 13).

5) I have woken with a sore throat and slight temperature. I've got a lot of mucus and phlegm. After work I feel very tired and get a bit tearful. I am short-tempered with my son – not able to cope with his noise. I feel I need rest and am anxious about work tomorrow. My head feels achy and hot (Day 19).

I have a lot of mucus and my head feels hot. My throat is also sore. My mood is calmer and I do not feel tearful today and my mood is fine towards my son (Day 20).

I still have my flu symptoms. I feel emotionally/mentally that I have definitely come through a change. Looking back over the pages, I felt very confused and clumsy. My writing is full of spelling mistakes, and I felt as if I was revisiting old anxieties. This feeling has passed now and I feel mentally alert again (Day 21).

6) Slight sore throat (Day 2).

Sore throat on waking, as if a lump in my throat (Day 3).

Woke with a sore throat (Day 4).

Sore throat again, lump sensation (Day 37).

7) Dose 1. Throat dry > drinking water (B). 7.40 p.m. Unusual feeling in throat; not a sore throat but more a constriction, as if the throat was closing up, > drinking water (A). I felt a bit panicky; this feeling subsided after a while (Day 1).

7.30 a.m. Dose 4. Throat constriction still present.(A) Feel really thirsty and a little dehydrated with it, > drinking water.(B) (Day 2)

As a result of the proving discussion I realized that I have suffered from sore, restricted throat sensation intermittently during the last month. > drinking water (Day 22).

Throat constricted, > drinking water; also feeling wobbly emotionally (Day 25).

Anxious about intended meeting so rang a friend for emotional support and felt she was not able to give it. Feeling rather angry with my friend as if this has thrown into relief my issues over friendship. Is this an old issue which has never been confronted? Almost feel that this is the last straw if she does not come to the meeting. Feel rather angry and irritable and feel that this mood has descended since the college weekend.(B) (Day 26)

I dreaded the meeting this afternoon. However, my friend came and was very supportive. She seems to have responded to the plea for support. The meeting was difficult and potentially very conflictual, and I was worried beforehand that I was angry and might explode, but I managed to release this anger in a measured and assertive way.(B) On reflection, I feel as if a weight has been lifted from my shoulders (Day 27).

Still very dry mouth. (Day 32)

(No further report of the sensation of constriction in her throat after Day 24. Ed.)

Still rather thirsty (Day 37).

Sore throat. Sneezing with runny nose. It feels like the beginning of a heavy cold – the first this winter. A good clear out before the spring (Day 47).

Energy gradually returning after this time of cold and fever (Day 57).

8) Catarrh stuck in back of nose/throat (C) (Day 6).

Catarrh in back of throat < morning (Day 8).

Throat feels dry and little sore at back in mornings (Day 10).

10) Mild headache on and off all day in frontal lobe and slightly sore throat; also a feeling of a lump in my throat (Day 2).

Persistent asthmatic cough most of the day, triggered by very cold air cycling to the station in the morning. It feels like a return of the chest infection treated homoeopathically prior to the proving. Maybe it is caused by my emotional state regarding my mother. My sense of the proving is that it is bringing up old issues, so could it be bringing up old physical symptoms too? (Day 9)

Very cold morning; I inhaled icy air on my cycle ride to the station which triggered an asthmatic sensation; there was no coughing fit but I was left with the familiar metallic sensation at the top of my lungs that gradually wore off over the course of the day (Day 12).

Rubrics

Throat

Constriction, throat-pit 1818

Lump, plug sensation 1825

Lump, plug sensation, swallowing, on 1825

Glands

Swelling, neck 822

Cough

Dry 335

Tickling 356

Skin (and respiration – Prover 6)

1) 12.30 p.m. Still hot flushes, waves of heat, all over but especially on my face. Face also very itchy.(B) (Day 1)

7.30 a.m. My hair has gone really dry, drier than usual. It feels almost brittle, as if it could break. The skin on my legs is dry, especially the shins, almost flaky.(A) (Day 5)

9.15 p.m. Had an itch on the left side of my head, and when I scratched it, it hurt like a burning sore. It remained sore and painful for a few minutes even after I stopped scratching it and even though there was nothing there (Day 6).

10.45 p.m. I noticed the skin on my face feels very dry and taut, so much so that I had to put extra cream on it to relieve the dryness.(A) *Fifteen minutes later:* I had to put even more moisturizer on my hands and face, as they felt so dry.(A) (Day 7)

11 p.m. Both shins very itchy.(B) > aloe vera. Skin on my hands feels very dry, especially the palms. (A) Severe itch on base of left foot, right in the centre.(A) This lasted for about one minute (Day 8).

2 p.m. Noticed a spot on my chin that has been there for about three years has gone down. 6.30 p.m. Really itchy shins again.(B) It's probably the sugar. 7.30 p.m. I had that itch on my foot again, but right foot this time.(A) Since about four years I have had a 'deep' spot where I put a pin in. At the time I put a hot compress on it and scalded the skin. It scarred. This week since the proving began it has gone down. I wonder if the spot was hormone related? (Day 9)

I've still got dry skin on my face, hands and both shins.

Hair better; I've not noticed it being dry (Day 10).

Day 12 *(See her supervisor's notes for this day. Page 264)*

9.30 a.m. My face and hands felt really dry again, almost like you're out in the wind and it's pulling your face back; it's taut.(A) My daughter complained of an itchy left foot, in the arch underneath. It was driving her potty. She had to take her shoe and sock off to scratch it (Day 14).

9 a.m. Had a very itchy right palm, lasted one minute.(A) (Day 15)

Afternoon: I had an itchy tummy (like I'd been bitten). It was under the rib cage, centrally. It just stopped suddenly – it had been intermittent during the afternoon. There was nothing to see.(A) In the evening my shins were really itchy again.(A) I have a spot on my chin, which keeps coming and going. It flares up then practically goes (Day 21).

My shins are itchy today (Day 22).

No itchiness, but my skin is dry, in funny places like my arms and tops of legs, and my neck; and dry looking too (Day 31).

I had very itchy legs (all over) in the morning.(B) I can almost feel the remedy working downwards through the body. (I discussed this with the co-ordinator.)

My back's got very spotty.(B) All over, like pimples. Little red raised spots. There are ten or so in number and three on the tops of my legs, inside my thighs. The ones on my back don't itch. The ones on my legs are aggravated by water; it makes them a bit itchy. My skin's really dry all over, including my hair. I'm putting more cream on than usual. My neck looks really dry (Day 34).

My skin is very dry. I have a very dry patch the shape of an oval under my left breast. It feels slightly scaly and dry. It doesn't itch and looks a bit like eczema.(A) I have never had eczema (Day 37).

2) Whilst lying in bed, I realized that my psoriasis hadn't itched much since taking the remedy. This is unusual; it tends to itch a lot, especially at night (Day 3).

My psoriasis is now itching as usual (Day 4). *(There were four days of improvement.)*

I noticed a small mark on the side of my right hand approx halfway between my little finger and wrist. It was about 0.5 cm long, slightly raised, itchy and looked like a welt of some kind. I didn't notice cutting or scratching myself. I've never had this before (Day 6). *(Added subsequently: in reflexology this location relates to the liver & gallbladder.)*

Psoriasis very itchy (as normal). (Day 10)

I noticed a small, red spot on my left cheek approx 2 cm from my left nostril. It doesn't hurt or itch and there is no pus visible. I rarely get spots (Day 12).

The spot on my cheek is still the same (Day 15).

The spot on my cheek is smaller (Day 16).

The spot is tiny now (Day 18).

The spot on my cheek has gone. There is a new spot on my forehead, quite big and blind, hurts if pressed (Day 19).

I have a new spot on my neck with a white head (Day 22).

I popped the spot on my neck, which was filled with white pus (Day 28).

3) I've noticed two spots under the skin – one above each eyebrow, an unusual place for me to get spots (Day 7). The spots themselves are normal for me. *(Later on, when reading through the co-ordinator's proving diary, he describes a pink spot at the 'third eye' point, a similar area to my unusual spot.)*

6) *I have eczema and asthma, sometimes in alternation. During the proving my familiar skin symptoms got worse, and my breathing better. Since the proving (July '06 report) my skin condition is back to what I know as 'normal' but my breathing seems to have improved substantially.*

Skin

Dry skin (Day 1).

Sore, itchy skin (Day 2).

Skin 'angry', < warmth, < creases, burning sensation after scratching, scratched until bleeding during sleep. Affected areas: groin, arms, wrists, calves, face, forehead, neck, ears – splits at top and bottom of both ears (Day 5).

Skin very sore (burning sensation.) (Day 7)

Skin calmer (Day 8).

Skin burning, neck and chest (Day 9).

Morning. Calmer again today. *Evening.* Even although I'm feeling uncomfortable in my skin, I feel very happy in my mind. This is unusual for me (Day 10).

Skin itchy and irritable (Day 13).

Evening. Skin irritable (Day 16).

Neck area sore (Day 17).

Skin like sandpaper (Day 19).

- dry and scaly (Day 20)
- dry and sore (Day 23)
- dry and sore (neck area) (Day 24)
- dry and itchy (Day 25)
- sore under arms. I don't like touching it where it is sore (Day 26).

Very uncomfortable in my skin, itchy < evening (Day 27).

Skin sore and dry (Day 28).

Skin symptoms still present, very dry lips as well (Day 29).

- itchy and irritable, body, eyes and face (Day 30).

Skin extra crispy today, lips very sore and cracked, cannot smile (Day 31).

Feeling raw all over torso and arms (Day 32).

Less inflamed today, not as itchy. I feel as though I am healing now (Day 33).

Skin feels bumpy all over (Day 34).

- dry and itchy, hands as well (Day 38)

Hands itchy all over (Day 39).

Days 40–49 Skin continues to be sore, dry and sometimes scabby.

Respiration

I have noticed that my asthma is better at the same time as my skin symptoms getting worse (Day 6).

Asthma not too bad (Day 9).

Nausea (I thought I might be sick), then coughing as it rose up into my throat, then a pounding headache in temples < light (Day 24). *Sounding wheezy. (Supervisor's observation.)*

(See her review. Page 257.)

7) My skin is extremely dry on my hands, faintly cracking, like a map with lines over hands; they are very feint. Still very dry and I am drinking lots.(B) (Day 16)

Dry hands still – put lots of cream on. I woke up in the night with a dry mouth, and thirsty again (Day 17).

Hands are still dry. Despite putting on moisturizer and drinking lots.(B) (Day 18)

This was just before her period began. See her entry Prover 7 in Female section.

8) 8.50 a.m. Itchy left foot, inside on underside by heel. Nothing evident to cause the itch, but lovely to scratch. Not easily satisfied. Itches again very soon once you stop unless you scratch until it is slightly numb. 12.50 p.m. Itchy foot again – scratched a lot – feels numb now (Day 11).

Verruca appeared on left foot.(C) Three smallest toes on right foot itching at night, woke me up, scratching doesn't ease it (Day 18).

9) The sty has gone. On my left forearm I have a spot that's slightly itchy and raised. It feels as if it is an infected pore. When I squeezed it clear pus came out. Actually feels like a hard lump under the skin. It's been coming up for two days (Day 6).

The spot on my arm is going down and the lump under it (Day 7).

Skin – dry patch under my lip, similar to when I was a teenager/early twenties. Often used to get this in very cold winter weather. I keep getting small spots on my face – chin and hairline, which is unusual for me. It is as if I can re-experience various aspects of this period of my life (Day 13). *(See teenage section. Page 168.)*

There's a small patch of eczema at the top of my right arm – dry, raised, only occasionally itchy. Never had this before (Day 25).

Rubrics

Skin

Dry 1644

Sore, pain 1665
Itching 1657
Tension 1667
Skin/Chest
Tapping sensation NR
Popping sensation NR

Heart

1) 2 p.m. Began to have palpitations, < exertion.(C) This lasted for about fifteen minutes intermittently. I wondered if it was because I had been drinking tea with caffeine (Day 7).

1.50 p.m. Heart flutterings as before that lasted for about two minutes.(C) This made me feel slightly anxious – I felt aware of breathing and my heart beating fast. It made me feel a bit anxious – I felt short of breath (Day 9).

11 a.m. I ran upstairs and had a heart flutter – left-sided. It only lasted a second. I wasn't short of breath this time, and it didn't frighten me.(B) (Day 10) *These flutterings started up since I began the proving. Ten years ago I had inhalers for asthma, which caused similar palpitations.*

7.15 p.m. I sat thinking about my heart again. I only had one tiny heart flutter today.(C) (Day 11)

1 p.m. I had a couple of palpitations, and my period started today. But it was unusual. I have been tired and irritable, but my mood was better instantly, rather than in a few days of my period starting, as it normally is (Day 17).

I did homework until 12.30 a.m. By then I was overtired so when I eventually went to bed I was very restless, my mind was spinning. I had thoughts of not feeling happy and confident with my homework. I couldn't switch my mind off; it was racing with thoughts about the remedy *Mercury*. I had to lay down and do relaxation techniques to calm myself down. I had a couple of palpitations and then started getting anxious: worried in case I have something wrong with my heart. I was very aware of my heart beating, aware of palpitations. It took a good hour to get to sleep (Day 18).

On waking I still had the pain in my left leg on waking (the same as the darting pain yesterday), but it wore off quickly. I'm very tired but was up late. I was still feeling anxious/aware of heart flutterings. They've all stopped now I've finished my homework (Day 19).

Any palpitations? I've cut out tea and I've been fine (Day 22).

The palpitations have stopped completely – I just have tea in the morning now. That seems to make a difference (Day 26).

I've been in a bit of a state today because I've still been aware of the odd heart fluttering. My dad's been bad recently – I was really anxious it was to do with his heart. Then I found myself last night wanting to read up all the remedies, looking for a remedy for my dad. As I was reading I felt really negative, thinking I'll never remember all these remedies.(A) (Day 28)

8) 8.45 p.m. Sensation as if heart being squeezed. Muscular type contraction. Didn't last long, not alarmed but new symptom (Day 10).

12.45 p.m. Sensation as if heart squeezed again. Aware of faint pounding. Had this on and off throughout afternoon (Day 11).

Days 12 to 14. Same heart muscle fluttering/palpitations throughout day.

Heart palpitations/flutterings (again the sensation as if being squeezed); < when anxious (Day 16).

Heart palpitations/flutterings as before (Day 17).

Muscle by heart feels stiff. Under bra strap. Getting concerned about this now; < pressure (Day 18).

Heart – muscular stiffness on and off a lot during day. 8 p.m. Pain developed in heart area, sharp pain, moved to right towards sternum then back to left side. Came and went a few times for an hour then stopped (Day 19).

Heart – feeling stricture on and off all day (Day 24).

- palpitations still there but not as strong (Day 28).

Slight heart palpitations still, but faint, throughout the day (Day 30).

Palpitations still there on and off all day (Day 31).

- Heart pain still there on and off (Day 34).
- Heart pain feels more like burning pain now (Day 35).
- feeling burning again today (Day 37).
- pain on and off all day, less intensity than before (Day 38).
- pain like burning muscle pain now. On and off all day; always < leaning forward (Day 40).
- pain like burning muscle pain, on and off all day (Day 41).

Same heart pain on and off all day (Day 42) February 25th.

Retrospective entry after twelve week scan in hospital (March 27th). As a result of my scan at twelve weeks, I discovered that I was carrying twins, which died at nine weeks and two days (March 7th). I wasn't aware of this as no spotting occurred until 25th and only on 25th. Scan showed two embryos and no foetal heartbeat in either. Termed as incomplete miscarriage. Subsequently didn't miscarry naturally; had to have D&C to abort foetuses. (Day 53)

Rubrics

Heart

Burning, pain burning 1018

Fluttering, of heart 1019

Heartbeats, general, increased 1020

Pain 1026

Pain, region of heart 1027

Palpitations, general 1028

Palpitations, anxiety 1028

Palpitations, tea drinking agg. NR

Squeezing, sensation 1036

Back, neck and shoulders

2) I had a muscular twinge in my left knee and right lower back. It lasted a few minutes (Day 14).

4) Pain in neck and shoulders, shoulder blades. < stress, e.g. from my daughter having a tantrum, > hard massage. I've had this symptom for approx one week (Day 9).

8) Dose 1. 6.30 a.m. 8 a.m. Pain in left side of neck on cervical vertebrae nodule of neck extending to under left shoulder blade then disappearing and extending down anterior of left arm to elbow. Continued for half an hour.

Dose 2. 1.10 p.m. Numb sensation down inside of right arm. Tingling on tip of tongue before the remedy dissolved. End of nose numb. Sensation as if coming round from numb as in after anaesthesia at the dentist. Numbness in nose lasted two and a half hours (Day 1). *I became concerned by this numbness in my nose, so I stopped with this second dose. It was an uncomfortable numbness and I was worried that it might extend to other areas of my face.*

Woke up with pain running from vertebrae on back of neck down neck on left side (Day 33).

Pain in neck still there. (Heart pain still there on and off.) Strange feeling driving back from tutorial 10.15 p.m. Moved my neck to look at back of car and it felt like I was going to pass out/black out. Frightened me a bit because of driving so kept looking ahead. Afraid to move neck till I got home! OK when I got home. Must have been trapped nerve in neck (Day 34).

Neck pain gone (Day 35).

9) *Four days before the proving:* 9 p.m. I get a sense of hilarity about this remedy. Overwhelming laughter, bubbling up from my throat, irresistible need to laugh. I see this as the potential for this remedy. 10 p.m. I had a sense of my spine concertina-ing down, slumped, no inner strength.

Upper back ache all day (Day 3).

No more back ache (Day 4).

2.30 p.m. When swimming I felt physically very clear and fluid, with no aching in my shoulders/neck. I've realized today that the tension in my shoulders has reduced greatly recently (Day 13).

Rubrics

Shoulders

Pain, shoulders 1629

Tension in 1636

Neck

Pain 1461

Pain, extending to arm 1461

Pain, extending to shoulders 1461

Pain, left 1462

Arms

Numbness 90

Nerves

Fainting, faintness, head, on moving NR

Numbness 1487

Back

Weak, slumped, no inner strength NR

Extremities – limbs

1) *Seven days before the proving:* Feeling tired. Achy all over. Limbs feel heavy. Felt slightly nauseous. Appetite less than normal. Felt better about 7 p.m.

4 p.m. Pain in right kneecap area, < moving, especially up and down the stairs. This lasted for about five minutes.(A) (Day 4)

11.30 a.m. Feet cold today.

10.45 p.m. Generally my feet had felt icy cold all day but not sure if that is because I was out most of the day.(B) It took me a long time to warm up when I came home. My hair had felt dry and brittle.(A) Husband had noticed that my hands felt very dry.(A) (Day 7)

6 p.m. Itchy shins; it drove me mad. It came on so suddenly. It

was like a burning itch.(B) > aloe vera ointment. When I used to have sugar I used to get very itchy legs. 7.30 p.m. I had a really itchy left eye, again with a slight burning sensation.(A) 11 p.m. Both shins still very itchy.(B) > aloe vera. Skin on my hands feels very dry, especially the palms.(A) Severe itch on base of left foot, right in the centre.(A) This lasted for about one minute (Day 8).

6.30 p.m. Really itchy shins again.(B) It's probably from eating sugary foods. 7.30 p.m. I had that itch on my foot again, but right foot this time.(A) (Day 9)

6 p.m. Feet: icy cold again.(B)

8 p.m. My face felt really hot and flushed again.(A)

9.20 p.m. I had my warmest socks on my feet, but my feet felt as cold as ice – they were not cold to touch, except my toes.(B) (Day 10)

11 a.m. My right hand is really cold when using the computer keyboard.(A) Just the one hand, and one cold area. I am right-handed. This lasted approx half an hour (Day 11).

8 p.m. Feet icy cold again.(C) I was OK earlier, much better (Day 12).

9.30 a.m. My face and hands felt really dry again, almost like you're out in the wind and it's pulling your face back; it's taut.(A) Today my daughter complained of an itchy left foot, in the arch underneath. It was driving her potty. She had to take her shoe and sock off to scratch it (Day 14).

7 p.m. I had very cold feet today. They were literally icy cold, as if I had no socks on. I used a hot-water bottle to warm them up but it still took a good few minutes to warm up.(C) 10 p.m. I had a very cold body; I had to put on my dressing gown in bed, and have a hot-water bottle, but felt I had a cold coming (probably from getting a bit of a chill that day.) (B) (Day 15)

8 pm. My arms and legs just ached and I had darting pains in all my limbs on the outside areas. (Not hands/feet.) I had exactly the same kind of pains in my arms and legs. It could have been referred pain from my back from sitting in a bad chair doing my homework. It lasted most of the evening, on and off (Day 18).

On waking I still had the pain in my left leg (the same as the darting pain yesterday), but it wore off quickly. I'm very tired (but was up late). I was still feeling anxious/aware of heart flutterings. They've all stopped now I've finished my homework (Day 19).

7.30 a.m. I had a pain in my right knee, on the left inner side, < bending knees, going up and down stairs. It lasted for an hour and then just went.(A) In the evening my shins were really itchy again.(A) (Day 21)

My shins are itchy today (Day 22).

I had very itchy legs (all over) in the morning.(B) 1 p.m. I had a slight pain in the left, lower abdomen, the area where the ovaries are. I was not peeing so much and it was a normal colour – it had been cloudy.(C) I can almost feel the remedy working downwards through the body. (I discussed this with the co-ordinator.) My back's got very spotty.(B) All over, like pimples. Little red raised spots. There are ten or so in number and three on the tops of my legs, inside my thighs. The ones on my back don't itch. The ones on my legs are aggravated by water; it makes them a bit itchy. My skin's really dry all over, including my hair. I'm putting more cream on than usual. My neck looks really dry. Temperature? A bit of both. Real hot and cold spells. More cold flushes – the cold starts in my hands, then a shiver goes all through me and my whole body feels cold. My feet have not been cold recently though. I had to stand by a radiator or put on an extra layer of clothing. I get that if I haven't eaten.(C) So I'm > eating (Day 34).

2) I noticed a small mark on the side of my right hand approx halfway between my little finger and wrist. It was about 0.5 cm long, slightly raised, itchy and looked like a welt of some kind. I didn't notice cutting or scratching myself. I've never had this before (Day 6). *(Added subsequently: in reflexology this location relates to the liver & gallbladder.)*

I had a muscular twinge in my left ankle (Day 13).

I had a muscular twinge in my left knee and right lower back. It lasted a few minutes. 2 p.m. I had a piercing, throbbing, radiating pain on my left upper arm. It lasted approx five minutes (Day 14).

I had a muscular twinge on my left knee whilst driving. It went away when I got out and was walking (Day 18).

3) 8 p.m. Dreadful toe cramps. They go when I apply pressure and hop around on my toes. I haven't had toe cramps for around six months and they haven't been this bad for over a year or more (Day 12). *Return of old symptom first experienced in my late teens.*

Occasional toe cramps – very mild – have come and gone all day (Day 14).

Really itchy – between the right big toe and the next one; small red bumps on the skin. Never had this symptom before (Day 25).

Toe symptoms have gone (Day 27).

4) *Numbness.*

Six days before the proving: My legs have no sensation from below my knees; it felt numb when I got out of bed.

Two days before the proving: Pains in the right hand, outer edge. Dull numbing pain. Sensation like writer's cramp. Intensifies occasionally, < every half hour or so, also < as day progressed.

Pins and Needles in Hands. Four days before the proving: Pins and needles in hands, both sides, each at separate times from each other. This persisted for three days, at sporadic times.

Hands feel a bit numb, no pins and needles or cramps though (Day 1).

Hands: I've not remembered to note it before but over the past couple of weeks I've fallen asleep with my fingers crossed together, joining my hands, usually above my head. It felt relaxing to stretch the fingers while crossed or linked as well. This has happened about four or five times now (Day 11).

7) My familiar chilblains on my feet have got a lot worse in the last couple of days. Red, burning, throbbing and irritating (Day 5).

My hands have become very dry, despite putting extra moisturizer on because of the cold weather (Day 16).

8) Dose 1. 6.30 a.m. 8 a.m. Pain in left side of neck on cervical vertebrae nodule of neck extending to under left shoulder blade then disappearing and extending down anterior of left arm to elbow. Continued for half an hour.

Dose 2. 1.10 p.m. Numb sensation down inside of right arm. Tingling on tip of tongue before the remedy dissolved. End of nose numb. Sensation as if coming round from numb as in after anaesthesia at the dentist. Numbness in nose lasted two and a half hours (Day 1). *I became concerned by this numbness in my nose, so I stopped with this second dose. It was an uncomfortable numbness and I was worried that it might extend to other areas of my face.*

Sleep less broken last night – woke only once. Difficulty sleeping on right side. Woke feeling very cold, despite the weather being very mild. I was OK once I got moving. Numbness in left arm throughout the night extending to fingers. Woke with total numbness and loss of sensation in my left hand. I shook my hand hard to get it to come back. It took a while though. Sore throat left side. After breakfast felt tired – laid down and went to sleep. (Unlike me.) (Day 2)

Right knee, ligament inside of knee feels pulled and twisted, < long period sitting (Day 8).

Ligament in right knee, inside of knee painful to touch. OK to walk on (Day 9).

Knee bad today. Kneeling down strains it. When I go to get up it is painful. OK when sitting or walking (Day 10).

8.50 a.m. Itchy left foot, inside on underside by heel. Nothing evident to cause the itch, but lovely to scratch. Not easily satisfied. Itches again very soon once you stop unless you scratch until it is slightly numb. 12.50 p.m. Itchy foot again – scratched a lot – feels numb now (Day 11).

Verruca appeared on left foot.(C) Three smallest toes on right foot itching at night, woke me up, scratching doesn't ease it (Day 18).

Morning: Pins and needles in left arm despite not laying on it.

Evening: Cramp in both feet. Feet felt cold but when wrapped in duvet they cramped. Had to put feet in sink in hot water to relax the muscles (Day 24).

Pins and needles suddenly came on whilst sitting on settee, left leg, unable to shake it off or alleviate by movement. Rubbing helped (Day 26).

9) The sty has gone, and on my left forearm – I have a spot that's slightly itchy and raised. It feels as if it is an infected pore. When I squeezed it clear pus came out. Actually feels like a hard lump under the skin. It's been coming up for two days (Day 6).

The spot on my arm is going down and the lump under it (Day 7).

There's a small patch of eczema at the top of my right arm – dry, raised, only occasionally itchy. Never had this before (Day 25).

Rubrics

Arms

Numbness left 90

Numbness, left, night NR

Tingling, prickling 105

Feet

Cold 608

Icy cold 609

Cramps 611

Cramps, toes 612

Cramps, toes, pressure amel. NR

Hands

Numbness left 845

Numbness, left, night NR

Coldness 828

Coldness, computer keyboard, when using NR

Legs

Itching, burning 1139

Knee

Pain 1094

Pain, ascending steps, on 1095

Pain, bending on 1095

Pain, descending steps, when 1095

Pain, knees, kneeling, when 1095

Pain, move, on beginning to 1095

Pain, knees, right 1095

Pain, knees, touch, on 1096

Sleep

1) *The day before the proving:* In bed I was restless before falling asleep. Unusual for me. Woke at 4 a.m. to pee. In the morning woke very awake, and energetic. This is very unlike me.

Day 2 of the proving. When I went to bed, I felt wide-awake, as if my brain was over-stimulated. Then, all of a sudden, it was like a switch and I went tired, and soon went to sleep.

I feel alert; my eyes feel really wide-awake. I'm not usually a morning person at all (Day 3).

I awoke about three times last night for no reason and had awful trouble getting back off to sleep. This morning: eyes, wide-awake feeling again; and full of energy all morning.(A) (Day 4) *(Four wide awake days followed by four days tired, not feeling like getting up. Ed.)*

7.15 a.m. Felt I couldn't get out of bed. Feeling so tired physically and mentally.(A) (Day 5)

It was an effort to get up: it took a good ten minutes for my eyes to feel properly awake. I couldn't get up when the alarm went off – normally I'm straight up when the alarm goes off. I kept dropping back to sleep (Day 7).

7 a.m. This morning when the alarm went off, I kept turning it off. I couldn't get up at all, I was really tired; I just wanted to go back to

sleep.(A) (Day 8)

After this day, lively again.

7.30 a.m. Awoke feeling very awake. My eyes felt wide-awake.(A) 11 p.m. Felt like doing homework, so did so until midnight.(B) Went to bed, felt restless, tossing and turning. Didn't sleep until about 1 a.m.(A) (Day 9)

7.15 a.m. The alarm went off and I literally jumped out of bed. I sprang up and felt really wide-awake (including eyes).(A) (Day 10)

7.30 a.m. I jumped out of bed, my eyes feeling wide awake but my body felt tired.(A) (Day 11)

I woke up at 3 a.m. and had real problems getting back to sleep again. I kept clock-watching until about 5 a.m. I felt really wide-awake and could have got up.(A) 7.15 a.m. My eyes are very awake although my body is a bit tired and heavy.(A) (Day 12)

8.30 a.m. Woke from a horrific dream. *(See her dream diary.)* Very tired eyes, and I had a headache over my left eye area.(C) Didn't have it when I woke up (Day 13).

I can't remember any dreams. It's the first time for the last few nights I've not woken between 3 a.m. and 4 a.m. and been wide awake.(A) 8 a.m. I felt really wide awake but very cold. I felt cold for most of the day.(B) (Day 14)

1.30 a.m. I woke up with a very sore throat and blocked nose. I managed to get back to sleep quite quickly.(C) 3.30 a.m. I woke up. I'd had another strange dream. I was wide-awake after this.(A) 7.30 a.m. I got up, but my eyes were tired and heavy. 2 p.m. I was very tired. I could have gone to sleep.(B) 3 p.m. More awake, but I could nod off if I sat down.(B) (Day 16)

I have been very restless at bedtime. I've been fidgety for a good twenty minutes. The bed doesn't feel comfortable and I take ages to settle.(A) (Day 35)

2) I felt very tired and lethargic all day despite getting a much-needed lie-in. I just wanted to lie on the sofa and watch TV on my own all day (Day 16).

5) 9 a.m. Woke having slept very well, took remedy. No dreams to remember (Day 2).

7.40 a.m. I woke having not had a good sleep – as was the case a few days before. I felt as if it hadn't been deep. No dreams to remember.

8 p.m. I feel very tired and sleepy. I still have a slight headache, which seems to have moved forward and is more around the temples (Day 3).

I have had an un-restful night. I had a very vivid dream (Day 4).

Another night of waking and vivid dreams. I feel tired and un-refreshed (Day 5).

Another poor night's sleep. Vivid dreams. Again in the evening I feel tired and my mood is low (Day 6).

Bad night's sleep. Feel as if I'm not in a deep sleep at all (Day 7).

Again bad night's sleep (Day 8).

Still sleeping not very well, but last night was a bit better. Realize I seem to properly fall asleep around 5 a.m. and today slept in until 9 a.m. (Day 9).

A good night's sleep was had! I know I dreamed but I can't remember what? I have had lots of energy today – perhaps a result of having had a good night's sleep (Day 11).

Slight nosebleed. I realize my nose was also bloody before going to bed yesterday. I've slept badly for most of the night but slept better in the last few hours (5–7.30 a.m.). This on retrospect has been the case a few times before (Day 12).

I am sleeping more deeply now. I cannot remember my dreams (Day 17).

I have slept well, but woke feeling very fluey (my son has the flu and a cough). The back of my throat feels irritated ad blocked. I have a hot head and am very sleepy (Day 18).

I have had a bad night's sleep due to stomach cramps. I am windy this morning but still have a slight stomach-ache and constipation (Day 33).

Bad night's sleep – kept waking and needing a pee (Day 34).

I have slept better. My mood has been more relaxed and I feel more hopeful about the future. Less anxiety. I have been very calm (Day 36).

I've slept badly with broken, interrupted sleep. I have had such vivid dreams (Day 37).

I've realized I'm sleeping better at night again (Day 45).

I woke feeling very un-refreshed – as if I hadn't slept (Day 47).

Slept well last night, realized I haven't noticed any vivid dreams lately. Feel very happy and calm (Day 48).

6) Days 1 to 3. Slept very well – like a log.

Very restless sleep, after speaking to co-ordinator (Day 20).

Restless sleep again (Day 21).

Very restless night. I did not get to sleep until very late, I was still awake at 5 a.m. I feel this was the effect on me of the energy of the proving group at college today (Day 22).

8) Sleep less broken last night – woke only once. Difficulty sleeping on right side. Woke feeling very cold, despite the weather being very mild. I was OK once I got moving. Numbness in left arm throughout the night extending to fingers. Woke with total numbness and loss of sensation in my left hand. I shook my hand hard to get it to come back. It took a while though. Sore throat left side. After breakfast felt tired – laid down and went to sleep. (Unlike me.) (Day 2)

Sleep: broken several times in night. Slept deeply early hours till 6 a.m. (B) (Day 4)

Last night: Interrupted sleep. Husband had emotional crisis at 1 a.m. Just got off to sleep about 2.30 a.m. Broken again. Slept very deeply till 6 a.m. Very difficult coming to, to get up when alarm went off. Felt tired through lack of sleep. Irritable, short fused (Day 7).

Night: broken sleep (returned). (Day 18)

Woke OK, 5.50 a.m., but was in deep sleep as late to bed. Went back to bed at 7 a.m. Went into deep sleep, woke with start as I thought husband had overslept (Day 20).

9) I found it very difficult to wake. I felt very groggy and slow. All day I wanted to take things very slow and gentle on myself. I feel subdued and want to do the minimum required. Going to see my supervisor on her houseboat brightened me (Day 28).

Tired, because only got five hours sleep, but went for a swim – desperate for a swim (Day 30).

10) Very tired around 3 p.m. Possibly normal for me, but I felt it more so than usual. I slept for about one and a half hours (Day 1).

Very sleepy around 3 p.m. again. This is not unusual for me at this time of year (I find the cold and dark difficult to tolerate), but this seems more extreme than usual (Day 3).

Slept very deeply and woke not remembering any dreams but feeling rested (Day 4).

Aware of half awaking several times during the night and woke feeling tired (Day 5).

Slept well and woke feeling rested (Day 7).

Slept late, no dreams (Day 8).

Slept very deeply, woke early (early start for work). Generally, I sleep well, most of the time. However, during this period, I have found that, even if I have a disturbed night, I feel OK and as if I had slept well. Late night working on computer at home (Day 9).

Woke feeling sleepy but rested, no dreams. Sleepy again after lunch (Day 10).

Slept well, no dreams (Day 11).

Broken sleep – woke a couple of times for no reason and went back to sleep again. Dopey in the morning (Day 12).

Broken night – woken in early hours by shouting in the street. Woke very tired in the morning (Day 13).

Tired on waking, despite sleeping well (Day 16).

Rubrics

Sleep

Position, arms, head, over, fingers, crossed NR

Position, hands, head, over, fingers, crossed NR

Falling asleep, restless before NR

Waking, general, alert on waking NR

Falling asleep, suddenly tired, like a switch NR

Waking, general, difficult 1714

Waking, general, night 3 a.m. 1717

Waking, general, night 3 to 4 a.m. 1717

Sleepiness 1703

Sleepiness, general, afternoon 1704

Sleepiness, general, afternoon 2 p.m. 1704

Sleepiness, general, afternoon 3 p.m. 1704

Un-refreshing 1713

Restless 1701

Waking, general, frequent 1715

Interrupted 1698

Waking, difficult 1714

Waking, general, feeling as if has slept well, even after a disturbed night NR

Dreams

1) I had a vivid dream last night. I used to have a phobia of cancer. I was at a hospital or a huge doctor's surgery and I was told that I had been diagnosed with cancer of the teardrops! Bizarre. (A) (Day 3)

4 a.m. I woke up having had the most horrific dream. I dreamt I was in a kitchen and there was a lady a bit like an old neighbour (but it wasn't) and I saw her stabbed to death. I woke up and I thought, I hope I didn't do that. I'd watched a programme on Jack the Ripper – so perhaps it was a mixture of that and homework: on 'Delusions, had committed a crime'. (A) I felt slightly anxious for most of the

day. I even looked it up on the Internet to see what it meant – when there are so many obstacles in your way and you've lost control. When I went back to sleep I had another dream. One of the college teachers was in it, telling me I had to sit all my Materia Medica tests again and do all my homework assignments again (Day 13).

I can't remember any dreams. It's the first time for the last few nights I've not woken between 3 a.m. and 4 a.m. and been wide awake. (A) (Day 14)

Early hours. I dreamt that somehow someone had driven into the front and back of my car, where I park for school. I can remember feeling, 'Oh my God, everyone will think it's my fault,' as there was no one around. (No cars nearby.) (A) (Day 17)

My dreams are still vivid but I can't remember them. I did rack my brain. I dreamt what the remedy was the other night, but I've forgotten. (A) (Day 22)

Over the last few nights my dreams have been vivid but I've not remembered them.(A) (Day 31)

2) Generally I have lots of dreams, hectic, busy and action-packed. Lots of excitement and running around. Recurring dreams of my dad. He died aged forty-eight of a heart attack. Undiagnosed arteriosclerosis. I was twenty-three at the time. My psoriasis began a year later.

Six days before the proving: I had a hectic night of dreams about being chased by gangsters whom I had overheard discussing something illegal they had been involved in. They kept catching me and I kept managing to escape or convincing them that I hadn't heard enough to pose any threat to them. I felt frightened; it was a fear of being caught and killed.

Five days before the proving: I had hectic dreams again. They had something to do with being chased by an unseen monster – a bit like the one in the film *Predator*.

Four days before the proving: I dreamt that I was at my mum's home in Norway and it was as if I lived at home again. I felt at ease.

I dreamt that one of my neighbours' houseboats was moored next to mine. It broke a mooring and I managed to grab a rope, then others got hold of it and we were able to pull it back in place. Although the boat is huge, I didn't feel particularly frightened, it was more exciting than anything else (Day 2).

I dreamt that my supervisor for the proving had some cream with the potentised remedy in it, which we decided to rub into my cheeks to see if it had any effect. It did – I came up in a red, pimply rash, which was not sore. I also dreamt I was with my mum and brothers. We were trying to work out why my dad had died. Somehow we discovered that he was one of twenty-nine people who died for a particular reason (which I cannot remember). It was something double top secret! At some point, we all woke up in the morning and one of my brothers had a hangover. I really wanted to give him *Nux vomica 200* but didn't have any with me. This troubled me greatly (Day 4).

I dreamt that I had some temping work at an office I worked in four years ago. It was surprisingly enjoyable. I had a laugh with my old workmates, my old boss was keen for me to come back and do some more temping and I enjoyed it, knowing I didn't have to stay if I didn't want to. A pleasant dream, quite light-hearted (Day 11).

I had a dream about another Predator type monster with an ominous presence. I was in a huge building with lots of levels. Some were offices and some floors were derelict and dark. I was trying to escape the creature by getting the lift to other floors, but never knew where it would be. It was invisible except for the eyes. A couple of times I saw its eyes in the dark. They were two lights (electronic looking) and almond-shaped. Toward the end of the dream, I turned into a Predator-type monster myself and began contemplating trying to catch and kill other people!! (Day 14)

I had another dream about a building with lots of levels. I was working in a school/nursery. There were lots of us working there. About three or four of us discovered secret hatches in the floors, hidden under layers of carpets, floorboards and other bits and pieces that we could get through and hide. We felt that as there were so many of us, our employer wouldn't notice we were missing (Day 15).

I slept heavily and can only remember one snippet of a dream. I was talking to some people from college and said my/our experience was mainly related to coincidences. They said theirs was mainly about sarcasm! (Day 18)

3) *The dreams I had during the proving reflected themes linked to family, insecurity, anxiety and difficulties. They were often upsetting and disturbing causing me to wake up in the night.*

Coincidences. *Four days before the proving:* I dreamed that I was talking to the detective sergeant who is investigating the robbery that I walked in on at my ex-partner's house. In the dream he sat me next to the criminal who they'd caught. I knew it was him and confirmed this to the detective (but it didn't look like the burglar I saw in real life). I remember feeling worried that this guy had seen me identify him to the police.

Three days before the proving: Today I got an unexpected phone call from the police requesting I do a photo fit on the man I saw in the burglary. (This is real life not a dream!) I thought it coincidental that I had dreamed about that the night before.

Unresolved issues. *Now during the proving:* Last night I dreamed that I was living with my family in our old house. My mum had decided to leave my dad and I was really upset, I felt all the security had been knocked out from under me (Day 3).

My analysis: I think this may be old issues re-surfacing going back to where I used to live with my mum and dad. Mum and dad did used to argue badly for a time when we lived in that house but they never split up. We all used to argue and freely express our anger with each other! My family are all pretty close and we know we are a bit dysfunctional but we all love each other. This dream was very unusual as the house in the dream was my actual old house that we all used to live in: our main family home that I grew up in. Normally in my dreams, the location does not reflect reality.

This seemed to be a dream about losing that security I feel I have with my family.

Last night I dreamed I had these long artificial nails on and I was trying to fight a witch who was sitting next to me. She looked exactly like me and I scratched her across the face. I woke up very upset (Day 4). *My analysis: Reflecting on this dream, I think this may be an old issue rearing its head that I have not yet been able to deal with. This is about me disliking parts of myself and fighting with myself.*

I dreamed that I was at college last night although it looked nothing like college in real life. I was reading a novel about a horse that got measles and a teacher had set us homework about remedies for horses. A colleague (a project manager I work with in real life) was at the college too and we worked on this homework together. She managed to book a room at the college for us to go in and do this work. In the college room there were no lampshades and so I recommended that we just buy some cheap ones before using the room. *(In real life I do need some lampshades in my new flat.)* The lecturer showed us a video of himself on a trip in the artic or somewhere snowy. He was snowmobile riding through the snow and skiing. There were lots of big bubbly clouds all over the snowy landscape. My sister was also somewhere in the dream but she wasn't my sister. She was dressed very alternatively and walking around a cool part of town going to a cool bar (I think). Also I dreamed that I was in my flat and there was this pile of black bits on the bedroom floor in a circle. When I went to Hoover them up I realized they were little flies. *In real life, I have some flies like this on a houseplant in my flat but there are only one or two and they don't lie in circles on the floor!* (Day 16) (*See also quote no 497 in Part Six Page 382. Ed.)*

I dreamed I went to work and they'd put all these balloons hanging from the ceiling together with a cardboard box on each desk. *The box on each desk is part of a real internal marketing plan that was to happen today.* I was at work but in my pyjamas and then decided to ring in sick (but was already there). I had this crusty slimy mucus in my mouth, which meant I couldn't speak properly when I was explaining why I was sick. I started to pull it out of my mouth and was aware it looked disgusting so was trying to hide it from others. Anyway this thick, white mucus came out and the crusty bit on the end was the tail of a brown snake.

Anger unexpressed – Then I was sitting next to my assistant at work and she asked if Jim had bought me a Christmas present. *Jim is a senior manager at work and is a friend of mine.* I remember being surprised that she knew about the present so I lied and said 'no' and asked her why she's asked. She said it was because when she worked for him she was ordering music CDs and he kept asking how much they cost! There was also a bit at some point in the dream where another girl who works for me told me very accusatorily that I was going to get a £2K pay rise as were all the managers (Day 17).

In mid March six weeks after this dream, we had our pay review and I had a letter through saying I was to be given a pay rise of £2,000. I had no idea that I would be given this sum and was not expecting to be given quite as much.

Dreamt about my dad. He was ill and wanted to talk. I can't remember much else. Dad and I were pottering about in this village somewhere. It didn't look like my dad. Nausea on the train to work again this morning – 8.45 am to 9.10 am. Funny sour taste in my mouth. I cannot stop thinking about that mucus snake thing from my dream the other night. I can almost feel it in my mouth again when I think of it (Day 19).

Confusion and clumsiness. I dreamed a couple of us went to my friend Ruth's place. *In the dream it wasn't where she lives in real life – was a flat not a house.* We arrived at hers floating on a table (like a magic carpet but a table). We hovered outside the flat window, which she let us in through. It didn't occur to me, or anyone in the dream that the mode of transport was in anyway unusual. I didn't even think about it. Then I was clearing up with her and she was annoyed because I'd used extra baking trays to put the food out which she had specifically been trying to avoid. I felt guilty – I was trying to be nice and didn't want to upset her. I then was trying to be over helpful to compensate and I fed the cat but dropped my cornflakes and milk in its bowl so I was quickly trying to repair the damage by scooping them out with a spoon (Day 20).

Last night I dreamed that my ex-partner bought a very modern, small, neat, modern three-bedroom house on the outskirts of everything, in deepest suburbia. I had bought a beautiful but run-down flat in the centre of town. It was full of period features and some furniture had been left by the previous tenant. When I looked out of my window I could see the previous tenant – a pretty Spanish girl with her boyfriend in a studio flat. The whole side of her studio flat opened up so that you could see everything inside. She was arguing with her boyfriend. I could see he was being a pain. I also found her diary in the flat I bought. It was together with other bits and bobs she had left in a chest of drawers. I can't remember what it said but I did read some of it. I knew she should dump her boyfriend, I could tell he was no good for her. She didn't see that though. I could also sense that she was somehow restricted by staying with him (Day 22).

My analysis: This dream has some parallels to reality. I split up with my ex last February because I felt restricted in that relationship. He stayed in the house we'd bought together on the very outskirts of Brighton in deepest suburbia, while I moved out and bought a new flat which is the top half of a Victorian house and is much nearer town. I'm also friends with a man who I don't think is very good for me and I think I should end our friendship. I think that this dream is symbolic of certain issues in my life that I need to deal with, resolve and move on.

Day 30. Reading back over the dream where the mucus/snake in my mouth prevents me from speaking, I wonder if this is symbolic of unexpressed anger. When I let the mucus out of my mouth, I am worried that people will see it and it's disgusting. I wonder if this is all wrapped up with concerns that people will not think I'm a 'nice person' if I am expressing anger. Also Sue – a woman who works for me is in the dream and I have a lot of pent up anger towards her. She is very negative, tries to do as little as possible at work and takes long breaks and doesn't respect me. I don't think I'm dealing with the situation very well. Also Jim, the friend I'm angry with, is talked about in the dream. These are two people with whom I have not fully been able to express my anger.

4) *Five days before the proving:* First dream: about an ex I saw in a shopping mall with his friend – he was standing around in the shop and I went to say hello. He didn't recognize me even after I told him my name, so I said hello to his mate who I also hadn't seen in years, hoping he would recognize me. They both didn't and I felt hurt and confused. I turned my back to look at the clothes further down the shop, then turned to find some police standing where they had been. I thought perhaps they'd done a runner after nicking something. I then thought maybe they'd recognized me but didn't want me involved in the scene of their crime, which made me feel better.

Second dream: I was in a supervision class at college. My supervisor told me I needed to take *Phosphorus 200*. I took it, then I felt myself falling off my chair, a sinking sensation, I thought I'd fainted. I was aware of people around me, yet unable to move or open my eyes. I thought this must be the *Phosphorus* burned out state. It felt very real.

The first night of the proving. Dream: About being in East End of London, at a music festival. It was grey and a bit dark. I was on the top deck of a double-decker bus looking down at the streets. I saw the music festival on a big screen and tried to see if I could see myself on the film (I didn't). Then I remember trying to walk home (I used to live in the East End). I got caught up in a wind, which was like a vortex. It spun me around in circles, really fast. I felt dizzy and passed out. I then got up to try and get to a tube station. I was taller than my boyfriend who is 6'3"; I think I was wearing very high boots. I had trouble keeping my balance, holding on to stair rails. It felt good, being taller than everyone despite this. He disappeared from my dream and then I realized I was on a high unicycle, which spun around, a bit. I managed to get off easily, though I felt a bit panicky that I'd not be able to. I had bought a return ticket at the tube station, was holding my unicycle and going down an escalator. An old lady walked past and said she liked to keep fit by going to the gym, which I said was 'good for her'. I decided I needed to get back out of the tube station to buy something, possibly tobacco and then found myself in a café amidst some women. I sat down at a spare seat at their table and got the feeling they'd been victims of abuse and were having a refuge meeting. Unable to stop myself, I fell asleep in my chair and woke up realizing I'd lost my daughter (who appeared in the café when I walked in there). I panicked a lot, running to a lift to see if she'd got in there and gone to another floor. I found her on the sofa in the café, tucked behind a big cushion and all right. I was so relieved as I thought she may have been snatched. I left the café and bumped into an ex-boyfriend who was flirting with me. I wanted him to go away.

Dreamed about a big manor house I used to live in as a child. There was a wild party going on there and lots of people I didn't know; some people were dressed up in slightly kinky outfits. It was my mum's ex-boyfriend's house and I wondered if he was there (in reality he sold the house years ago). I have dreamed about this house before, having secret corridors and rooms and I went to look for these again. I managed to find a secret passageway by pressing books on a bookshelf (like something I've seen in a film). I entered the corridor, saw some lights on and felt scared and anxious. I turned around and quickly shut the shelves up again. There was a sexual element to the theme of the party, which made me feel uncomfortable (Day 2). *I'm feeling strange as I write this and tearful. I don't know why. I just know I was very unhappy living there as a child. My mum's ex-boyfriend was an alcoholic and they used to fight a lot. I'm wondering whether the private/secret rooms represent something I've repressed in my subconscious, not sure though. It seems as though I'm revisiting places in my dreams that I have bad associations with. My dream about the East End of London and sitting with women who I felt had been abused has made me think about the time I was beaten up really badly by an ex-boyfriend when I was living in the East End with him. These are just speculations, and I think possibly I'm analysing things too much. I'm OK within myself; just feel as though something has been stirred up within me.*

First dream: My boyfriend suddenly turned against me, told me he had no feelings for me and I felt rejected and really upset.

Second dream: I was arguing with my mum and sister about what café we were going to go to. We ended up splitting up and I felt hurt and rejected (Day 3).

Dreamed I was lost in London, not sure where I was going. I found myself in a carnival, walking through people's houses, lots of music and parties going on. I walked past a young man on the street, who was sat at a table, rolling a joint. He was beckoning me over and I was tempted to share the joint with him, then I realized he was cutting up lines of cocaine as well. I looked at him, he was a mess, really out of it and I decided to walk on. Then I remember jumping over walls, running through peoples' houses, unsure of where I was going and feeling anxious. I ended up in a music festival in a field, enjoying myself. I saw some young Can-Can girls being a bit obscene, they threw up their skirts and there was a small dog between their legs. I then realized they were little girls and this disturbed me a lot. I tried to find my way out and get to a couple of my friends' house, people I know in London (Day 19).

5) *Six days before the proving:* Dreamed that the proving had taken place. I was in a castle and all the participants (who I didn't recognise – but knew them in the dream) were sat at a table each taking sips from a vial and then swallowing their remedies. The person before me got up to go and fetch the remedy they'd forgotten in their bedroom and then I went to my room also. Upstairs there was a frightening looking man and I suggested we alert someone, but was told that this man was some kind of security guard. I felt afraid. I woke up.

Night of Day 4. I have had an un-restful night. I had a very vivid dream. I remember a part about opening up my flesh with a scalpel (it didn't hurt and there was no blood) and extracting a small hair, which shouldn't have been there, with a pair of tweezers. I felt relief to get the hair out. A face of a man appeared in a window and it gave me such a fright, I woke up with a start. That is all I can remember. I then went back to sleep much more deeply for an hour before the alarm went off.

Review: Proving relates a lot to early teens (clumsy, low self-confidence). The hair represents an impurity, something 'yuck'. Does the man represent Stuart, the proving co-ordinator? (Relates to my night journeying? Ed. See Page 22).

Another night of waking and vivid dreams. I feel tired and unrefreshed. I dreamed I was at a huge ball and my body started to swell. I swelled up like a balloon and a doctor was called. I urged myself to sort out my stomach problems (Day 5).

Another poor night's sleep. Vivid dreams, I can only recall one. I had to attend a homoeopathic clinic sitting in session. It was night time and raining, when I got there I was late and I had brought my son as the case study and he was not in a good mood (Day 6).

I've had vivid dreams in the night. All I can remember is that I was meeting up with homoeopaths from college. I feel very unrested (Day 10).

I woke up having had dreams all about cleaning. I felt I immediately wanted to go home and clean my home (even though I did before we left!). (Day 16)

I've had a dream that I had just had a baby. Myself and my sister were choosing a name for the baby. That's all I remember (Day 21).

My sister told me she was pregnant a week after this dream.

(Compare Prover 1 feeling broody, Page 200.)

I've slept badly with broken, interrupted sleep. I have had such vivid dreams, and found them so disturbing that I do not want to write them down. They were sexual and very unpleasant (Day 37).

7) I dreamt last night that my children were left alone, asleep during the night in a building. They awoke and I was not there. I was in another building, struggling to get to them but something was stopping me. I awoke very distressed (A). (Day 5) *As an afterthought, and as a result of a discussion with my supervisor, I wondered if this dream links with a feeling of constriction of being hemmed in, as if can't break out.*

Dreams of confrontation and conflict –

Nightmare, awoke at 3 a.m. with a start. It concerned an issue of confrontation with a teacher at my son's school. I felt really disturbed by this since parents' evening the night previously was at my daughter's school and it was exemplary.(A) The sense of feeling disturbed and concerned stayed with me all day (Day 12).

Unsettled night. Dreams were full of anxiety about an impending event that I am about to organize. I feel that some conflict may lie ahead (Day 21).

Woke at 3.30 a.m. after awful nightmare, was shouting and shrieking. Nightmare concerned a move to a new house, which turned out to have awful neighbours who were violent and cruel. I was shouting, 'Have we exchanged!' since I had changed my mind and wanted to move back to my old house (Day 39). *This doesn't really 'speak' to me or resonate with any reality. I am not moving or even thinking of it.*

8) Dream: Dirty stagnant pond, very dark. Overwhelming fear at something nasty coming out of the pond to get me. The fear was so real and I became conscious and could feel my heart pounding with the fear so I got closer to my husband for protection. Daughter climbed into bed at the same time; I'm not sure if she picked up my fear, but we all hugged tight under husband's protection (Day 9).

Dream: Came out of work (not current work) – large building. Walking down road with colleagues to go out for lunch or dinner – not sure which. Felt I didn't know these colleagues that well and that I was in a strange place like London and didn't know the area, almost like I was new in the job. It was summer as I was wearing summer clothes. I stopped to do something, can't remember what, while others went on. When I got to the location restaurant/pub, my colleagues were all sat down drinking and, by now, they were colleagues from a job I did six years ago. Not same people I came out of the tall building with. Needed to go to the toilet, realized was in an Indian restaurant because could smell curry. Toilet was a room upstairs and was disgusting. It was just a room with plastic bags full up with black excrement and tissues. Was busting to go to toilet so urinated in a plastic bag, had no toilet paper so used my knickers and threw them away. End of dream. I don't remember any more (Day 10).

Dream: about sister getting married. Couldn't be bothered to get ready, so didn't go. No evidence of who she was marrying. She was dressed like Carmen Miranda in blue sequined cloak and wrap type hat! (Day 35)

9) *The day before the proving:* At bedtime I prepared myself to be aware of any significant dreams for the proving. I wake at 5.30 a.m. with this dream – I felt imprisoned, possibly in a prison, sitting on the floor with someone standing over about to shoot me. Somehow I broke through the floor to my left and dived through the hole to arrive outside. I felt sullied and had the thought, 'I am no longer the Virgin Queen.' *Retrospectively I now see this relates to my first experience of sex, how I lost my virginity against my will.* I took the first tablet two hours later.

Night of Day 2. Dream: Saw two old school (girl) friends in bed together as a couple. One, E – I always saw her as beautiful, elegant and played the piano well; she needed crutches in the dream – she always had weak ankles. The other friend, A, was heavier built, quite plain, very down to earth, very funny, brilliant sense of humour. In the dream I was surprised at witnessing them lying together. Retrospectively I see these two characters as representing two aspects of myself, and connecting them within myself. Later in the dream my husband and I were about to have sex in a shower only to realize that we could be seen through an opaque glass window, behind which was a canteen full of people.

After taking the three doses yesterday, I didn't take any more, because the remedy seems to have taken effect through my dreams (Day 2).

Dream: Something ominous in dark water (Day 3).

5.30 a.m. I woke again with a significant dream: I was cycling up a very steep hill, finding it difficult, arduous. I thought I knew where I was going because I had to return to somewhere I'd just come from, but got lost. I feel very low, tired and like I can't cope with all the continual family stuff. Like the dream I feel like I've gone back to where I've already come from, I recognize this state from times when I have really struggled with my children and had little support in caring for them. *Sepia* was very helpful at those times (Day 4).

Dream: I was at college, although a different layout of rooms. We all left the room to get a drink at tea break, going through corridors with friends. I craved coffee so I went back to class with a mug of coffee. I'd got lost on the way so I was not only lost but found it difficult to get to my desk. I then realized my dog was charging around the room excitedly. I got him by the collar and tied him to a chair outside the room. I was embarrassed at wanting a coffee. The lecturer asked me if I was enjoying the music. I realized that I hadn't been listening and had only been vaguely aware of it in the background. I was embarrassed that I hadn't taken note of it before and realized I'd been missing the point so far. Then I was on a small rowing boat with my advisor and supervisor for the proving. It was a dark night, starry skies, clear water. I wanted to cry but couldn't. Looking into the water I was moved by its tranquillity and serenity. A sense of emotion swept through me, I was pulled to my right, almost pulled off the boat towards the water. My advisor said to my supervisor jokingly, 'Bloody Nat murs!' (Day 6) *(This refers to a personality type associated with the homoeopathic remedy Natrum muriaticum. Ed.)*

Dream: With a friend. I knew her from age three to fifteen. I always saw her as slightly haughty, very knowledgeable culturally and politically, quite serious. We were in London on a river trip. I wanted to see the light, things on the surface around us, she wanted to go down into and explore some dungeons. (Day 8) *Retrospectively I view this as my resistance to delving into the issues at stake, which are at this point still dark and buried, deep.*

I get a sense that this remedy affects the heart and sacral and crown chakras. The words amethyst and quartz come to mind, but I do not know about them for their possible relevance. I have a sense of calmness, love, serenity, clarity(Day 11).

6 a.m. Dream: In a large house, possibly there on holiday, it's spacious, clean, tidy, overlooking fields and bright open space, with a stream at the bottom of a hill. Beyond I was aware of two volcanoes that were smouldering with lots of smoke.

(Several dreams featuring water, and now fire. Ed.)

There was also to my left a patch, which appeared to be volcanic mud very close to the house. There were two men present who seemed to be two teachers of homoeopathy of some importance to me. I pointed out the volcanoes which by now there was very little smoke coming from them. What had been dramatic and painful was now only a signal of what had happened before (Day 26). *Generally I feel really slowed down, calmer and not stressed. There appears to be a link that when I have vivid dreams of some significance, there is some sort of resolution and I am much more relaxed about everything.*

Dream: I was cycling to Chichester along an easy path near the coast but through fields. My husband was with me but walking, so sometimes he was with me, at other times behind me. We got to Chichester (others were ahead) in a really short time, and I couldn't understand why it takes longer to drive there. We were then in a building of which I remember very little. I'm left with a sense of slight darkness and confusion of what was in the building (Day 27).

I found it very difficult to wake. I felt very groggy and slow. All day I wanted to take things very slow and gentle on myself. I feel subdued and want to do the minimum required. Going to see my supervisor on her houseboat brightened me. (Day 28)

I've had strong realizations throughout the day of where some of these patterns come from – memories of feeling different from everyone else, that

I was abnormal. Also realizations that other people's perceptions are very different to one's own mindset about oneself. I saw my family today, and chatting to my dad said that I'm revisiting past stuff, of which he was at the time painfully aware but unable to do anything. He told me a way of massaging the forehead whilst accessing these memories and exploring them, but maintaining objectivity. Then going back further in time to see where these fears come from, still maintaining an objectivity to enable releasing these fears. (Day 30)

Dream: I was with my first boyfriend (true love at fifteen/sixteen!). It was a very sweet, romantic, innocent relationship, which never progressed far physically. We remained friends for years after. I remember very little of the dream, it just seems to be part of the flashbacks that are taking place. Retrospectively I now see this as the oldest flashback, and the beginning of where healing needs to take place (Day 32).

Woke with a dream: 1. I saw two birds in a niche in the wall. They were soft, grey, black and white with long beaks. I didn't know what they were at first and then suddenly realized they were kookaburras. They were sitting together looking down on myself and others.

2. I was on a very steep hillside with other people. There were some craggy rocks and two of the people broke off a rock each. Then coming up the hill, across from another hill, came what appeared to be two park rangers saying that the people couldn't take the rocks away. 'You can't run with those.' (Day 38*) My impression is that it is not possible to change our physical body.*

I've been feeling slightly resentful of the proving over the last couple of days. I'm not quite sure if what's taken place has been necessary and what, if anything, I've learnt from it. It has been very uncomfortable to dig up stuff that I'm very aware of, it's not denied; I just had hoped that over these years I really had moved on.

Dream: mainly anxiety about getting enough study done to meet college expectations. *Later that day:* I've been slightly detached all day, very relaxed, almost dreamy. I feel relaxed about my studies, being with the children, with enough time for everyone and everything (Day 39).

10) Running through undergrowth in a wood, chasing and overtaking ten-year-old boys. I feel I am playing but also protecting/helping them (paternal role). We are racing to climb an embankment, which turns into a tree. Climb to the top of the tree where I find a note telling me to meet three people with Indian names, in a place I remember as 'Chromoland'? *(I am a photographer.)* The names and place seem very important in the dream and I am sure I will remember them. I wake up and write down the details, but on really waking I find that this is also part of the dream and cannot remember any details other than that two of the names were male and one female (Day 1). *(I have two sons and a daughter)*

Aware of dreaming during the night; but left with one abstract image on waking of a very perfect jet black brick shape object, with no purpose, or none that I could remember (Day 2). *To me this has connotations of perfection and serenity focussed in one place. This seems to be a reflection of how I find myself: solid. I feel that my dreams are currently more abstract. Usually they would be of my attempts to sort out work issues or life issues. Just now they are not related to either.*

Strange dream starting on the top deck of a London bus, an attractive young (twenty-ish) oriental girl attaches herself to me just wandering around central London. I am aware during the dream that there is an element of infidelity here, I am attracted and flattered by the girl's attention but it is more a romantic than sexual experience and I know I am not going to take it any further. The girl is not anyone familiar. I wake feeling a little guilty but glad about my marriage. The dream reminded me of my life before marriage when I was more emotionally hungry (Day 13). *(Stuart and Prover 4 also had dreams of being on London buses, red buses.)*

Rubrics

Dreams

Firstly rubrics as in Murphy's Materia Medica

Amorous, sexual dreams 451
Bicycling 453
Buildings 453
Chased 453
Cleaning 454
Crimes, accused wrongly, that he might be NR
Difficulties 455
Disgusting 456
Escape 456
Excrements 457
Family 457
Frightful 458
High places 459
High places, falling from high places 459
Monsters 461
Pursued 463
Shooting, being shot, of 465
True, dreams come true 466
Vivid 467
Waking, the person 468
Water, dreams 468
Water, dreams, rowing on 468
Way, losing 468
Sex, dreams of 464
Vertigo 467
Birds Kingfishers/Kookaburras NR

Dream Themes

- of a feared disease – a prover had a dream of cancer, a phobia of hers
- of difficulties, arduous tests and trials, a very steep hill
- of confrontation and conflict
- of constriction and being hemmed in, prison, of escape – of

being chased by an unseen monster, and trying to escape – fear of being caught and killed – of police pursuing criminals – of being frightened – of the need for protection – anxious that she would be wrongly accused – of maybe knowing too much, and gangsters/criminals would harm me for that?

- of secret, hidden illegal things, secret corridors, getting lost – fighting a witch, old issues, parts of myself that I dislike – of places with bad associations – of something ominous in dark water – of one person wanting to see the light, things on the surface, the other wanting to explore some dungeons – resistance to dealing with deep buried, dark issues
- of a houseboat losing a mooring, then pulling it back in place
- of clumsiness, then quick to try and repair the damage
- coincidental dreams
- of relationship issues that need to be dealt with, shifted and resolved – of past intimate relationships
- of smouldering volcanoes – difficult things of the past that have been dealt with
- of childhood home, of losing secure family feeling – that daughter had been snatched – of my children asleep in another building, struggling to get to them, but something stopping me
- of being caught in a vortex – being on a unicycle, spinning around, fear that I couldn't get off but did – of being on the top of a London (red) bus – of wearing high boots – of cycling
- of a disgusting toilet, black excrement in plastic bags –of cleaning, of extracting impurities – of a dirty, stagnant pond, something nasty coming out to get me
- disturbing, sexual dreams – dreams of marital fidelity
- of kookaburras
- of perfection and serenity – tranquil, serene water, in a small boat, a dark night, starry skies, clear water, almost pulled into the water – of a sinking sensation

Provers' Reviews (at the time and later on)

Prover 3 – Summary

July 3rd 2006 – five months on

My thoughts and reflections on the proving are as follows:

Mentally –

Confusion/clarity: Initially the remedy brought out a mental confusion, clumsiness, although at the tail end I felt clearer mentally. I had a couple of clairvoyant dreams during the proving. This is not something that has happened to me before that I've noticed. I have always had a slightly clairvoyant sense in that I get a feeling that something is going to happen. This intuitive feeling seems to have intensified since taking the remedy and it somehow seems clearer, and more specific. Before it was very vague.

Anxious/calm: When first taking the remedy, I had this calm feeling at points where I would normally feel anxious and stressed. Then towards the end of February, I had this feeling of 'indifference' about things I would normally worry about. This was actually quite pleasant and liberating. It hasn't lasted and I now have my usual worries about deadlines and things I need to get done.

Unresolved issues with –

1/Anger: I noticed that I was very angry with certain people in my life. I'm not sure if I was angry with them before but didn't realize it and the remedy brought the anger to the surface, or if the anger wasn't there before. Anyway, it had the effect of highlighting issues that had been dragging on for some time and forcing me to resolve them. The anger was linked to me judging these people wrong for how they were behaving.

Situation 1 was a friend/colleague of mine who is married and yet pushes for an 'on-the-side' relationship with me. I felt very critical and angry with him after taking the remedy, whereas before I had always reasoned that these things happen, he is confused, has feelings too and is not to be judged or blamed.

After several attempts to resolve the issue, I have finally come to a resolution within myself with this and now have a better relationship with him that makes working together a lot easier.

Situation 2 was a colleague who works for me who was not working very hard and taking long breaks. She also seemed to have slipped into a very negative state. I had known this for some time but was resigned to think that as long as she got what she needed to get done I wasn't going to worry. However, the remedy seemed to bring up a huge amount of anger and judgmental criticism in my head of this woman and her attitude. It made me face the situation head-on and reprimand her, which was actually a bit destructive at first. Things have now moved on and we have a better working relationship. She is working harder and has a much more positive attitude than before she started to slide.

2/Guilt: The other issue that I seemed to be carrying around, which I dreamed about during the proving and suddenly burst into tears about one evening at home alone without having even been thinking about it, was my break-up with my ex-partner last year. I suddenly seemed to realize I had been carrying a ton of guilt about ending the relationship and was still concerned that I had hurt him badly. Before, I had always justified to myself that my ex had not given me my freedom and was controlling, and by being critical of his behaviour to me I was avoiding facing the guilt inside me. Having realized this and talked it through with my ex, I seem to have come to a better place in myself. My relationship with my ex, which was good anyway, is now much better as I feel we have now moved to truer friendship.

Dreams: On the first night following taking the remedy, I dreamed I was in a family house I grew up in with all my family there and an upsetting situation. The fact the house was the actual house we lived in is unusual for my dreams normally the location may represent an actual one but is a fictional one. General dream themes were about family, insecurity, anxiety and difficulties.

Physical Symptoms: Hot flushes starting around stomach abdomen and rising up across face and chest and up the back and back of the head.

Nausea in the mornings and while travelling.

Itchy, red rash across chest/heart area.

Abdomen – gripping pains in waves, < pressure, < doubled-up, > stretching out. This was a return of old symptoms but it was very intense and interestingly, I have still not yet experienced it since.

January 26th 2008- two years after

Teeth. After the proving my teeth became very sensitive and I went to the dentist and he said I had receding gums and this was a genetic condition. He said proper cleaning would help slow down the condition and prevent soreness. I do clean my teeth in the way recommended by the dentist now, but I had never had this problem prior to taking the *Amanita rubescens* in the proving. The tooth sensitivity has flared up on and off over the last eighteen months with little correlation to the cleaning regime, although diet definitely worsens things, e.g. < sugar. That said, it was not always worse for sugar and sometimes would happen during good diet and teeth cleaning periods. I would say though that for the last three to four months, my teeth seem to have settled down and I have not experienced the extreme sensitivity.

Unresolved issue – During the proving, I became aware that I was carrying a lot of guilt and pain for finishing a relationship with my ex-partner. I had not even been aware of this until taking the remedy. Since the realization of this, I have been through a long period of worrying about him and the hurt I caused. The stupid thing is that he is fine and has moved on to a new and happy relationship. However, I could not seem to shake this feeling of sorrow for what I had caused. It has been rattling around in my head until about two or three months ago when I heard a radio show. A woman, whose partner had left her, rang in to explain it was the best thing he'd ever done for her and she was now happy with a new partner. She said she was devastated at the time but is now so glad it happened: he did her a favour. I felt a sudden release and completely changed how I viewed walking out of my relationship. I realized my ex probably would say the same. So I finally feel that I have come to terms with this and have let go of the guilt and sorrow.

I'm not sure if this is relevant to the proving or not but I seem to have become more aware of the importance of my family relationships. I have strengthened the ties with my family (Mum, Dad, brother and sisters) that I love but have not always prioritized. I was always putting work, college and friends above them. (Perhaps because I feel they will always be there for me regardless?) Again, I seem to have come to this realization and changed my priorities to include them and spend time with them. This has had a positive impact on me and I feel I properly appreciate them now.

Prover 4 – Since the proving

February 6th 2008

After the proving I found a tremendous amount of enthusiasm for my dissertation on the AIDS miasm. I found similar themes in the AIDS nosode remedy to *Amanita rubescens*. Dreams of houses, responsibility for children and feeling detached and rejected being some similar themes.

My life changed dramatically when my daughter's father came back into our lives in February 2007. This was the biggest unresolved issue I felt I had and would never resolve. My daughter is now much happier and her constipation has disappeared, a condition she had since she was a baby. We are still together, though I feel there is a lot more work that needs to be done in order to keep our relationship strong. I have told him I need space and we are living separately, in the hope that we can grow stronger before making any big commitments. He wants to marry me but I haven't been able to contemplate this yet. However, I feel optimistic that whatever happens, things will work out for the best.

April 12th 2008

Since typing up notes on cases and people's experience with this proving I have felt the effects, as follows.

My tooth on the left side, second from the back has an abscess on the gum just below it. It has been there on and off for more than a year. *Mercury* the remedy helped a bit. I had not been able to find an NHS dentist until recently (when I started getting involved in working on Amanita again). It was a pleasant surprise to find one, two weeks ago.

Been very tired by 5 p.m. Just want to lie down, curl up and go to sleep. Get irritable that I can't do this, having to tend to my daughter's needs. However my relationship with her is excellent at the moment, I am cherishing every moment with her; we are very close.

A few days ago my boyfriend left a coffee filter on the stove without realizing that the ring was on, and the plastic part underneath melted completely; we only became aware of this from the toxic smell. I have spilt several drinks again, mostly on my desk where I'm typing these notes.

While typing Stuart's case notes (I had almost finished), I had a strong urge to take another *Amanita* tablet. I took this five minutes ago. I now feel very focussed, but also a little tearful after having a row with my boyfriend. It was about unresolved issues on his side of the family, affecting not only me but my daughter as well.

I have recently become very focussed in getting my career in order, as a homoeopath and also teaching relaxation classes for kids. I have also given up smoking dope (again), which I have had further problems with in the past years since getting back together with my ex (the father of my daughter who abandoned me when I was pregnant). He has always smoked a lot, however, he is resolute now that he wants to give it up as well, not prompted by my input, which is very unusual for him.

Something I didn't note before: my right hip has been very painful since the proving. My osteopath tells me there is some disintegration of the tissues between the bones; this has worried me a lot.

It's usually worse when I'm under stress, especially emotional stress. Also worse in the mornings upon getting up from bed and wears off during the day. Yoga helps loosen the stiffness. (I've had scoliosis since I was born and this contributes to the problem. My right leg is slightly longer than the left and I have a tilted pelvis because of this.)

My relationship with my mother and sister has improved dramatically. I had felt totally neglected by my family to the extent that I almost wanted to disown them during the time of the proving, and for some time afterwards. My sister had a terrible breakdown last year. She attacked me in my home at one stage, pushing me towards an open window, which was three floors up. I had witnessed a murder from this window outside my house a few weeks beforehand, which possibly made me insecure about this.

As I write this about 20 minutes have passed since taking the remedy again. I feel focussed on getting this work done. My eyes are awake and I am focussed to the core of my being. It's late, 11.45 p.m. but I want to get this done. I have put my emotions aside in order to do this. This may appear as detachment to my boyfriend, after our earlier row, but I hope to resolve things between us tomorrow. I had a few drinks tonight, but the remedy appears to have sobered me up. I am feeling a lot warmer too, especially in my cheek. I'm not feeling so emotional as before. About an hour has passed and my right foot is tingling, like pins and needles.

November 25th 2010

Coincidences. I had been discussing the new remedy *Amanita rubescens* with a friend of mine approximately two weeks prior to receiving a phone call from Stuart asking me to write a review of my experiences since the proving. I had thought of the remedy on and off since discussing with my friend and it seemed a bit coincidental when I got the call soon after that. Around this time I had a premonition about a very old friend I hadn't seen for almost fifteen years. It was just before Halloween and I was leaving a pub with a friend when I bumped into him. Again, I'd only been thinking of him approximately two weeks beforehand when I was thinking of the days I used to practice judo. He was my old judo instructor. It was probably the first time I'd thought of him in about ten years.

My life over the past couple of years has generally improved in that I now feel things are finally taking off with the homoeopathy and reiki. I've had more new patients over the past five months than I've ever had since I qualified as a homoeopath back in June 2007.

Until around May this year I experienced a lot of family dysfunction at home, with my mother's boyfriend causing most of the disharmony. Trying to communicate with my mother was like talking to a brick wall. I managed to deal with this by keeping up my Buddhist practice on a daily basis. It helped me find an inner strength and clarity to see the whole picture with my part in it. By June, my mother finally split up with her boyfriend after approximately twenty years of a very dysfunctional, on/off relationship. I live under the same roof as my mother, although I have my own kitchen/living area; her boyfriend still managed to encroach on my life making it very unpleasant to live there. I felt violated and wanted to move out, but my financial situation wouldn't permit and I wasn't keen to uproot my daughter yet again having got her into a very good school nearby a couple of years ago.

I also split with my daughter's father in June 2009 after my 40th birthday... we had been arguing mainly about unresolved issues concerning his side of the family but affecting us, and despite going to a couple's counsellor we seemed unable to resolve anything as he refused to go to a group the counsellor advised him to. I felt like I had nowhere to turn, as it seemed I had no support at all from the very people who should be there for me. I finished with him after we rowed on my 40th birthday. It felt like the last straw that broke the camel's back and I decided to concentrate on my career and my daughter's welfare instead. I met someone else, a musician who I dated for a few months but finished with him as this proved to be dysfunctional too and I didn't wish anymore dysfunction around my daughter. Since then I've had no real interest in forming a relationship, almost to the point that I have an aversion to men in general. My friends have been more of a support than my actual family during my times of crises. However, things have improved a lot over the past six months with my mother and my sister, and my daughter's father wants to try and work things out again. He is also expressing an interest in Buddhism and I'm taking things very slowly. We're more like good friends than lovers at the moment, which is about as much as I can handle for now.

My libido is extremely low, has been for approximately six months… it seems I have no desire at all for sexual pleasure. I find my energy more directed towards other creative outlets. After splitting up with the musician, I bought myself a good violin around March last year and started playing it for the first time in decades. It felt good to be back in touch with that part of myself again. I generally feel stronger within myself and more independent, focussed and driven.

September 2011

I still have a low libido, find it hard to relax with sex. Have also discovered lumps in my breasts, they both feel sore and tender at times to the point where I don't like wearing a bra. Worse on the left breast, where I had a cyst drained approximately two months ago. I had been drinking and smoking a lot, earlier this year after losing a very dear friend who died suddenly in India in May. He was an ex-boyfriend dating back to the early 90s, who had tried to get back together with me last year after we bumped into each other on the street (I hadn't seen him in about fifteen years).

Work is slow and I have lost my slot at a health and fitness centre after it was taken over by a new owner. I'm trying to work from home instead. However, I realize I shall need to find another job to make ends meet. Worried about finances and security issues generally.

On a good note things are going well with my family, getting on better with my mother but I do still have issues with my sister who has always been disrespectful towards me. My partner is naturally upset about my lack of libido but he's been fairly understanding considering. We do seem to be getting on well in other ways and generally quite happy as a family unit.

Prover 5 – An overall review to date

March 14th 2006 – two months from the beginning

From the week before the proving until only a week ago, I feel I have been on quite an intense emotional and physical journey. I'm certain this is proving related and not a coincidence. This is because of how dramatically I have felt symptoms since the time the proving started and how clearly an 'end point' was reached. Currently I am feeling really happy, much more detached from unhealthy family relationships. I have always had a very fast energy, rushing around doing many things, but in the last ten days I feel a real calm and slowing down. I have visited an acupuncturist twice and organized babysitters to give myself time to relax around other adults, rather than always being at home on my own. I'm even feeling excited about my home move and new possibilities this could bring. Subsequently my stomach problems are improved. I have no cramping, am not constipated and want to eat healthily. I haven't smoked a cigarette for ten days and this time found it easier to quit.

This positive relaxed mood is in huge contrast with how depressed I felt during the proving. Anxiety and foreboding were my general feelings daily. When visiting family I felt particularly fragile and lacking in confidence. The feeling of clumsiness and stupidity, which I felt throughout the proving, was even more acute around my family. I felt I was being oversensitive and too needy of their affection. My usual tougher exterior was not there. Now the proving is over for me I feel these family issues are not necessarily resolved, but I'm calmer and more grounded in dealing with them.

I am glad to have been a part of the proving and for the changes which have taken place since, but I did struggle at times with what I feel was a total lack of support. At times the intensity of my sadness and stomach/bowel problems were a lot to bear on my own. I'm not sure I'd ever want to repeat being part of a proving again. I wonder if other provers also found this? I am really interested by the fact that what some provers found to be cured (such as sleep problems) I developed as a problem. I know the proving is over for me as my old habits – e.g. good sleep – are back to how they were before. Time will tell how else this proving has been of effect.

One Year On – Spring 2007

Looking back over my diary, I'm really struck by how miserable I was at that time and how fragile and unsupported I felt. I am in a completely different state of mind now. I feel very strong and rarely get 'down' on myself. I cannot say this is totally down to the proving, as I associate giving up smoking with my mental state changing for the better. However, I definitely feel the proving kick-started my giving up cigarettes.

The main emotional change I attribute to the proving is a positive detaching from my son. Our relationship was far too intense and I felt I rarely had an 'adult' life. After the proving I organised babysitters much more without worrying if this would upset my son – it didn't! A few weeks after the proving I also took the decision to live above my workplace, a pub, until I'd found the right place to live long term. Living with lots of my friends above a pub with my son proved to be a lot of fun for us both and I think before the proving I would not have taken this decision, as a pub would have seemed too inappropriate for a child. What I'm trying to say is that since the proving I have felt more relaxed about recognizing my needs to not be 'Mum' all the time, but also have adult time.

I have grown so much in confidence in the last year, but I have ongoingly seen my homoeopath and have had other remedies, so I feel that I can't put that solely down to the proving. My overall reflection when looking back is that the proving was the catalyst for many changes within me, particularly affecting relationships in the family.

Prover 6 – Overall thoughts on the proving.

I was amazed at the feelings of excitement that I had prior to taking the remedy. At first I put this down to the energy of us as a whole group, and then I began to think that it was me that was going mad. I found myself wanting to do things like windsurfing (I would probably drown), and sky diving. (I would never contemplate doing anything like this; I hate heights.)

After taking the remedy I just seemed to be experiencing physical symptoms, and nothing on a mental level until the co-ordinator phoned me to hear how it was going for me. After speaking to him all of the excitement seemed to return briefly – I thought he was 'zapping' me down the phone line! Very strange. *(Another example of the 'spreading' quality of this remedy. Ed.)*

I am pleased I took part in the proving. It has been a very interesting experience for me, and as a group I think that it has been good for bonding and the making of new friendships.

And in July 2006

Breathing has been good this year – not needed inhaler at all. I think the proving made a difference. Before had to take a puff every night.

And more recently – December 2011

Apart from being dryer in the winter my skin has been pretty much clear since the proving, as well as my breathing, and I have not used much homoeopathy around it. Before the proving I had suppressed both the skin and breathing symptoms for so many years. I remember having a big aggravation of both during the proving then it all calmed down.

Prover 7 – Summary and Overview

My own feeling is that the recurrent themes running through my proving are perhaps more apparent in the first few days of taking the remedy. I feel that the centrality for me related to a sense of constriction that seemed located in the throat. I am not sure if this is related to the feeling of mental constriction that I have felt. For example, from nursing sick children I did feel a sense of being constricted, of being hemmed in. There was a sense of needing to break out, and it was definitely alleviated by fresh air and exercise. This is generally a feature of mine. In the first hours of taking it I did have a sense of 'lightness', a sort of otherworldly experience, a sort of timeless, suspended sort of feeling. I did wonder subsequently now that we know it is a fungus whether this could be linked to its toxicology. This could also be linked to the panicky feeling.

To return to the throat and the voice: I wonder if the anxiety or dread were relieved by vocalization. That is a sense of release of the blockage in the throat. Speaking, talking things through was definitely linked to a sense of alleviation, but that is not surprising. I did feel that at some level it did make some old issues return, and maybe it made me see some old issues perhaps more clearly, or at least to revisit some issues.

Overall I felt a general sense of well-being during the first month – that is the period from taking the remedy to the February college weekend but this seemed to wear off. Friends did say that I was looking better in myself and I felt more energized even with periods of tiredness. This did coincide with a period where I was detoxing my body which I always do every January. Tiredness and lethargy, which also seemed to figure in the picture, I do not see as significant because, although I was tired at the beginning, I was exercising more and found that I had the energy and great desire to do so. I believe that from the February weekend until now this has not been the case and that the sphere of influence of the remedy lessened.

Prover 8 – Review

February 11th 2008 (In response to my email enquiry as to how things were since the proving.Ed.)

I guess you need my reflection on the proving?

To be honest I haven't given it much thought and the reason for that is, for me, the proving brought out my syphilitic side very heavily and I have struggled, even with good homoeopathy, to move away from it.

My teeth are still playing me up two years after the event, something I never had prior to the proving. Despite good dentistry, I still suffer with pain in my teeth. I will never know if my miscarriage was related to the proving or something that would have happened anyway. I have had another one since and I have not been able to conceive so far. I am now 43 and I feel it's probably unlikely that I will have another child, which is a great disappointment to me and for my daughter who would love a sibling. I believe in fate and that may well have been my life map anyway, who knows.

I personally dislike revisiting the proving because it brings a heightened awareness of the issues of the time, especially my teeth and emotional side and this is quite upsetting for me, even now as I type this. The post-proving meetings you arranged I wanted to attend initially but even the email giving the dates kicked off stuff for me again.

I know you are coming to college to finalize the proving and I will do my best to be there but please understand if I feel I can't be as I find this emotionally distressing.

Prover 9 – Synopsis

October 2011

My personal journey with this remedy was to uproot something which had been holding me back for a very long time. This remedy enabled me to recognize the specific event at which point I had lost my sense of myself. It was a situation that had left me feeling totally degraded and outside of myself. For several years I lived with feelings of absolute self-disgust and repulsion. The remedy's action restored my sense of integrity by bringing to the surface exactly what I needed to see and deal with. I re-lived through a dream the painful experience that completely altered how I perceived myself and how I believed people wanted me to be. Although I had been given many homoeopathic remedies over the previous few years, which helped me along my journey of healing, it highlighted exactly what was causing me to remain stuck. Since the proving I have been able to completely let go of my negative attitude towards my body and have completely left behind destructive eating issues. I feel released and that I move forward in my life on my correct path with much more clarity.

I feel that the kookaburra/kingfisher theme amongst a few provers symbolizes diving into the depths of oneself to catch and bring up to the surface something specific, the piece of information that is needed to restore oneself. Kingfishers have an absolute precision in their flight and what appears to be an intuitive ability to catch their fish in the dark water. It is interesting to me that several provers felt their intuition became clearer than usual.

Prover 10 – Review

On Day 17

At this stage I stopped taking daily notes as I had the feeling that the immediate effects of the remedy had passed.

Physically I feel perfectly normal as before. Emotionally I feel I have retained a better perspective than before, and I am more tolerant and forgiving. I have been able to improve the level of anger in the house and we are working better as parents than before. This is particularly apparent in the behaviour of the two boys, who seem happier and calmer of late. Our two-year-old daughter still has a terrible temper though but maybe this is more a part of her age.

I have found myself less judgmental recently (one of my worst character traits) and have been able to enjoy the company of groups of friends amongst whom I had felt uncomfortable and hypocritical recently.

Supervisors' Reports during the proving (and other parallel experiences)

Supervisor of Prover 1

I was forgetful today and had one episode of giggling whilst speaking to my prover. It was not because what she said was funny, more silly giggling and a release of tension.(A) Very tired today. Have had three episodes of cramp in right hand (below little finger) during the day (Day 2). I did have episodes of cramp in hand, probably right one, approx nine years ago.

Our house alarm went off spontaneously. It only does this very occasionally – once a year perhaps. Mid morning: I had to eat two chocolate bars, one after the other (unlike me). 7 p.m. I was singing a line of a song I know well, but the words came out wrong – one word rhymed with the correct word, but was wrong. I remembered this had happened earlier in the day too.(A) 9.15 p.m. I had a strange twitching in my left lower shoulder blade. It felt like someone was tapping me (fairly gently) from inside. It followed an irregular beat. It seemed a bit like something 'shorting-out' electrically.(A) 9.40 p.m. Still twitching as above. NB see my prover's notes for Day 3 at approx 7.30 and 9.30 p.m. She had similar tapping sensations!

One further episode of cramp in right hand (same place) whilst using computer keyboard. All day, on and off: my knees ache; they did yesterday too. But my knees do give me trouble at times; however, today I had great trouble getting up from kneeling. My legs seemed not strong enough to get me up. I've just realized there seem to be a lot more emails flying about between year two students this month. Mainly suggestions for helping each other – the group seems more cohesive. Very itchy lower leg towards left ankle when undressing to go to bed. Then the same on the right but less intense. The itching was relieved a bit by scratching (Day 3).

Tired today. Limbs, especially legs, felt stiff and heavy when I got out of bed, > continued movement. (This is not an entirely new symptom, but I've not had it this severely before.) If I get down near the floor, either crouching or on my knees, I have to really push myself with my hands to get up again. It is the reoccurrence of an old symptom, but it has not been this bad since pregnancy.

I had a headache after meeting with my prover at her house. I had to rest on my bed for half an hour, using a crystal on the tender spots on my forehead and the back of my head. It felt better for walking in the fresh air.

Is my perception of distance changing? I tried to park the car in too short a space.

Numbness in limbs again. Limbs feel weak and heavy. Is MS like this? (Day 4)

Overnight: I found myself half-awake several times, trying to get myself to remember in the morning, that I'd thought about horizontal bands of a dull golden yellow colour, like a bee.(A) 8 a.m. After I'd washed my face and neck, I noticed the sensation of the flannel on my skin stayed there for a while. My prover had a similar sensation one day – a feeling of something on her face that wasn't there.(A) I couldn't park the car again. I couldn't judge the length of it or the distance from the kerb; I even got the angle of the car against the kerb wrong (Day 5).

9.30 a.m. I noticed 'pimples' with tiny white heads on front surfaces of both thighs – a symptom I'd had in the past infrequently, but more prominent than I'd ever had before.(C) (Day 7)

7.30 a.m. I awoke with puffy eyes – both upper and lower lids were swollen and red. Both cheeks and nose are also swollen and red. I had a little 'pouch' of swelling under left lower lid.(A) 4.30 p.m. onwards: had slight abdominal pain, just below the umbilicus, over quite a wide area. I want the warmth of a hot-water bottle against it. 6.10 p.m. Face still red, and feels hot, but most of swelling gone (Day 8).

Awoke with swollen eyelids again, and red face. Redness has continued all day, extending to neck, and at times both ears have been hot, red and burning. Cheeks also burning. I feel conspicuous. *Evening:* cheeks itching a bit, and scalp. 'Spots' on thighs are lessening. I have put on weight (about six pounds since the proving started). I have been hungrier, eating chocolate at times, but feel some of it may be fluid retention. Generally I feel a little less tired and a bit more relaxed today about things. Strangely, I hadn't noticed I was 'uptight' until I stopped being so. However, events seem to conspire against me getting my homework done. 11 p.m. When I undressed, I found a red area on the back of my left upper arm. It was swollen and the tissue felt hard, like a cellulitis. I had to scratch it – I couldn't not!(A)

Face still hot/red, slightly tingly and numb. Neck still red, bit blotchy. Ears less red. I feel these could be old sunburn areas (Day 9).

11 p.m. I've got a red area on the back of my left upper arm, much the same as yesterday. It was 'quieter' during the day when it was covered and I couldn't get to it, although still warm. It was < getting undressed and < scratching. Right arm affected too, but to a lesser extent. I had lots of itching, changing places – scalp, back, left lower leg at back just below knee, left hand etc. Face still a bit red but less than yesterday. Feels burning and is hot or warm to touch. I spoke to the co-ordinator on the phone and felt I was rambling to him (Day 10).

7.30 p.m. I woke up to find a red area on the inner back of my left ankle (no longer on arm). This had gone by the evening. 8.45 p.m. When undressing for bed, I was very itchy, especially my palms and soles, but was itchy all over too. (Slight return of old symptoms after allergic reaction to antibiotics.) I had to scratch myself violently – could have scratched myself raw. The itching even woke me up three times or so in the night to scratch (Day 12).

I got the urge to clean out a cupboard and throw old things away. Once I started, I couldn't stop. I was late to bed. I felt I could do anything, if only I had the time. Tasks which have daunted me sound easy at the moment – just need time (Day 13).

Towards the morning, I had a dream where I was struggling to find a room for the night in a hotel, which was like a very tall, narrow, bouncy castle. I was afraid to go up to higher floors to find a free room because I thought it would tip over. I felt frightened (Day 15).

Prover 1's advisor's symptoms during the proving.

Advisors are homoeopaths who undertook to check through the proving material with a prover and his/her supervisor. Information obtained during meeting with advisor on March 23rd 2006, Day 66.

Felt emotional over things, such as family matters, which usually would have been detached about.

Breast pains.

Catarrh – sounded 'nasal', nasal congestion.

Abdominal pains – stomach cramps, like labour. (These started the day following a tutorial group meeting of Year Two students who were involved with the proving.)

Often things (symptoms) lasted for twenty-four hours.

Felt tired 4–5 p.m. (not usual).

Impaired spatial awareness – damaged car bumper.

Need for sugar. 'Just awful. I never ever buy chocolate bars, but I did.'

Nervous cough.

Floater noticed (eye).

Itchy shins.

Light bulbs went.

Supervisor of Prover 2

In college, a week before the proving began. Atmosphere of group – I felt there was an air of excitement, giggly, with a sense of anticipation about the proving. Everyone seemed light-hearted and animated. People were giggling. I noticed people being more clumsy than usual and a bit scatty. After circle time I felt grounded and centred. It was a pleasant feeling. I felt intuitive and trusting. I still felt giggly.

Three days before the proving began: My partner and I went to Bristol for the operation on his jaw. When they took him down to theatre, I went for a walk in the hospital grounds where I found a nice woodland. I came across an opening and stood facing the sunshine and closed my eyes. I felt an immense feeling of peace and I could hear the birds singing; the smell of the dew on the grass was overwhelming. When I opened my eyes I could again hear traffic and the peace evaporated. I checked the time, 11.15 a.m. Later when talking to the anaesthetist, Dan went under at 11.15 a.m. After walking around I went back to the same spot but could not recapture the feeling.

The day before the proving began: I dreamt last night that my prover and I were at a party where lots of people were taking ecstasy. We were trying to convince them to take potentised ecstasy, as it would be much less harmful to their bodies but also a much better high. Everyone thought we were mad. We then approached friends that were not taking ecstasy but knew about homoeopathy, they also thought we were mad because of the link to class A drugs.

Feel very positive. Lots of energy, yet calm and centred.

Day 1. Felt irritable all day, felt like everyone was out to attack me, very sensitive. I then realized that it is a full moon and became aware of the cats doing their usual full moon scattiness. I felt as if I could have a good cry in evening, but didn't because it doesn't feel real. Instead watched television and felt much better.

Have felt positive all day (Day 2).

I dreamt last night that I had a big mole type growth on my cheekbone and I was acutely aware of how disgusting it must be for others to look at it (Day 3).

Feeling wobbly emotionally, hassled and tired. Angry that my ex is withholding my money even though courts have ordered him to pay it two months ago. It's unfair that there is nothing I can do. I am noticing that although I want to be and am trying to be organized about the proving, every time I go to do something i.e. find a pen or make a phone call, I am being scatty and clumsy and unorganized. I am usually an organized person. Met up with prover.(T) (Day 4)

Feeling giggly all day since seeing T last night (Day 5).

Woke feeling scared, I think it was a bad dream but I cannot recall it, felt exhausted (Day 9).

Woke from a dream feeling scared as if I had been trying to escape from somewhere; can not recall it though (Day 11).

Woke scared and anxious as if bad dream although cannot recall it (Day 12).

When meeting up with T, I mentioned something about children; a mutual friend said exactly the same earlier in the day. I was discussing with my partner that when he went to Brighton what food he could buy from the Indian food store, Taj. (We were talking about olive oil particularly from there.) Later when I was at friend's birthday someone gave him some olive oil from Taj (Day 13).

Cycling to the gym, I witnessed a car accident where lady wrote off five cars (luckily no one was hurt). I felt very lucky to be alive; if I had been cycling a few seconds before or after the incident she could have knocked me off my bike. When I was at the gym, one of the cars that had been hit belonged to one of the girls that work there, which was some way away (Day 14).

After talking to T, she mentioned having eaten a box of Maltesers with her husband. My partner, not knowing this, went out and came back with a box of Maltesers (Day 16).

Came to light at college weekend that I have had clumsy speech, as lots of others have (Day 22).

Day 52 *Reflection after college weekend:* There has been a real apathy about the whole group. People that usually contribute and ask questions were quiet. A few people appeared very pale and dazed and there did not seem to be the normal light-heartedness amongst us. Life seemed to be an effort without much motivation. It was agreed that this time of year brings that out in people when we have all had enough of winter.

Supervisor of Prover 3

Strange dream last night about the cat getting the goldfish and biting their tails off, and although we rescued them they were so injured that they were unable to swim. Started clearing out cupboards and re-organizing them, and throwing away the clutter (Day 1).

Desire to clean out cupboards and de-clutter continues. Feeling frustrated and irritated. Very short-tempered. Emotional and weepy. *(See also Day 22 below.)*

9 p.m. Coughing and clearing throat. It felt as though there was mucus rising at the back of my throat, but I couldn't clear it. *Prover has tickly, dry cough at this stage.* (Day 2)

Mild headache developed in the afternoon, across the top of my head. Also a feeling of nausea (Day 4).

Today my prover has a little bit of a tickle in the throat and a little bit of mucus.

I felt quite nauseous today from 7 a.m. to 1 p.m. approx with no appetite (Day 5).

Slight nausea, coming and going in waves, and only lasting for a few seconds (Day 6).

Prover has very mild nausea – fleeting (Day 7).

I was shocked to pass a worm this morning, approx six to eight inches long. It was completely painless, and has never happened before (Day 10). *(See Prover 9, Page 162)*

Still possessed with a desire to spring clean everything. I keep cleaning out and re-organizing the kitchen cupboards etc. Almost like a nesting instinct. This is a very strong almost manic desire (Day 12).

I have been experiencing, slight and fleeting periods of nausea, once every two or three days (Day 18).

Further to college meeting on 4th and 5th February.

I realized that I forgot an important appointment on 13th January, the day the proving started. I didn't even remember, until I heard others recalling the same thing, that I had forgotten the appointment. Even though I reminded myself about it in the morning (it was my son's friend's birthday party from 4–6 p.m.), by the time the afternoon came I had completely forgotten it! I was even wondering what myself and my son were going to do all afternoon! I am not normally this absent-minded.

Also after hearing my fellow students talking about confronting long-standing issues I resolved to confront my husband about a disagreement we were having and to forcefully state my case. Around the time the proving began I had felt unable to do this. I did speak out on the 6th February, and though the outcome was not as I would have wanted, I felt better for stating my case and getting it 'off my chest'. We had been having the same disagreement and discussion over and over again. I felt as though my wishes and desires were being totally ignored, and that I wasn't strong enough to stand up to him and win the argument (Day 22).

Today I noticed a strange sensation around the area of my right kidney. It is sensation of pressure, coming from both the outside and inside. It is not painful, just uncomfortable and I am constantly aware of it (Day 27).

Themes and symptom areas. These are the general themes that come out in the proving: the desire to spring clean and reorganise cupboards and throw out clutter can be seen as analogous with the feeling of wanting to confront and clear out old issues, which some of the provers have been experiencing.

Her review of the proving to date, a month later. March 7th 2006

This has been an interesting process to date. As a supervisor I expected to have little input, and have been surprised to find myself writing pages in the diary.

Interesting themes have come up from both of our experiences, themes that have been identified either by the co-ordinator, or other provers in the class.

For my prover the hot flushes and confusion/mental dullness I think are significant. Also resolving old conflicts, or at least confronting the issues.

For me, I think the forgetfulness and perhaps the kidney symptoms are important. I also resolved to confront an issue, which had been bothering me for some time.

We both experienced nausea and coughs.

Mental Symptoms	Physical Symptoms
1. Desire to clean, re-organize, and get rid of clutter.	Hot flushes, ascending to between breast and head. Onset sudden.
2. Confusion, mental dullness, almost childlike.	Irritating cough, constant clearing of throat, mucus rising to back of throat.
3. Concentration difficult.	Tickly, dry cough, a little bit of mucus.
4. Frustration, Irritation with family.	Nausea and felt sorry for self, fresh air amel.
5. Weepy and emotional.	Headache across top of head, with mild nausea.
6. Forgetfulness – forgets important appointments.	Fleeting nausea.
7. Feels weak-willed and weary unable to stand up to others.	Worm in stool.
8. Unable to express one's point of view clearly.	Tickly cough, sounds like a bark.
9. Point of view not being understood or appreciated.	Pressing sensation in right kidney.
10. Resolve to confront issue and act on this resolve.	

Supervisor of Prover 6

These notes have been written at the beginning of April 2006, that is, at the end of the proving, and therefore come with the benefit of hindsight. I was a supervisor and had just started a new remedy myself (*Calcarea carbonica*). Changes that I noticed (and there were not many!) I put down to that remedy, rather than the proving remedy. However, I must say that at college weekends I felt the group dynamic, as if we were all energized by the remedy, or, more likely, the proving process. Otherwise, I do not feel the remedy resonated with me at all.

Seven days before the proving: I felt – and also felt that year group as a whole did so – very giggly in class, with lots of jokes and easy laughter. It was nice, and on reflection, I think it has bonded us more as a whole group, rather than a few little grouplets.

Day 20. My period starts – heavier than usual, and lasted about three days longer than usual.

End of February – Day 45. I experienced 'hot flushes' during the night for about three to four nights in a row. It felt like warm water being poured down my back, like a cape. *(Compare case example No 4 date 27/02/06 – around the same time as this happened! Ed.)* It was strong enough to wake me up, but not enough to look at the clock at check the time! At the time I didn't think anything of it in relation to the proving. I am at the right age for hot flushes and it had been very cold and so I wore pyjamas those nights and may have become hot as a result. It was not until the college weekend that I realized this had been a theme of the remedy, which is why I mention it now. I have not experienced it since.

Supervisor of Prover 7

College day – seven days before the proving: After the remedies were given out at college I suddenly started to feel really tired and weak. I put this down to the fact that my period had started the night before as I often get similar problems, but not usually that sudden. When I got home from college I felt really ill, I had aching, shooting pains all down my legs and I was shivering all over. I could not eat the evening meal, as the thought of food made me feel worse.

Day 2. I had a croaky throat that I kept having to clear, when I was on the phone to the prover. I have had a cold with catarrh and a dry night cough anyway, so I thought it may be part of that.

I woke up very tired which is normal for me, but then mid morning I suddenly came over very tired and my head felt woozy, this tiredness then remained for the rest of the day. I noticed a pain in the small of my back as if I'd lifted something too heavy (Day 3).

Evening: On the way home from meeting up with my prover I started to get aches and pains again; they were in my legs and once again I felt shivery too. The symptoms seemed about 50% less severe than they were after the college day (Day 5).

I have a sore throat that came on after waking up. It is a sensation of a lump in the back of the throat on the left-hand side, which is the same side I had dental treatment on yesterday. I had two teeth filled with white fillings, but I did not have any injection. It seems worse when I swallow (Day 19).

Menses is unusual: rather than the usual dark red blood, it is bright red. The clotting and the pain are as normal for me, and I am experiencing dizziness and weakness which is as normal. I woke with the sore throat this morning, which then got more severe as the day went on. It hurts to swallow and it's worse with liquids, better with solids (Day 20).

I woke with a sore throat in the night and needed to drink lots of water before I was able to get off to sleep again (Day 21).

I was early to college this morning. In fact I realized that I've been more organized and early for things since we started the proving. This is very unusual for me. I am feeling much more alert and awake today at college, which again is unusual. I normally have trouble keeping focussed, I feel much more clear-headed. The only thing that I'm having trouble with is appointments; I keep forgetting them. I missed my homoeopath appointment and when I spoke to him I said, 'I feel like I have someone else's head on, I forget appointments but I am still able to remember and do everything else.' I have still got the sore throat and the constricted feeling, but it doesn't seem to be so bad during the night now (Day 22).

I had a big argument with my husband tonight. Things are really not good at the moment between us, I'm at my wit's end and do not know how much more of this I can take. He's been really abusive and angry since he gave up smoking in October. I'm really worried about the effect this is having on the children as they are witnessing these outbursts. I feel I am getting very angry back at him at the moment, which is unusual and is making the situation much worse as then neither of us cools down easily (Day 23).

The arguments between my husband and I came to a head today when he stormed out of the house, upsetting our daughter in the process. I have spent a lot of time thinking about the problem over the last twenty-four hours and when he got back I insisted we talked things through. We were really able to clear the air and he was able to take a long look at himself and admit he has a problem; I even got him to agree to see a homoeopath (which he had said in the past he would never do) and a counsellor. Making these decisions has really helped as we are both much more relaxed in ourselves and with our children, we feel more positive about the future.

I've been urinating a lot more frequently and yet have not been drinking anymore; there is no change in the colour of my urine (Day 24).

I'm still urinating more frequently. I've been feeling very breathless for the last twelve hours and also suddenly feel very tired and weak this evening but this could be down to the release of so much built-up tension and stress. My throat is still very dry and sore; it feels like there's a lump in it. It's worse first thing in the morning and last thing at night and what is strange is, I'm not thirsty with it. We are all much calmer and relaxed in my household since we cleared the air yesterday, it's like a cloud has lifted from over our house and everything seems much brighter (Day 25).

My general experience over the first 24 days:
I have been getting very short-tempered and tearful, losing it over really silly things and crying over the least thing. This seems to be much worse than normal, I am usually only this bad before and during my period, but this time it has carried on much longer.

I realized that as well as sorting out emotional stuff we have also spent the last month sorting out the house, clearing clutter and purchasing many more storage units.

All the way through this proving I have been emotionally up and down, I felt at one point as though the depression I had three to four years ago was returning. I felt as though I have had little or no energy left to get on with the day-to-day stuff: that once I have dealt with the emotional stuff, I felt as if I just wanted to run away from the rest.

All of these symptoms seemed to lift and clear away on Day 24. This was after the day was spent confronting our issues and working out what to do about them.

The effects on my family of the proving?

My youngest daughter has had a return of old skin symptoms from when she was younger; she has had eczema on her face in the exact places she had it before. It does not seem to be itchy; in fact it doesn't seem to bother her at all.

My husband, children and mum have all had the left-hand sided sore throat, which feels like a lump or constriction in the throat. They have all had a lot of dryness, which is worse at night and first thing in the morning.

Both my children also had colds with this, with lots of green discharge from the nose, but this is quite normal for them.

The calmness continues in my household, despite having one of my children off school with her sore throat. We have all still got the sore throats; they only seem to be there first thing in the morning and last thing at night now. Otherwise feeling generally OK in ourselves. I'm still urinating more frequently (Day 26).

The calmness continues… It feels like a huge weight has been lifted from my shoulders. We have all still got the sore throats (Day 27).

It's only me with the sore throat now. The rest of my family seem OK (Day 28).

My sore throat is better on waking and does not come back today, but I still have a sensation as if there is a lump on the left-hand side (Day 29).

I have the lump in my throat on the left-hand side (Day 30).

There has been another confrontation in my family – between my mum and her boss. She has put up with unreasonable treatment and harassment by him for the last two years and she finally bit back. She has had no success discussing the problem with him so went above his head to personnel. Now things are looking much better for her and she is enjoying working there again (Day 32).

I made a very spontaneous decision to go and visit a friend up North, leaving tomorrow; this took a lot of very quick organizing. This was very out of character for me, as usually I have to plan things well in advance and be very sure of all my travel plans (Day 36).

I am very relaxed about my last minute travel plans, which is unusual as I would normally be worried it would all go wrong (Day 37).

I spent a very relaxing day with my friend. I'm not even worrying about how I'm going to get home tomorrow. This is not like me. What's going on here? (Day 38)

My journey home was a bit of a nightmare but I didn't get stressed like I would normally, I feel so chilled out (Day 39).

Days 40 to 44: I still have the lump in my throat on the left-hand side.

The lump in my throat seems to get worse throughout the day and by 5 p.m. my ear starts popping. Within an hour of this I had gone deaf in that ear and it had got very painful, throbbing and shooting pains (Day 45).

I had severe earache all day, sharp stabbing pains with a popping sensation and my ear still feels blocked. I had a very bad night's sleep last night due to the pains in my ear (Day 46).

(From this day on no further reference to the throat pains. There is a sequence showing up here: location of symptoms passing up the body along with the shifting of unresolved matters. Solar plexus, throat and now ears and sinuses. Ed.)

Once again I had a very bad night's sleep, due to the pains in my ear. My ear still feels blocked and painful, the pains are stabbing and shooting and there is a popping sensation (Day 47).

My ear is still painful but I had a better night's sleep last night. The ear is still blocked. I feel that this could either be down to the fact that I have been drinking too much milk recently, or it could be to do with the proving, as it is a reoccurrence of an old symptom from ten years ago when my ear got so bad that the eardrum burst (Day 48).

My ear is still blocked but the pain has gone; there is now a constant buzzing sound in my ear. My sinuses are twingeing and aching as well. I am still cutting out all dairy products and now have a constant headache, but this is more than likely due to the fact that I have also stopped drinking coffee at the same time (Day 49).

My ear is still blocked and buzzing and my headache is still very bad, its pounding. My sinuses are still twingeing and aching and my eyes feel sore – both when open and closed (Day 50).

My ear and my headache are the same as yesterday. My sinuses are still twingeing and aching but my head feels clearer now, not so woozy with the headache. I have been very emotional this morning; I had a very long cry (Day 51).

I'm feeling a lot better, my headache has gone and my head feels a lot clearer and my sinuses are OK. I feel very emotional today, still very angry; I just want everything to get better. My ear is still blocked but no longer painful, it's still making a buzzing sound (Day 52).

Overall review of the proving:
I feel the proving has had a profound affect on my emotional state, and things that I thought I had dealt with are coming up again. I feel very down, and my confidence is at an all time low. I feel out of place among my college group, as if I shouldn't be there. I'm not good enough. I had a time like this about six months ago, which I worked through with my homoeopath. I feel out of place with my partner, taking things he says as a joke to heart. I feel very tearful and can't stop thinking about things people say or the way they are around me. I feel like I've done something wrong all the time. These feelings are not as bad as they were before, they seem to be up and down: one day I will feel like this, and the next I will feel OK again. I am finding it very difficult to talk to anyone about all of this.

I am walking on eggshells around my partner because he is trying to work through his problems; he is confronting some major issues from his past, which have come up since this proving started. He has such buried grief, anger, guilt, rejection and hate from events that have happened to him in his life which he has not dealt with and now he is starting to, it's a step forward but it's a long struggle.

He is not working at the moment so he is feeling very low and he loses his temper very easily. We are under each other's feet all the time so we are constantly arguing. I feel angry at him because he is not out of the house at all and I can't get on with the things I need to do for college. It makes me feel like he's not really trying to get a job, although I know he is.

The proving is making me feel like I'm back in a space I don't like very much, heading back towards the depression I had three to four years ago. At the moment there are a lot of good days, but I feel like I'm teetering on the edge and absolutely anything could send me crashing back down again. Could this be the remedy bringing this all out again to clear it once and for all? How long should I give it? Or should I go back to see my homoeopath?

This remedy seems to have brought a lot of things to a head for me, my partner and my mum. They seem to be getting their issues sorted out so maybe I will too. It seems as though it clears away the emotional clutter, enabling you to deal with things and move on.

Extra note. There has been 'transference' of this remedy's energy even further than my immediate family, which is amazing considering I was only a supervisor anyway.

I sit in a Healing Meditation and Psychic Development circle with another eight ladies; we meet up once a week. When we were chatting this week they started to talk about things which were unusual that had been happening to them over the last few weeks. I was amazed when they all reported that they had been clearing away the clutter in their houses, dealing with emotional issues, and had also been more clumsy than normal. They did not know about the proving and when I explained it to them, they were amazed. We deal with energy all the time with the healing, but they had never experienced anything like that before.

Supervisor of Prover 8

During the proving

Right leg/nausea: I have a cramping feeling in the back of my right leg and I don't know what might have caused it. It feels like the muscle is in a cramping spasm, ongoing but quite a gentle one. I've also been feeling quite nauseous.

Feeling of insecurity from my past: I also felt a strong surge of a feeling that comes from my past that makes me feel uncomfortable. It's one of the strongest surges of that feeling I've had in a long time and it was not in a situation that I normally would have felt it in. It's a sort of insecure feeling that I've always found difficult to describe (Day 1).

Feet: The cramp feeling cleared up today but I have started to get quite swollen feet. They feel very hot and puffy (Day 2).

Womb: I've been having some twinges in my womb almost like period pains. I don't think it's ovulation because I've only just finished my period. I still have puffy feet (Day 3).

Some twinges in my womb and the same feeling of nausea (Day 4).

Abdomen/Bowels: I've been really windy in my stomach today. My stools were squirty with a lot of air in them. The wind was quite rumbly through my stomach. I don't think that I have eaten anything that might have caused this (Day 5).

Another rising sequence of symptom locations. Here we see the expression of held in anger (Day 7) as part of this – solar plexus releasing. Ed.

My stools have returned to normal today and the wind has died down. I have some more period type cramp pains, quite mild. It is starting to feel like the energy of this remedy is beginning to affect me in a hormonal way. I wouldn't normally experience this amount of 'period feelings' after my period; I don't normally feel nauseous either. I haven't taken any homoeopathic constitutional remedies for a while and I know I'm not pregnant (Day 6). *Several parallels with her prover who was pregnant. Ed.*

Moods: anger expressed – I've been feeling angry about the person I'm working with. Yesterday I finally told someone and I couldn't hold it back. Today I said if it's not sorted or if I'm not happy then I will leave. It wasn't a threat; I just thought that, after last year being so bad, I wasn't going to have another year like that. I felt very strong and clear about it (Day 7).

(Release of energy. Ed.)

Good energy, joking: I feel full of energy. Went to parents for grandmother's eightieth birthday and felt that I dealt with it really well. Usually it would be more difficult. I was very joking and jolly (Day 9).

Anger expressed: Having some difficulties with person I work with, feeling a bit angry about it. Let some anger out again today (Day 11).

(On up to the throat now. Ed.)

Started to get a sore throat in the afternoon, very painful and it wouldn't clear. In the evening had a bit of a temperature and I was quite restless (Day 12).

Cold symptoms, neck: Woke up feeling ill. I have still got a really sore throat. Came home early from work with cold symptoms coming on. My glands were swollen and painful around my neck and chin area (Day 13).

Catarrh starts up, eyes – Morning: Throat still sore. *Afternoon:* Left work feeling very distracted because of cold but still restless and talkative. Started to get a huge flow of catarrh – very clear mostly from right nostril: burning catarrh, and my eyes are sore (Day 14).

Sleep affected: Didn't sleep very well; feel like I'm having delusions. Head is bunged up. Can't taste anything and still have huge amounts of clear catarrh from my nose. This is the worst cold I have felt in a long time. I don't ever remember having a cold this bad. Just can't rest and want to keep talking. Very difficult to do nothing; the worst time was in the night at 4 a.m. (Day 15).

Generally < with lack of sleep: Had another terrible night's sleep. Couldn't sleep for coughing and runny nose. Woke every hour. At 4 a.m. stayed awake for an hour, couldn't sleep. Fell asleep around 6–7 a.m. and could then sleep late into the morning. Feel even worse today; feel like I'm going to die. Maybe a slight exaggeration! It's weird though, because my skin, hair and eyes all look good. I don't look that ill from the outside, apart from my nose where the catarrh has burnt my nose and it's all scabbed (Day 16).

Not feeling much better today, maybe a little less catarrh, but not much else is better. Still feeling very restless although very ill. Off work (Day 17).

Advised by my homoeopath to take *Lachesis* for my cold. It seems to have slowed me down. I feel more sleepy.

(I am not sure if there was there a distinct shift in her changes/realizations after the Lachesis, or whether she felt that the proving remedy effect was continuing. Ed.)

Emotional: I had a big emotional outburst over something – it seemed to be an overreaction to what had happened – I'd got a second parking ticket outside my house within a couple of days (Day 18).

Still feeling quite emotional today like I'm going to cry over anything if it goes wrong (Day 19).

Started crying whilst doing some work at home today. Felt angry that I had put up with my dad and my mum, walking on eggshells around them. Cried when my husband came home, and talked about it. I felt that I was no longer going to be so careful with what I say and how I say it, just be me (Day 20).

Cold symptoms reducing: Cold is starting to feel a bit better. I feel a bit stronger about dealing with my family, stronger in myself and in being myself around them (Day 21).

College weekend: This time, when we linked our hands together at college in the circle, I felt dizzy as if I couldn't stay still, like I was swaying on a boat (Day 22). *(Compare Prover 9's dream. Page 242.)*

Cold > Starting to feel better from the cold (Day 26).

Saw my homoeopath. I explained something from my past: how my thirteenth birthday *(puberty onset? Ed.)* had affected all my following birthdays. (It is my birthday soon.) This time I managed to calm down after a couple of days and accept it as it is, in respect of who would come; bit of a move on for me! (Day 27)

Taking new remedy from my homoeopath (Day 28).

Had people over for my birthday today. Didn't worry about whether everyone would turn up, like I normally would. Had a good healing therapy from a friend. It made me feel really tall, almost like my legs were really long, and more grounded (Day 36).

My husband gave me my presents when I got home from work but I didn't get excited like I would normally, I just got disappointed that I didn't get what I wanted. I felt really bad about feeling like that (Day 40).

> *Realization about family situation:* I got talking with my sister-in-law about my brother and how he felt about how he grew up. I had wanted to talk to her for years about this but had not had the courage to talk about it. I was too scared. I explained how I felt

about how I grew up and she said she would talk to my brother. It was the first time I had thought of my brother being in and going through the same stuff as me. The rest of the afternoon I was crying on and off. She suggested we meet up, and I would like to. I feel scared about meeting up, but I feel lighter around my heart, almost relieved.

In the afternoon I saw a kingfisher. I have not seen one for years; I thought how rare it is to see one. It flew straight over the estuary. It is the only bird I know that flies like that and is that beautiful blue/green colour (Day 41). *(See her notes about kingfishers, below.)*

Childhood associations: I had strange thoughts when we were driving around Lymington and nearby places today. I kept thinking about time and how in one way or another I could still be on the road we were driving on from when I was a child. As if both my husband and I were there at the same time as I was as a child with my parents.

Delayed menses: I have been a little worried about my period being late. I haven't had much of a libido lately (Day 42).

Menses starts. Hot flushes: My period finally came today. Light at first. I feel emotional, that's as usual for me. I have had a couple of hot flushes. I thought I might have early menopause because of this light period with hot flushes (Day 48).

Menses: Period is slightly heavier and getting quite painful. The blood looks slightly brighter in colour than I am used to. *Magnesium phosphoricum* taken today (Day 49).

College weekend: Period very heavy now although not so painful.

Grounded but 'floaty' mind! At college standing in group circle my feet were firmly on the ground; I didn't sway this time. I felt very grounded. *(Compare with Day 22 above.)* My mind was a bit scatty though. In a good mood but didn't really want to concentrate. A kind of apathetic feeling like I have felt all week about doing my college work, and about weekday work! (Day 50).

Very spaced out again in my mind: distracted easily. Didn't feel like speaking up at college like I would normally. Felt a bit nervous about making comments in the group like I did when I first started at college. I saw two large bits in my period that looked like a tiny miscarriage, which is odd for the third/fourth day of my period. *(Compare her prover's experience, very close to this time. Prover 8 Day 53. Page 141. Ed.)*

I haven't been paranoid about illnesses for quite a while. I think I may be being a bit paranoid again.

Throat: Have had a burning in back of throat for a couple of days – not acid reflux (old symptom) but burning, no bile (Day 51).

Menses: Have finished my period for just over a day but I'm still having some twinges in my uterus.

Realization about expression of emotions, and other changes: I feel open to a more spiritual way of life; it feels more than just 'what will be, will be'. Things between me and my husband have been really good and very loving. I now have a clear understanding that some of my emotions around one part of my life are completely suppressed, and I need to find a way to release them. Still some burning at the back of my throat (Day 54).

Have been having tingling down my left arm, mostly, but also my right arm and the rest of the left side of my body; it feels like a gentle pins and needles (Day 55).

Tingling sensation seems to have mostly gone now. I decided to get up and exercise before I went to work today. I managed quite easily to motivate myself to do it, which is quite unusual. I felt really good after it (Day 56).

Haven't been feeling myself lately. I have been numb to my feelings and emotions and even my husband has noticed that I have been 'indifferent' (his word). It feels to me like I am dumbing down my major emotions so that I can deal with some deeper stuff.

Theme of resolving issues with a family member: I dreamt last night that my brother had died and I phoned C his wife to ask if she knew, which she replied, 'Of course I do, I'm his wife.' The comment upset her, as she was grieving. Then I got upset because I would never be able to resolve things with my brother. The whole dream was very family orientated, and even in the dream I didn't have that much emotion to get hold of. Some tingling in my nose today (Day 60).

Proving Summary

My experience with the proving so far has been very interesting. Although I was supervisor and did not take the substance, I still noticed some things happening on a physical level as well as a mental and emotional level.

I do believe in the 'energy' of the substance and picking up energies from others around, and I had heard previously about the supervisors also experiencing some of the remedy symptoms, but I don't think I would have expected to have had as many symptoms as I did have or for as many situations to arise that would seemingly be out of my control. An example of this was the discussion I had with my sister-in-law about my brother and how he had felt growing up. I know that I had wanted to speak to her about my brother for some time because I find it difficult talking to him, but the right time had never arisen. My sister-in-law had instigated the conversation that led us to that subject. It seems clear that the link between the proving and this happening now are strong, and I also know that similar events have happened to other members of the proving group. This makes it all the more interesting for me because it means that the effects of the proving are reaching a lot further than just our year at college, but out into our families and friends, and possibly further.

There were a lot of experiences that I had had over the past few months that, after reading Stuart's (co-ordinator) notes and talking to others in my year, I have realized are linked to the proving. The one that I find the most fascinating is that, when reading through Stuart's notes of his experiences, that he had seen a kingfisher whilst returning to a place which he knew well from childhood and being drawn to the blue/green colours and the flight of the bird. I have always been interested in seeing birds that are rare to catch a glimpse of, and whilst away in a town that I knew well from childhood, I also saw a kingfisher. I was surprised that I had seen it because I was a passenger in a car at the time and they are difficult enough to spot when you are looking for them. I got excited, as I normally do about things like that and then forgot about it until I read Stuart's notes. I immediately felt there was a relevance. I had not planned to revisit the place I knew from childhood, I had wanted to go to Wales, but ended up there because of financial restraints. It really felt like things outside of my control were making this situation happen. When I spoke to another person in my year about it, she said that she had had a dream that she felt was important to the proving. It was about a kookaburra; she had looked into it and found it was related to the kingfisher. I went on to look further into the meaning of the kingfisher and found some really interesting information for which again I feel is relevant.

The kookaburra is the forest version of the kingfisher and directly related. It is meant to be related to expressing one's self in a clear and concise manner. The relationship between finding them near water is also to do with the emotions, which is less apparent in the kookaburra. The kingfisher is meant to be a very spiritual bird and provides energy for accomplishments.

Another interesting experience – Whilst the proving was going on I went to see my homoeopath to continue my treatment with her. At this stage I did not know what the remedy was or a great deal about it, and neither did my homoeopath. She prescribed me a remedy. She did not tell me what it was at the time. Since then I have asked what the remedy was, knowing that it had played a positive part on the reduction of my fears. The remedy was Yellow – one of the colour remedies. The colour that resonated the most with the proving remedy was yellow. Again, this just shows me how far the proving 'stretched' and how it affects lots of people connected to it in one way or another on an energetic level.

I would really like to be part of another proving, to experience the symptoms and the positive changes that happened to me and to others involved in the proving and be able to see where a remedy like this might be useful.

The Kingfisher

Kingfishers are found worldwide but are mostly tropical. They are solitary birds that utter distinct rattling or piping calls that can be heard a long distance away. The ability to express oneself in a clear and concise manner is part of the teachings it holds.

Their usual nest is a burrow in a sand bank or in a hollow tree. Kingfishers have been known to tunnel several feet into sand banks. This indicates the need for sacred space around them. Those with kingfisher medicine will find that they must have time within their day for quiet contemplation where intrusions of any kind are not permitted.

Bold in its actions, the kingfisher will dive headlong into the water to catch small fish. It shows us how to plunge into the unknown with confidence and not with fear. Kingfishers have large heads, long and massive bills and compact bodies. Their physical appearance is symbolic of the challenges and opportunities relevant for those with this medicine.

A large head can indicate past life connections relating to the misuse of the ego. In this life a need to keep the ego in balance is mandatory. *(I find that interesting for myself. Ed.)* The long and massive bill of the kingfisher suggests a need to use one's words carefully and their compact bodies represent a need for regular physical exercise and the toning of one's muscles. This need is sometimes a result of a past life influence relating to physical health or structural imbalances that is present in this life.

Kingfishers are found near the water. Water is associated with the emotional body of man and those who have this totem will find a strong need to live on or near the water. An exception to this is the kookaburra, a forest kingfisher who is less associated with water.

The kingfisher is a bird that holds many teachings. Most of its teachings relate directly to the spiritual, emotional and physical growth of those that hold this medicine. When growth is achieved, prosperity on all levels is attained. The kingfisher has the energy to accomplish various tasks in an efficient manner. It is a powerful teacher and those with this totem would be wise to call upon it when the need arises.

Supervisor of Prover 9

My thoughts about the proving two years on – March 2008

Looking back it all seemed a very unsettling time; at the time that the proving began I also began developing a new show with my theatre company. Early on in this process the father of my business partner died which then meant that she needed time off work. The working process became hysterical at times and was very funny but in quite an out of control way. I would come home feeling very drained and I became very protective of my sleep. Following this intense period my business partner and I both experienced some major resolutions within our families. With her family it was to do with the unequal sharing of her father's will; he did not divide things equally amongst her identical twin sisters and this caused a lot of upset, as it echoed past unfairness in the family. This has since been resolved amongst the siblings and they have agreed to even things up a little.

My own father died many years ago when I was six and my sister twelve. We were never allowed to go to his funeral and he was never talked about after that; however, out of the blue my mother rang me to say my dad's best friend (who died two years previously) wished to have his ashes scattered with those of my dad, and would I come, along with my sister. There then followed an informal ceremony with my mum and sister, my godmother, her daughter and son-in-law. I never knew where my dad's ashes were previous to this, although it has in fact always been a very special place to me, and somewhere I often played as a child. This provided great resolution within our family. Both of these things happened about seven months after the proving.

Supervisor of Prover 10

Due to acute illness, my prover entered the proving approximately one week after the rest of the group. My timings all relate to his time of taking the remedy, so Day 1 would be Day 7 of the proving for the rest of the group.

One day before the proving:
6.30 p.m. Very sudden and very sharp pain in my head, right side. I felt it right inside my head radiating out to right temple. Lasted just seconds but made me clutch my head and wince in pain.

(Her sequence – Head, cough, ankles, fingers, shoulders. Then diarrhoea and nausea, and skin. Ed.)

Day 1. Very happy during day and feel very motivated to exercise, but tired and irritable before bedtime at 10:30 p.m. 11 p.m. I woke coughing and retching. Had to sit up. No expectoration and no cough afterwards. No experience of this before or since. Period 27/28: Very quiet for me. (I usually bleed for seven or eight days, very heavy for two days.)

Saw a friend of mine and felt that she was cool towards me. Complete paranoia that I had done or said something to upset her. Although it is normal for me to worry about what people think I would not normally ask them – I asked this friend directly. The answer was 'no' – in fact she was feeling extremely under the weather, and run down. Felt guilty about asking her and causing her more angst and grief (Day 3).

Very tired but had a disturbed night. Mild headache for most of the day, across forehead. Not bad but just there (Day 4).

Very unfocussed today. I was meant to spend the whole day studying and did everything but, despite being time pressured to fit everything in (Day 5).

Very, very busy but very calm. Lots of running around, but felt very happy and calm (Day 6).

Busy day but felt quite energized. Felt particular closeness to my husband. Although we are very close and content anyway, this just felt different (Day 7).

Strange sensation that my ankle hurt as if sprained or strained it;

the right ankle. It just came on suddenly and not as a result of activity. It was worse, much worse for walking on it. Very tired in morning and struggled to get up. *(Alternations of lively and energised with being tired. Ed.)* Had acute anxiety attack due to my son having the start of a cough. This is normal for me, due to his history of asthma (Day 8).

Have an odd pins and needles sensation in my right index finger. Seems to be linked to my shoulder, perhaps like a trapped nerve. The sensation seems to come from my shoulder down. It lasted all day (Day 13).

This is the first weekend that the college has met together as a group. *(See Observations following college weekend below.)* Still have pins and needles sensation in right index finger (Day 14). *Note – symptoms seem to me to be very right sided!*

Woke up and pins and needles sensation has gone.

Came home from college and felt fine – had dinner with family. 7:30 p.m. – Very acute diarrhoea and nausea. Extremely painful stomach cramps. Digestive problems are extremely rare and uncommon for me. Took a dose of *Arsenicum album* (Day 15).

Still some stomach cramps and feel washed out and weak. Feeling improved as day went on (Day 16).

Had a lot of emotional problems offloaded on to me from various friends today – spent at least three hours on the phone listening to other people (Day 17).

Observations following college weekends – February and March 2006.

After the weekend at college and listening to the experience of others, I noticed that I had been slightly clumsier than normal – more physically than mentally. Was surprised to hear of other experiences of pins and needles, following the unusual experience that I had had.

Update May 2006

I had one further episode of pins and needles.

The biggest thing for me is the very noticeable improvement in my 'normal' skin symptoms. I normally suffer from very itchy and inflamed dermatitis/eczema on my hands. Whilst I have been having ongoing homoeopathic treatment for this, which has improved things beyond what I thought possible, I was still having the following symptoms regularly:

Extremely itchy flare-ups – mainly between fingers and up the sides of my fingers, eruptions like little blisters. My hands (only) experienced what I imagine a hot flush would be like – they would feel like they were on fire and be extremely itchy. This would mainly happen at night whilst I was asleep and I would wake up with my hands burning and me frantically scratching them, sometimes until they bled. The only thing that would break the itchy and burning cycle would be to get up and place my hands under running cold water. It seemed to be linked in some way to my cycle too and the rise and fall in hormone levels. Since the proving I have had a marked improvement in these symptoms and have experienced the very distressing hot flush sensation only once and mildly. However, my hands have been very dry.

Menstruation – I have also found that this month, my period symptoms have also improved significantly. Period arrived 27/28. Although the first two days were still extremely heavy, they were manageable. However, the biggest thing to note was that there were significantly fewer clots and the duration was shorter than it has been of recent years.

The remedy I have had recently was *Sepia 200*, having benefited from *Sepia 30* for quite a long period of time. I feel that my own treatment had been making huge steps in improving these symptoms for me, so it could easily be a continuation of the work of the *Sepia*. However, I was interested to learn of the experiences of heat and itchy hand symptoms that others described.

Incidentally, there does also seem to be some mental and emotional symptoms around family and unresolved issues, especially in relation to recently deceased. I have also experienced a fall-out with my brother, which again is not a normal occurrence thankfully. However, although we are talking, I do feel that we have not cleared the problem and there are now unresolved issues, which will need to be addressed at some point. Whilst I feel ready to address these issues and think that it will have a positive impact on our relationship together and with other close members of the family, I do not think that my brother is there yet and ready to do this. It is worth noting that the disagreement involved my late grandmother, who died in July 2004.

Later review – The issue was never resolved with my brother although our relationship remains close and has not been affected by the earlier disagreement.

I have recently been able to move on from a very hurtful experience that happened about two years ago, where a friend continually criticized my children to me and in front of others. Not only was I hurt by her comments but also hurt that she had not tried to make amends, despite me providing ample opportunity and it impacting hugely on our families (our husbands are long-standing friends and we have children of very similar ages). I feel that I have drawn a line underneath and no longer worry about it.

Rubrics List

Energy and temperature fluctuations. High energy then burnt out. Libido

Chills

Beginning, in hand 294

Chilliness, body, night 295

Chilliness, body, perspiration, with 295

Chilliness, heat, alternating with NR

Chilliness, waking, on 296

Generals

Cold, body temperature 756

Cold, body temperature, low vital heat 756

Heat, alternating with chills 763

Heat, flushes of 763

Heat, flushes of, emotions from NR

Heat, flushes of, exertion from least 763

Heat, calmness, with NR

Heat, flushes of, perspiration, with 764

Heat, flushes of,, with stomach pain NR

Heat, flushes of, upwards 764

Heat, flushes of, upwards, from stomach to back of head NR

Heat, flushes of, waking, on NR

Warmth, desire for 801

Warmth, desire for warm clothing 801

Head

Heat, sensation, 881

Heat, sensation, rising up, chest, from 883

Heat, sensation, occiput 884

Heat, sensation, occiput, flashes of 884

Vertigo

Intoxicated, as if 1882

Eyes

Open, eyelids, sensation as if wide NR

Enlargement, sensation 540

Enlargement, sensation, morning, on waking NR

Face

Heat 583

Heat, burning 584

Heat, cheeks 584

Heat, flashes 585

Heat, flashes, cold feet, with 585

Heat, flashes, itching, with NR

Heat, flashes, sunburn like NR

Heat, sudden 586

Heat, sensation of 585

Heat, toothache, with 586

Shoulders

Perspiration, axilla 631

Hands

Coldness, hands 828

Coldness, hands, right 828

Feet

Coldness, feet 608

Coldness, evening 608

Coldness, warm, become suddenly, after getting into bed NR

Coldness, hot, face, with 609

Coldness, icy, cold 609

Perspiration 626

Stomach

Nausea 1748

Nausea, vertigo, with NR

Nausea, vertigo, during 1755

Food

Appetite, general, increased, hunger 725

Appetite, general, increased, hunger, waking, on 726

Chocolate, desires 732

Generals

Contradictory, and alternating states 757

Energized NR

Energized, exertion, by NR

Energized, exertion, mind, body exhausted with NR

Energy, lots of, anything feels possible NR

Energy, alternated, switch like NR

Energy, increased NR

Energy, decreased NR

Energy, decreased, no inner strength NR

Energy, high, waking, on NR

Energy, Kundalini, internal circulation, raising of NR

Energy, switches on, light switch, like NR

Female

Sexual, desire, increased 684

Generals

Weakness, Diarrhoea, from 804

Weakness sensation, rest, desire to NR

Weakness sensation, eating after 804

Weakness sensation, exertion amel. 805

Weariness, aching, with NR

Weariness, sensation 811

Weariness, sensation, evening 811

Weariness, waking, on 812

Mind

Exhaustion, mental 1323

Exhaustion, mental. Burnt out NR

Exhaustion, mental. Burnt out, after a period of high energy NR

Exhaustion, mental, waking, on 1324

Confidence, lacking, no self-esteem 1290

Alert, mentally 1265

Fastidious 1326

Fastidious, with desire to clear clutter NR

Housework, aversion to NR

Intoxication, sensation, as if 1356

Laughing 1363

Laughing, desire to 1363

Lively 1366

Positiveness 1381

Tranquillity 1416

Tranquillity, with lots of energy NR

Sleep

Sleepiness 1704

Sleepiness, sudden 1710

Sleepiness, sudden, like switching off a light NR

Waking, energy, with lots of, immediately NR

Waking, sudden 1717

Waking, sudden, as if flicking a switch NR

Left and right sides

Generals

Sides, left 787

Eyes

Itching, left NR

Feet

Itching, soles of, left NR

Itching, soles of, right NR

Head

Itching, scalp, left NR

Itching, scalp, left, painful NR

Headaches

Extending to, head pain, eyes, left 924

Forehead, extending to eyes, left NR

Forehead, extending to eyes, left, above 928

Left-sided headaches 936

Sharp, pain, vertex, left NR

Vertex, left NR

Knees

Pain, right, inner side NR

Pain, right, inner side, stairs agg. NR

Legs

Pain, walking, left leg NR

Nose

Discharge, watery, left 1507

Itching, nostril, left 1513

Modalities: Time. Environment
Time of day

Face

Heat, afternoon, 2 p.m. 584

Generals

Afternoon, agg. 750

Energized, amel, morning NR

Energy, decreased, agg., 2 to 5 p.m. NR

Energy, increased, 5 p.m., from NR

Mind

Depression, afternoon 1308

Exhaustion, afternoon, 2 p.m. 1324

Irritable, afternoon, 2 to 4 p.m. NR

Weary, of life, afternoon 1418

Sleep

Sleepiness, afternoon, agg. 2 till 4 p.m. 1704

Stomach

Nausea, afternoon 1748

Vertigo

Afternoon, agg 2 p.m. NR

Fresh air

Environment

Air, gen, indoor air, agg. 517

Air, gen, open air, outside amel. 517

Air, gen, open air, outside, desire for 518

Warm, warm, room, agg. 525

Mind

Confusion, walking, amel. 1293

Fear, claustrophobia, closed places, trains of 1328

Walking, amel. 1417

Direction of action of the medicine, and significant locations

Back

Spine, inner strength, sinks down NR

Female

Sexual, desire increased 685

Generals

Energy, inner strength, sinks down NR

Heat, flushes of, upwards 764

Heat, flushes of, calmness with NR

Heat, sensations, rising up, chest, from NR

Sensations, direction, downward NR

Electric lights and switches

Environment

Light bulbs, flickering NR

Light bulbs, blow, suddenly NR

Mind

Depression, happiness, alternating, like a switch NR

Sleep

Sleepiness, sudden, like a switch NR

Sleep, Waking, sudden, like a switch NR

Burning

Nose

Smells, burning, something 1523

Suddenness

Generals

Light bulbs, blow NR

Feet

Coldness, feet, warm, sudden, like a switch NR

Female

Pain, uterus, sudden NR

Menses, stops and starts, sudden NR

Generals

Heat, flushes of, sudden NR

Headaches

Sudden pains NR

Hearing

Noises, shrill sound, sudden NR

Mind

Crying, sudden NR

Depression, alternating with happiness, sudden NR

Exhaustion, sudden NR

Suddenness, behaviour in NR

Suddenness, emotions NR

Suddenness, physical ailments NR

Nose

Coryza, watery discharge, sudden NR

Skin

Itching, sudden NR

Itching, stops suddenly NR

Stomach

Cramping, sudden NR

Sleep

Waking, sudden, like a switch NR

Other miscellaneous symptoms

Skin/Chest

Tapping sensation NR

Popping sensation NR

Sensitivity

Generals

Sensitive, energy field of others, to NR

Mind

Awareness, heightened 1281

Impressionable 1350

Sensitive 1393

Sensitive, mental impressions, to 1394

Sensitive, external impressions, to 1394

Sensitive, moods of others, to the 1394

Sensitive, sensual impressions, to 1395

Dangers and vulnerability

Mind

Sensitive, sensual impressions, to 1395

Awareness, heightened 1281

Fear, danger, of impending 1328

Vulnerable, feels 1417

Sensations: lightness

General

Lightness, sensation 767

Delusions

Floating in air 367

Body, general, lighter than air 362

Constriction – feelings of

Generals

Constriction, sensation, internal 757

Throat

Constriction, throat, external 1818

'Spreading' or distant effect of the medicine. Coincidences. Telepathic (?) links. 'Journeying.' Affected by others/provers' effects on others.

Mind

Danger, aware of NR

Synchronicity and coincidences, frequently noticed NR

General

'Astral' travelling, heightens potential for NR

Thoughts and prayers make an impact, heightened awareness, that NR

Interconnectedness of everything, heightens awareness of the NR

Reactions to remedy, wide-spreading NR

Mental and Emotional States
Excitement and exhilaration, uncontrollable or inappropriate giggling.

Mind

Cheerful feelings, happy 1285

High-spirited 1345

Elated, state of mind 1319

Excitement, excitable 1321

Excitement, excitable, alternating with sadness 1321

Exhilaration 1324

Mind, excitement, desire for 1322

Mind, excitement, throat area, felt in NR

Exhilaration, alternating with sadness 1324

Playful 1381

Laughing 1363

Laughing, serious, matters, over 1363

Laughing involuntarily 1364

Laughing, silly 1364

Mind, foolish behaviour 1337

Talking, excessive 1409

All these possibly alternating with feeling alone and insecure.

Symptoms without rubrics made.

Loads of energy, but like he is riding a bike with no brakes on.

'Delusion' – feels like he is on a roller coaster. Can't switch mind off.

Calm, relaxed, happy and secure, as if there are no time restraints. Mentally alert and clear thinking. Fastidious. Able to get on with things and show feelings.

contrasted with

Insecurity and low confidence. Self-conscious. Negativity and tearfulness. Depressed about health. Anxiety. Restlessness. Disorganized, unable to carry out tasks, clumsiness, bad writing,

spelling errors. Forgetfulness, repetition of words. Difficulties concentrating. Irritability and wanting to be alone.

Calm vs. Irritable

This section is perhaps encapsulated in this image (Prover 9).

'Lower heart – anger and frustration.

Upper heart – lightness and love.

There's a disconnection between the two and a need to find a bridge.'

Mind

Contented, feeling 1295

Tranquillity, serenity, calmness 1415

Tranquillity, serenity, calmness. Incomprehensible 1416

Capable, handle anything, feels she can NR

Clear, mind 1287

Impetuous 1350

Quick to act 1382

Anger 1266

Irritability 1357

Irritability, anxiety, with 1357

Irritability, alone, wants to be 1357

Irritability, children, towards, own 1358

Company, aversion to 1287

Company, alone, amel when 1288

Irritability, family, to her 1358

Irritability, remorse after outbursts NR

Conversation, averse to 1295

Crying, remorse from NR

Concentration, difficult 1289

Concentration, difficult, studying, reading while 1290

Confusion, mental 1290

Confusion, concentrate the mind, on attempting to 1291

Confusion, intoxicated, as if 1292

Confusion, mistakes makes 1292
Memory, forgetful 1370
Memory, forgetful, words while speaking of, word hunting 1371
Memory, weakness of 1371
Memory, weakness of, done, for what he has just 1372
Memory, weakness of, said, for what has 1372
Memory, weakness of, say, for what he was about to 1373
Mistakes, speaking, in 1374
Mistakes, writing in 1375
Awkward, mentally 1281
Awkward, drops things 1281
Anxiety 1270
Anxiety, future, about the 1275
Vulnerable, feeling, with need for protection, or reassurance NR
Apathy 1280
Indifference, apathetic, struggling, unequal, adverse circumstances with 1352
Fear, opinion of others, of 1333

'My fault.' Judgments. Reconciliation within families. Return of old symptoms. The need to sort out unresolved issues. Clearing out junk: 'yucky things'.

Fault and Judgment

Delusions
Delusion, wrong, he has done 380
Mind
Reproaches himself 1385

The following in italics should all be considered or made into rubrics.

Dislikes himself, or parts of himself
Blames himself

Dreams – Crimes, accused wrongly, that he might be
Forgiveness – need to forgive himself
Clutter, desires to clear
'Negative' aspects of himself, has to clear these
Personal issues, need to confront and deal with
Unresolved issues
Family, needs to distance himself from
Reconciliation – need for
Acceptance of a situation – need for
Insecurity, loss of sense of security
Protection, and reassurance, need for

Critical, censorious 1296
Critical, censorious, disposed to find fault 1296
Critical, censorious, disposed to find fault, and feels bad about this 1296
Anger, absent persons, while thinking of them, at 1266
Anger, about something that has needed to be said NR
Tolerance – need for NR
Will, loss of willpower 1419
Tranquillity, serenity 1415

Anxiety about health. Fears.

Mind
Anxiety, health about 1275
Fear, cancer, of 1327
Anxiety, palpitations with NR
Anxiety, heart condition, about NR

Claustrophobia

Mind
Fear, phobias, claustrophobia, closed places 1329
Fear, phobias, narrow place, in 1333
Environment

Air, open air, outside, desire for 518

Body Parts and Functions

Head/Headaches/Vertigo

Head

Heat, sensation 881

Heaviness, sensation 885

Heaviness, sensation, headache from 885

Headaches

Dull pain 922

Forehead 925

Forehead, extending to temples 927

Forehead, extending to vertex 927

Sore, vertex 975

Vertigo

Vertigo 1878

Vertigo, afternoon 1878

Eyes + vision/nose + smells

Eyes

Alert, sensation NR

Alert, sensation, suddenly NR

Ecchymosis 540

Enlargement, sensation 540

Heaviness, sensation 543

Itchy 546

Pain, 550

Pain, light 552

Pain, pressure amel. 553

Sore pain 563

Tired, sensation 568

Wide-awake, sensation NR

Vision

Foggy, suddenly NR (original word was bleary)

Nose

Coryza, watery 1502

Coryza, watery, suddenly NR

Obstructed 1517

Smell of burning, something 1523

Sneezing, general 1524

Face

Pain, right 590

Pain, eye, below, right NR

Nose

Coldness, tip of 1497

Numbness 1517

Mouth/tongue/teeth

Teeth

Numbness of teeth, clenching, when 1800

Pain, teeth, toothaches 1800

Pain, hot face, with NR

Tongue

Taste, bad 1848

Taste, metallic 1851

Taste, musty 1851 (original word was fusty)

Food and drink. Appetite and thirst. Effects of alcohol.

Food

Appetite, increased, hunger 725

Appetite, increased, hunger, afternoon 725

Cheese, desires 732

Cold, drinks, water, desires 733

Fruit, desires 737

Meat, desires 739

Spicy, food, desires 743

Sugar, desires 743

Sweets, general, desires 743

Thirst, general 744

Alcohol, general, aggravates, easily intoxicated 724

General

Weariness, water, drinking amel NR

Stomach, nausea and feelings of intoxication. Abdomen and bowel movements. Urine and Bladder

Intestines

Flatus 1060

Flatus, evening 1061

Flatus, night 1061

Stomach

Belching 1723

Nausea 1748

Nausea, Coca Cola, drinking, amel. NR

Nausea, eating, after 1750

Nausea. water, after 1750

Nausea, faint-like 1751

Nausea, vertigo, with NR

Vomiting, morning 1777

Appetite

Diminished 725

Loss, food, thought of NR

Vertigo

Nausea, with 1884

Abdomen

Cramping, pains 11

Distension 16

Sharp, pains 54

Rectum

Constipation 1596

Diarrhoea 1601

Diarrhoea, morning 1605

Diarrhoea, waking, with urging 1605

Urging, sudden 1624

Urine

Colourless 1869

Pale 1872

Yellow 1877

Female Menses/feeling broody/libido

Female

Menses, bright red 665

Menses, dark 666

Menses, frequent, too early, too soon 666

Menses, late 668

Menses, scanty 672

Menses, profuse 674

Throat and /coughh/breathing

Throat

Constriction, throat-pit 1818

Lump, plug sensation 1825

Lump, plug sensation, swallowing, on 1825

Glands

Swelling, neck 822

Cough

Dry 335

Tickling 356

Skin and respiration

Skin

Dry 1644

Sore, pain 1665

Itching 1657

Tension 1667

Skin/Chest

Tapping sensation NR

Popping sensation NR

Heart symptoms

Heart

Burning, pain burning 1018

Fluttering, of heart 1019

Heartbeats, general, increased 1020

Pain 1026

Pain, region of heart 1027

Palpitations, general 1028

Palpitations, anxiety 1028

Palpitations, tea drinking agg. NR

Squeezing, sensation 1036

Back, neck and shoulders

Shoulders

Pain, shoulders 1629

Tension in 1636

Neck

Pain 1461

Pain, extending to arm 1461

Pain, extending to shoulders 1461

Pain, left 1462

Arms

Numbness 90

Nerves

Fainting, faintness, head, on moving NR

Numbness 1487

Back

Weak, slumped, no inner strength NR

Extremities – limbs

Arms

Numbness, left 90

Numbness, left, night NR

Tingling, prickling 105

Feet

Cold 608

Icy cold 609

Cramps 611

Cramps, toes 612

Cramps, toes, pressure amel NR

Hands

Numbness, left 845

Numbness, left, night NR

Coldness 828

Coldness, computer keyboard, when using NR

Legs

Itching, burning 1139

Knee

Pain 1094

Pain, ascending steps, on 1095

Pain, bending on 1095

Pain, descending steps, when 1095

Pain, knees, kneeling, when 1095

Pain, move, on beginning to 1095

Pain, knees, right 1095

Pain, knees, touch, on 1096

Sleep

Sleep

Position, arms, head, over, fingers, crossed NR

Position, hands, head, over, fingers, crossed NR

Falling asleep, restless before NR

Waking, general, alert on waking NR

Falling asleep, suddenly tired, like a switch NR
Waking, general, difficult 1714
Waking, general, night 3 a.m. 1717
Waking, general, night 3 to 4 a.m. 1717
Sleepiness 1703
Sleepiness, general, afternoon 1704
Sleepiness, general, afternoon 2 p.m. 1704
Sleepiness, general, afternoon 3 p.m. 1704
Un-refreshing 1713
Restless 1701
Waking, general, frequent 1715
Interrupted 1698
Waking, difficult 1714
Waking, general, feeling as if has slept well, even after a disturbed night NR

Dreams

Rubrics and themes

Firstly rubrics as in Murphy's Materia Medica
Dreams
Amorous, sexual dreams 451
Bicycling 453
Birds Kingfishers/Kookaburras NR
Buildings 453
Chased 453
Cleaning 454
Crimes, accused wrongly, that he might be NR
Difficulties 455
Disgusting 456
Escape 456
Excrements 457
Family 457
Frightful 458

High places 459
High places, falling from high places 459
Monsters 461
Pursued 463
Shooting, being shot, of 465
True, dreams come true 466
Vivid 467
Waking, the person 468
Water, dreams 468
Water, dreams, rowing on 468
Way, losing 468
Sex, dreams of 464
Vertigo 467

Secondly – dream themes

-of a feared disease – a prover had a dream of cancer, a phobia of hers
-of difficulties, arduous tests and trials, a very steep hill
-of confrontation and conflict

-of constriction and being hemmed in, prison, of escape – of being chased by an unseen monster, and trying to escape – fear of being caught and killed – of police pursuing criminals – of being frightened – of the need for protection – anxious that she would be wrongly accused – of maybe knowing too much, and gangsters/criminals would harm me for that?

-of secret, hidden illegal things, secret corridors, getting lost – fighting a witch, old issues, parts of myself that I dislike – of places with bad associations – of something ominous in dark water – of one person wanting to see the light, things on the surface, the other wanting to explore some dungeons – resistance to dealing with deep buried, dark issues

-of a houseboat losing a mooring, then pulling it back in place – of clumsiness, then quick to try and repair the damage

-coincidental dreams

-of relationship issues that need to be dealt with, shifted and resolved – of past intimate relationships

-of smouldering volcanoes – difficult things of the past that have been dealt with

-of childhood home, of losing secure family feeling – that daughter had been snatched – —of my children asleep in another building, struggling to get to them, but something stopping me

-of being caught in a vortex – being on a unicycle, spinning around, fear that I couldn't get off but did – of being on the top of a London (red) bus – of wearing high boots – of cycling

-of a disgusting toilet, black excrement in plastic bags – of cleaning, of extracting impurities – of a dirty, stagnant pond, something nasty coming out to get me

-disturbing, sexual dreams – dreams of marital fidelity

-of kookaburras

-of perfection and serenity – tranquil, serene water, in a small boat, a dark night, starry skies, clear water, almost pulled into the water – of a sinking sensation

Part Four

Thirteen Cases

To give examples of changes experienced by patients who have taken the remedy.

The third strand.

Cases 1 to 7 from Stuart Deeks
Cases 8 and 9 from Pauline Black
Case 10 from Roberta Young
Cases 11 and 12. Two reports on taking the remedy.
Case 13 from Ruth Radburn

Case 1 A.D.
Male 37 yrs
D.O.B. 03.12.69

07.07.05
He first came to see me because of recurrent difficulties walking, despite being physically robust. Numbness and loss of sensitivity in thighs, when walking. Would have to sit down to get the feelings back. He works in an office, lots of electrical charge. In general he would always feel much better when away from this kind of environment, for example on holiday in Southeast Asia.

Had immediate improvement with *Electricitas 30.*

Subsequently other remedies given – *Nux vomica. Thuja. Sulphur.*

23.11.06
Talks of teeth problems. Had them since a child.

Shoulder and neck blocked left side. Nervous. Stiff shoulders full of tension. One week ago couldn't move – turning whole body to look around.

Rx. Electricitas 30 b.d. 1/52.

30.11.06

More movement since. Still feels a nerve trapped. As if two nerves 'gone one against the other'. Injury as a child to head affecting neck and balance.

Tension anywhere else?

In abdomen. It started at time of father's death earlier this year. After he died, I have been examining the values I have. I was doing things I don't believe in. Angry with priest.

Martial arts grading brings on this tension too. I accumulate tension on my shoulder. Pain in shoulder was worse in the night. Waking about twice an hour. Having to change position. At end I was given to getting up at 5 am; > doing things. Pain in left shoulder feels tight, inflexible, trapped, vulnerable to left side.

When producing adrenalin feels effect in stomach.

Craving for sweets since April 2006. Biscuit and chocolate e.g. KitKat. If has some, will want more.

30.11.06 *Rx. Amanita rubescens 30* given.

Remedy effects in session –

1/ Shoulder loosening a bit. Heart sternum, energy going around. Front. Something active. Like something scratching skin. Pleasant sensation. Tension slowly going away from shoulders.

2/ Sternum sensation gone. Shoulder >, not trapped anymore.

Nerve still hurts. When puts head down feels something; muscles in area of back need a stretch, inflexible. Before left shoulder was trapped.

Mood changed. Relaxed more since remedy.

3/ Shoulder still fine, pain has gone. Neck a problem.

'Transformation.' Something moving. Painful but there is a movement, an activity as if two muscles are fighting.

We consider that the craving for sweets might be tension related?

Am. rub. 30 to repeat if pain returns after improvement.

Gap of three months

08.03.07
Five or six days after the last tablet the tension was completely gone.

Really blocked when last came. Then felt like block was moving like snaking in back, before it left. (He describes a horizontal figure of eight shape. *(See Prover 9's drawing in Part Six.)* Everything was moving as if something looking for an exit. Took it when pain came back and couldn't move and >.

Compared himself with a friend, who is attached to traditional thinking. After this remedy I realized I had completely abandoned the place I came from. Made me feel free. Realized I don't feel guilty about father's alcoholism. Wanting a precise idea why I left my family. Nothing to go back to, but OK about that.

Since remedy, constantly changing. Less importance on money and what it can buy. Free from so many things. Obligations that people place on you.

Moods – sometimes really up, sometimes down.

Realizing my personality was built as a reaction to my family I was brought up in. Therefore developed defensive personality. Don't show your feelings, won't be attacked. Silent. Distant. Now armour is coming down slowly; left to rebuild myself slowly. Many things that were buried are coming up. Living feelings that I had had long ago.

For the last month light sensitive especially right eye. Wakes with headache from light coming in, < close to sea reflection. Needs to wear dark glasses. Pain behind right eye, like a vertical line cutting eye in two. Headache in ocular area. Pain across and above eyes.

Headache > occupation.

Tense. Kung Fu grading, no headache. Attention focussed on something different.

Sometimes muscles feel inflexible and stiff. Generally. *Electricitas 30* ameliorates stiffness, so takes it weekly.

Sometimes I feel I have energy, in muscles in waist and upper body.

Sometimes feel very weak and have to go slow.

Light. Warm. Power.

'When dark goes away you discover things.'

Generally < closed places. Claustrophobic – needs light, at same time likes the dark.

08.03.07 *Rx. Amanita rubescens 30*

Effects in session –

1/ Eyes/vision. Colour of light has changed, becoming warmer more red, less grey. Pain that was there (across and above eyes equal on both sides) is going away. Still feels it on right side, but strongly reduced left side. Like switching from neon light to normal bulb. In right eye pain coming from behind. Light does not annoy me like before.

2/ Feels a bit cold, upper part and especially shoulder area.

Amanita rubescens 30 to use as required.

Gap of two months

02.05.07

Continuous need for sugars. Sometimes chocolate or spreading chocolate.

Craving after a week of gap, especially biscuits, chocolate digestives.

Light is especially difficult on cloudy days. Light is strong and grey.

Am. rub. 30 taken on the bright days. Still wears dark glasses – feels protected. With remedy all discomfort symptoms go.

I feel I need to renew/review everything. Thought about relationship with father especially and mother. Angry for a month with my father. Dialogue with my parents impossible. Little world as armour I built around myself; now it is coming down I'm feeling difficulties in relation with other people. Don't have external skin anymore; have to build up again.

Last two months full of memories, like a volcano erupting inside.

02.05.07 *Rx.* Re sugar, use *Am. rub. 30* when has craving.

Next report –

Reduced sugar craving when has *Am. rub. 30* – then doesn't think about it anymore. Collaboration between *Am. rub.* and personal will.

Re armour coming down, lots of things to understand, my personality and family. Difficulties of childhood – having to acknowledge these things. No sanity in my family at all. Father's death as catalyst for change in my life. Able to not hate parents but understand why they were the way they were. Memories that were buried are coming out.

Remedies that followed: *Buddleia* and *Tarentula hispanica.*

His review. October 2011.

(He is by now well acquainted with the remedy. He always refers to it as Amanita.)

Amanita – is strongly linked to the concept of sight… eyes… internal and external eyes.

It's a remedy able to help the patients to build a different life pattern, projecting their future in a new direction…

The remedy is able to open a channel connecting the inner core needs of the individual (what his/her subconscious really wants to be) to the everyday decisions. Everyday life and decisions are often far from people's real needs. They are frequently influenced by external people and previous conditioning; conditioning given by family, friends and society. Amanita is able to provide the person with a different type of awareness. They start slowly understanding their real needs. Their decisions in life change, shifting slowly but constantly toward their real needs. Amanita realigns everyday life to the person's actual nature, putting the person back at the centre of their life.

I started taking Amanita years ago and it took a while for me to understand how deeply the remedy was working on my mind, body and perceptions. Amanita really is, and I base this opinion on my personal experience, the medicine which cures the connection between your subconscious and your life; a gate between these two human dimensions… internal and external self. The changes that I have experienced have been slow and constant but the most important thing to say is that each change has been permanent.

The remedy helps and supports the person's needs of creating a 'tabula rasa' on which they can start re-building their life using new criteria chosen only by themselves. Amanita allows someone to re-build things the way they really like.

The 'tabula rasa' space becomes so important because it is something that is slowly, incessantly conquered back… that means the development of a strong awareness for any external factor or person which could bring unwanted changes, and fight back immediately creating protective boundaries of renewed strength.

Amanita rubescens came to be used in an office environment by this client, having experienced its benefits himself. Over several weeks he placed tablets of the 30 CH in flowerpots and other strategic places! Also on one occasion he diluted it in water and sprayed that around.

This is his report. *January 2012.*

The Amanita remedy acts in an office in a larger way.

An environment like an office where many people interact is comparable to a living structure with a bigger function. The Amanita would apply the same principles of harmony and change.

The medicine can transform the environment where it's used and eliminate or simply 'cure' disharmonic situations between human beings. The medicine would treat the humans and their interactions as cells of a complex body and would restructure the body itself replacing some of its components and changing its external environment.

Examples are listed below:

1) Some of the managers requested the furniture to be re-

arranged. The environment became more functional and each employee had more personal space.

2) The organization chart was changed due to internal restructures and unwanted people or difficult people were relocated in an area distant from the epicentre (the point where the Amanita was spread).

On a personal note, the Amanita in the office acted as a catalyst to reveal human attitudes that convinced me to start looking for a new job and change environment... in some ways the office discarded me as well.

The environment in the office found a renewed harmony and that does not mean that the place became an idyllic area. The office found its own harmony (which can be done) of elements suitable or unsuitable to the people who work and live part of their life in it. Amanita simply creates a new order in the office so that its reality is completely revealed and people (like me) are pushed to analyse if they can belong or not to such an environment. The choice between leaving and staying will be inevitable and in either way the result will be harmony.

Case 2 J.B.
Female 29 yrs
D.O.B. 28.12.77

07.11.07
Context. Had a severe knee injury six weeks ago. Coming to see me today – defiant to drive (to save money) when advised not to. Car wing mirror broken, therefore didn't and couldn't drive. She saw this as 'a universe protective thing.' Taxi driver turns up, at that moment. Coincidence.

Symptoms – Back hurts behind solar plexus, in the middle. Tends to hurt most of time. Headache more right side than left. Neck, base of skull, these days; before was in different areas in head.

07.11.07 *Rx. Amanita rubescens 30* given in session.

Remedy effects in session. *(The six entries here indicate the progression of the remedy action from taking it during the remaining part of the session.)*

1/ Sensation around eyes. Very aware of right eye, area around eye and my cheek. Sensation as if something on it. Keep going to brush it away. Heaviness around eye and forehead. Left side, headache, sharper pain. Temple, back from above ear. Painful to touch. Seeing the colour purple. *(Type went purple, unaccountably, in this paragraph. Ed.)*

2/ Now pain in vertex as if wearing something on top of my head.

Everything heavy, head. Pulling down cheeks below eye. 'Like on potter's wheel, water down on to clay. If chair was not here, I would slump.'

Feelings with this – idea of everything slowing down. Walking through treacle. Everything in slow motion. Struggle to speak.

Left knee gone numb, left foot tingling.

Headache, top. Struggling against it.

Recent image, world's strongest man in harness and pulling lorries behind him. Now physical sensation in body matching mental sensation. Image is of me with a big harness on pulling huge boulders in bag with long handles. Huge body with tiny legs. Still trying to pull.

Eyes really hurting.

Fighting for breath recently. Panic breathing a few times in past few weeks, as in the accident. Especially bad at top of chest near my neck.

Image of ripping skin from neck. Can't breathe.

3/ Eyes, can't look up. Even though everything feels heavy, can't blink. As if I'm on drugs: everything open. Eyes staring, like an anaesthetic.

Breathing, 'as if something catching instead of it being completely round like a straw – there are lots of things in the way, like branches.'

4/ Hands feel really cold.

Everything green seems a lot brighter than everything else.

5/ Feels quite solid, like swaying but being held. Like a dandelion swaying. Big puff of wind would make it fall over. Now it's a tree trunk, same wind; now swaying a lot, but not moving.

Feels like there's a weight at the bottom, anchored.

Eyes on the ground, looking at the grass outside in garden.

6/ Breathing – less catching.

Neck area feels normal now.

Knee – still numb, feet still tingling.

Feels very cold.

Head sensations all gone. Heaviness to cheek gone. Not swaying, not as tired. Had felt really ill.

Vivid green – has gone now.

07.11.07 *Rx. Amanita rubescens 30.* To take at bedtimes if difficulty sleeping. 1/52 max.

After two weeks

20.11.07

More positive after last session.

More down than up. Crying all the time, not being able to get out of bed to do anything. Breakthrough next day in counselling session – so low. Honest with counsellor and myself. Told her about alcohol, self-harming. Honest for having got it all out.

Allowed myself to be vulnerable, tell partner everything, about my finances (bankruptcy).

Sleeping one night of good sleep. If takes remedy dreams are more vivid.

Ovarian pains <

20.11.07 *Rx. Aurum muriaticum natronatum 200.* 4 doses a day for 3 days.

Nine days later

29.11.07
Gets a better quality sleep with remedies – not necessarily easier getting to sleep. Ovarian pains – no change

Thirteen days later

12.12.07
Went to court re bankruptcy. Have been going through life thinking I'm on death row. Going to see the judge was like going to face an executioner.

Now smiling, 'like a hot air balloon. Ropes have been cut and I can fly up.'

The following three cases provided my first experiences of the remedy in action. S.D.

Case 3 A.A.
Female 38 yrs
D.O.B. 29.05.68

08.03.06
No energy at all. Frightening being ill. Negative attitude to illness. Anger, resisting things, the way things are.

Anger – teenager in my head – irrational objections to things. Impatience (e.g. if too noisy, pissed off with children). Noise of children in the house.

Dream – father was being murdered, a big beast dressed in strange clothes lanced my dad and he died. Running away from the scene.

Physically – Stiff everywhere. A twinge in back.

Petty attitude in my head, e.g. my sister called – immediate response was I'm going to have to sort something out. Judgmental style, dominant now. But I don't need to judge, she's got a difficult life, I just need to love her.

Any bodily sensations just now?

Solar plexus – weak, watery, wobbly, no drive from that area.

My skin is sore; the rub of clothes is sore, raw. Top of back/shoulders down to waist is sensitive; it doesn't extend to front. Also scalp sensitive to touch when hair was being cut.

Much effort to do anything; gets hot mainly in my head and prickly skin. When it's like that I want to not have a body, not to be in it, it's a very uncomfortable feeling. I get hot and want fresh air; also if I get worked up thinking about things or resisting being looked after, or if there's a phone call about mum's place, stuff to get done. Don't want to deal with stuff.

If I go out, I get sweaty and dizzy.

08.03.06 *Rx. Amanita rubescens 30* b.d. 5/7.

Three weeks later

27.03.06

Remedy broadened things out, everything felt positive. Felt present and in my body, buoyant, able to transcend lethargy and negativity.

Solar plexus – before remedy – weak, watery, wobbly, no drive from that area; after > within three days of starting the remedy: 'wanting to come from that place.' Rediscovered innate enthusiasm.

Then stuff came up around health – about getting tired: I think if I'm ill I'm failing. Aware I can exercise to feel better. When tired, sliding back into looking at difficulty of things. Constantly worrying and thinking of what can go wrong.

Angry yesterday with husband: he didn't do something – it was an overreaction.

Lovely thing, friend had two dreams of me and my mother, like me and a little girl in a Persian garden. Also of releasing my mother into the sea as a sea lion. Others having dreams for me!

Things coming to me in relation to my mother – when I need to hear it.

(Her mother had died in the Thailand Tsunami of 2004.)

27.03.06 *Rx.* To take *Am. rub. 30* x 1 and keep other in pocket. Use if energy drops, more negativity, eruptive anger, or if overheated,

Eight months later

22.11.06

Remedy kept things at bay so could make the house move.

When anger and judgment thing returned in May and June, I started psychosynthesis sessions. It has been a time for separation between my mother and I. I was acting her out, couldn't separate from her; as if it's a betrayal to criticize her. It became clear to me that that trait of anger and judgment is hers. I don't need to continue, I have another way. It had to get so bad, for something to shift.

Threw up violently for hours after first session of psychosynthesis.

Giardia (return of old symptoms) purging in July for six weeks. Stopped dead in tracks, re doing or being over-responsible. After illness, conscious grieving. Since then energy has been pretty good.

Back, skin tingling, heat, all better now.

From remedy, stopped feeling over-responsible for members of my family. Can't carry that; big letting go of 'it has to be a certain way': let mother down if it is not as it was. Got free of the dynamic that my mother was in the family.

Not knowing what it was to be joyful. Since Mum died. Now more myself and self-expressed as a person since remedy. Generally very good.

Staphisagria followed – she had also benefited from it some years before *Amanita rubescens*.

Case 4 J.C.
Male 38 yrs
D.O.B. 04.05.67

Previous useful remedies –

Clematis – testicle pains. *Sulphur* – itching skin.

27.02.06

Cannabis habit – still wishes to break it.

Home life unstable. Some good times – then it breaks down so easily, expects further breakdown. Confused around whether he should be in this relationship. It could go either way.

Angry outbursts in last two weeks – around not being understood.

I don't fit in with her ideals as 'husband', father, provider – she feels like I'm attacking her all the time.

Holding on: What is the fear of letting go? At bottom: showing who I am – scared of who I am? Of releasing how emotional I am. What I do is bottle it. Need to open up more. Impatience, anger, frustration. Get confrontational and annoy people. Lack of ability to express in the way I want to.

Feels knotted up. In solar plexus and shoulders.

27.02.06 *Rx. Amanita rubescens 30*

+ one each night and morning for 5 days,

+ 6 more spares to take 'in place' of cannabis.

Remedy effects in session –

1/ Woolly layer over back – like a covering, an inch thick – slightly protective. It's a thick layer providing safety, comfort.

2/ It goes from the back of head to behind thighs under buttocks. Like a cape. Like a thick skin – not in the front at all. Like having a collar up. Half of tank top.

Back of head: feels more open. From back of eyes out, backwards and up.

3/ Body feels thicker. To do with abdomen. Holds solar plexus. Feels solid. Comfortable. Aware of thickness of abdomen.

4/ Shoulders looser.

5/ Mothers arms gesture. Support. More of a whole feeling, a circle. Slight warmth from waist up comes from middle of back below heart level. *(A release of held hurt in the lower back? S.D.)*

27.03.06

Remedy has helped me leave partner. Upset about this. Depressed. Accept I have to be upset. Before was not strong enough to move on. She phoned, sobbed on the phone. Didn't go to rescue her. I was just together.

In session – Again mother's arms position – arms rounded, hands in cradle gesture, one above the other.

Last night went to yoga. After that, took one *Amanita* tablet – seemed to do the job in this respect. Contributed to me not smoking cannabis, as I usually would of an evening.

27.03.06 *Rx. Amanita rubescens 30* to continue to take in place of (i.e. before) cannabis.

Eight months later

29.11.06

Muscular knots recently. Shoulders incredibly tense. All moved up to shoulders. Discomfort left side lower abdomen.

Pain/loss around father comes up. Highly strung. Learning how to hold anger. Letting myself feel it. Feels as if it could escalate – the aggression. Since remedy an ability to be more conscious about these feelings. Able to express myself more, letting myself be more confrontational – trusting myself more to be conscious in the moment. Is now being heard and acknowledged.

Excitement – shakes.

Aggression – held in shoulders.

These in combination – fear of breaking down and sobbing.

More happy with myself therefore refusing to argue. Not being confrontational. Can't argue anymore, I have a protective layer. Trust that I would be all right with decisions. I am all right. I've got nothing to prove. Gave more to myself – more time. Strong enough to face some emotional pain. My link to artistic things. Not selfish – it's the right path. Less guilt – about me living my life rather than guilty about leaving mother.

Security blanket, don't have to watch my back. As a shell – protective – useful at this time of moving house, being uprooted. Mobile protection. Sense of protection has maintained over summer.

29.11.06 *Rx. Amanita rubescens 30* given in session.

Response –

1/ Sharp pain dissipating, very slightly. Shoulders. Feeling of space under armpits. Front of chest feels open.

2/ Shoulders loosening. Right side is OK. Left side knot remains.

Earlier clenched fists. Not there at all now. Don't need to do it now. Links with open chest feeling. Front.

Tingling down back of arms. Back symptoms to do with arms and shoulders.

Wanting to be tearful, breakdown crying.

3/ Left side loosening now. Still knotted but more fluidity. Before couldn't move neck or around shoulders without it grinding/biting. Opening, as if it's pulling out at back (of head) making space.

29.11.06 *Rx. Amanita rubescens 30* night and morning.

29.11.06 *Rx. Amanita rubescens 30* night and morning.

Gap of three months

28.02.07

Has been going to hypnotherapy around not smoking cannabis, since last three weeks.

How have you felt since we last met?

Strong, good, real, frightened.

Tears, not so able to control. Mental state – like white noise. No clear thoughts about who I am and what I should be doing. Massive fear, whether my head works. Where does the fear arise from? Rolling feeling. Language I'm unfamiliar with in my head. Where is my head going? Lack of control over my thoughts. Sliding down a slope towards insanity. Falling through air – dropping into shit, the darkness, unknown territory. Insanity crept in, affecting sleep especially. Going a bit mad.

Shoulders, now less knots, more relaxed now in past month. Above sacrum, constant dull ache.

Dream. Of trying to murder an old man, to asphyxiate him with a plastic bag over his head. Next day distraught – knew it was an adverse effect of cannabis. (Has been taking cannabis with gin in these last weeks.)

Left side abdominal discomfort, surfaces around fear – less now. I realize that I am harsh to my body. I need to comfort my body. Fear of taking the remedy, and of giving me a ring, as it would stir everything up again.

Soreness in throat. Gums affected by Betel nut. Gums and jaw affected. Throat sore, especially right side behind right ear – sore. < evening to morning. Not before Betel nut – three days ago.

Huge rush to head of heat from neck, above shoulders up.

Neck bruised and sore. Palate bruised and sore.

28.02.07 *Rx. Amanita rubescens 30* given in session.

Response –

Instantly soothing it, altogether. Most affected in mouth area. Also lower back, more relaxed.

Thighs feel cold, top of thighs. Release of pressure on skull behind ear. Back edge of area of pain.

Fear around a worry. How violent I could be if someone presses wrong buttons. Fear of violence coming up links in with insane feeling.

More pain left side shoulder. Battered all over. Right knee, slightly more vulnerable. Jaw much better. Feel hungry, and like I could go to bed for a day.

Six more tablets given to use as required.

Six weeks later

04.04.07

Amanita rubescens 30 three times since last session.

Last one was two days ago.

Was angry about not being settled domestically. Remedy two days ago calmed me more than anything. Helped me let go re: something lost. Lessons coming thick and fast but readable and very clear. Now I understand what is going on. My actions are readable. Mentally looking at myself, watching myself behave, like being out of body, but not out. A lot of changes needing to happen – not worrying about when.

Not had craving for cannabis. The mad time was clearing of this. General happiness. Giggle to myself a lot. Shoulder, and neck symptoms much better. Can feel completely exhausted at times. Self-flagellation needs to be addressed – being hard on myself. Comes from beating myself up. Driven anger in there with that. I enjoy the hardness of life, 'get a kick from hard'. Humour has crept into the area of fear of how violent I might be if someone presses my buttons.

Amanita rubescens taken around heavy anxiety. Day after – eyes heavy and sleeps heavy. Sleeping well in new house.

Dream of beating a friend up with a baseball bat (after cocaine, dark things come up). What I want is to be strong, firm and not be guilty. Times of feeling very sure of myself, but guilty sometimes that I may upset someone.

Instinctive. High energy, raw energy. It's a ride. I'm on it and it makes me laugh – like most people laugh on a roller coaster. Running with the goodness – the way things work. Trusting my instinct. The joy of that. Less inhibited. Release. I seem to be jolting a lot of people. What makes me laugh and cry is that I'm able to be intense and it's all right.

Tooth problem, filling taken out.

Rx. Amanita rubescens 30 given to use as required

About this remedy, he said, – 'when I don't need it, something says I don't want to go near it. Don't think I could handle one!'

Other remedies given – *Nux vomica, Staphisagria, Ignatia.* During time of dental treatments *Am. rub.* ameliorated the pains.

Case 5 I.C.
Female 38 years
D.O.B. 08.02.68

Previous remedies:
Lycopodium – abdominal symptoms, pressure and gassy.
Pulsatilla – menstrual symptoms.

31.03.06
After *Lycopodium* wind > for a while. Belly not so noisy. Still gas, but not so painful/trapped, not smelly.

Seeing family relationships in a new and clear way – as if a huge abyss/space between us. Observed in a detached way what it was and made me really sad. Sense of isolation, indifference from everyone, lack of interest.

Gums fragile since three weeks ago.

Going to apply for a university course. One year ago I couldn't have done this. Feel like I have the energy – doesn't seem impossible or a struggle or big task.

Three days ago – thoughts, memories clogging up mind. Wish to clear this (like the flat needs clearing up). Sad memories – not heavy, not huge arguments; things mother said when I was fifteen. Would like to be clear of these things, even if no resolution.

'I need a remedy for clearing the mind.'

31.03.06 *Rx. Amanita rubescens 12* at bedtimes for two weeks.

Five months later

04.09.06
Amanita helped my state of mind. I feel less critical, petty.

Beginning of April, patches on left breast, and stomach, brown then red and then went.

Symptoms are generally now more left-sided than before. Painful places on shoulder. In last week, left-sided toothache. Sensitive gums and tense jaws. Gums have receded at back. Teeth sensitive to sweet, hot/cold. One tooth at back feels a bit infected.

Always had cold legs and feet. Going to sauna – crave heat to calm down. Hands warmer since the remedy.

Overall a bit tense – get stroppy with boyfriend for no reason.

Oversensitive and annoyed.

Breathing a bit constricted > *Pulsatilla.*

04.09.06 *Rx. Silica 1M* – 3 doses in 24 hours.

20.10.06

Felt good on *Silica.* Warm for a few days.

Teeth > with *Silica.* Infection >.

Sometimes get noisy belly at work but less than before.

Period OK. Pains > *Pulsatilla.*

Had a week when very upset with boyfriend, so getting at him, sarcastic to get his attention. Nasty to him.

20.10.06 *Rx. Silica 1M* – 3 doses in 24 hours.

Rx. Amanita rubescens 12 to take for difficult moods with boyfriend, for five nights, as needed.

Seven weeks later

07.12.06

Am. rub. > re calming mind down.

The latest *Silica 1M* ameliorated only for a few days, re feeling chilly. Feet cold, legs cold evenings, knee down.

Stronger gums and teeth.

Menses, last two months – *Pulsatilla 200* not working so well, but only small pains. >> warmth from saunas, wants the heat.

Mental effort – mind goes blank, e.g. meetings at work. Tense, trying to grab on to thoughts. Hold them. Mind goes blank. At work:

memory gone for what was going to say. Mental distraction. Not been like this since school days. As a teenager? I felt judged, under pressure to be a certain way I didn't want to be.

Recently physical symptoms: e.g. little verruca on left hand. Brown to red patches, like an old bruise. Left side. Looked like finger marks – from shoulder, down to breast level. Red and raised and itchy. Oval. Noticed after a shower.

Every two to three months anxious about situation with boyfriend – angry, insecure, doing wrong thing, waiting for something that will never be right.

Reflexology session – mind all over the place – dumping out a lot of stress. Then so depressed, weight on chest, hard to breathe. Anxious heartbeats. Bleak – all I could see was a harsh horrible world.

Amanita rubescens 12 taken 5.11.06 for five days. Next day belly noisy.

Dream (two days after starting to take remedy).

Moving to another city to study. Only a duvet in suitcase, had forgotten clothes. Unlikely, but very positive about starting all over again. Anticipation. Happy re being forced to start all over again. *(She would often have dreams of carrying suitcases and bags of her belongings, on station platforms etc.)*

Symptoms in session. Body relaxing, warmer.

Below sternum pain – had this as a child in stomach. Reminds me of when I was seven, and moved from a small town to a big city. Rigidity. 'I'm better than them, I've come from a better place.' Critical of others' attitudes, of town people.

Pain in stomach like eating a bit of apple without biting it and it gets stuck there. Pushing against stomach. Like ice, pointed icicles.

07.12.06 *Amanita rubescens 30* given in session, plus six spares to take before reflexology and in case of 'lump' in stomach.

Remedy effects in session –

1/ 'Got lost out there in the tree/the view. Moving out looking at the space. I think of focussing on things and getting angry with them.'

2/ Warming up feet; now warmth travels up to knees.

3/ Stomach a bit warmer/softening, a more subtle sensation. Feet and stomach – separately starting in both places, as if a line, central axis, warming up/traveling up.

4/ Relaxing brow centre.

5/ Aware of back of head, lower part.

6/ Brain feels relaxed. Feet still warm.

23.01.07

Cold body, but not feeling so cold inside.

Took the remedy at a time of swollen throat. When swallowed, pain throat and going into ears. Rx. amel. Like infections in winter, familiar from when little: ear infections, colds, flus. Can't drink, eat. As a child, ENT problems, and anaesthetics for operations. Otitis media.

Amanita rubescens taken when had cramp in stomach. Gradually longer periods without pains, so didn't need it.

Feels like taking *Amanita rubescens* when goes to sleep. 'Heals me at night.'

Also takes it when feels icy at night.

Blanks of memory for what was about to say and hearing is much better.

Right now – tension in heart area. Hardness, like a walnut size – something stuck. Where rib cage divides.

(Required location of action of the remedy seems to be moving up in the body.)

Rx. Amanita rubescens 30 given in session

Remedy effects in session –

1/ Loosening starting from centre and shoulders – lighter feeling.

Hands and arms feel lighter – less physical. Feel energy going into my hands.

2/ Noticing legs are cold, from knees down. Clearing small tensions in forehead.

3/ Now feeling heavy, wants to sleep.

23.01.07 *Amanita rubescens 30* to use as necessary.

Two months later

22.03.07

Feel stuck.

After last time I felt fantastic. Then after two weeks diarrhoea out of the blue, ate nothing bad. Woke with urgent diarrhoea. Felt a lot of nausea but don't like throwing up – so kept it down. Around two minutes after hot drinks I had diarrhoea. Had it for a morning. *Arsenicum album 30* helped this day.

Very cold, in blanket with thick ski socks on, felt feet were in the snow.

Five days before this session I felt anxious, emotionally stuck, not wanting to feel it.

Dream: One night of taking remedy: all about news, things happening, different colours.

Diary entry – 05.02.07 Irritable, impatient, anxiety attacks, stomach cramps. A lot of emotional tension repressed inside me. To do with holding feelings at work – unfairness at work, colleagues. Two days later to proper flu for four days. *Gelsemium 30* helped a lot.

Then *Amanita rubescens 30* taken again. Was feeling all over the place. It warms me up and makes me feel more solid. Solar plexus – really good feeling. As improved, began to feel cleansed and detached from this anger (about work). 'I see the flu I had as repressed emotions clearing out.'

Not digesting well. Taste, bitter/acid, especially on waking.

In a visualization – woods, cave, old 'priestess' woman took my clothes and I got into the water. Dark. The 'priestess' was there to protect the place and take care of me. She had a warm and comforting way. She gave me food.

Lot of times wakes with headache > *Bryonia*.

About every two weeks I take *Amanita rubescens* and feel more solid around heart centre and warmer. Feel more protected at work.

Strong wind agitates me. *Amanita rubescens* gives protection and standing firmer against the wind.

Sepia 30 helped before period. *(Gelsemium/Sepia relationship.)*

Saunas: have to be careful for example when getting up from sitting, can feel faint. Not experienced this since teenage time.

Remember teenage time – tired, not being able to study when 16–19 years old.

22.03.07 Continue with *Amanita rubescens 30* as required.

13.06.07

I have taken *Am. rub.* before going to sleep; it allows really good sleep if down or tired or anxious. When out of sorts, down or tired, it grounds me. Brings me back down to earth. Emotional sense of warmth, protected, stronger compact stability, focus.

'Now I feel stable, in a restful place.'

The remedy seems to bring dreams. I had a dream of sifting through old stuff, boxes of objects gathered from an old trip to Thailand fifteen years ago.

Now not feeling pressure of an academic exam. Before I was panicky – thinking I won't pass it, to protect myself from it going bad.

I have been reflecting on how father's side of family works. He is proud to tell people exactly what he thinks of them, and his ideas are always right. I have an instinct to prove people wrong – that's strong in me. Getting better about this since the remedy.

Dream early June – of evil angry mother. Out of control. I was male, the oldest of lots of children about. Concerned to protect younger children. In kitchen, I sense she wants to use knives to harm the children. Like my father being out of control, nasty.

Am. rub. seems to bring on big painful spots, which stay for a long time. On my face. Like a teenager. On ears, under armpits, on back, behind ear.

Continue with remedy as required.

30.08.07

Amanita used to open chest and lungs. If taken before bed, my breathing is wider, slower, deeper. Very nice.

Amanita pushing out stress to do with colleague.

Menses cramp bad. *Amanita rubescens* ameliorated immediately.

When taking exam, warmth around heart.

Amanita rubescens completed its use, for the time being.

Later remedies – *Sulphur and Sycamore seed.*

Case 6 S.D.

Female 36 yrs

D.O.B. 15.04.75

For her the remedy was the first, and so far only prescription.

Daughter is two years old

04.08.11

Presents with –

Heavy head, pressure middle of forehead. Foggy, confused, helpless. Describes the heavy mood – 'I feel I want to drive into a brick wall.' Intense since ten days ago. This was about a week before her period began.

Has times of very high energy, times of down. Her twenties were a time of never stopping. These days often has little energy. Exercise could clear her head.

When down, weepy, and can be verbally aggressive. Struggles with parenthood, feeling of wanting to explode with irritability.

Childhood – as a little girl, fear of what happens after death. Had a dream as a ten year old associated with this. 'In the dream I am a dot, like a small brain with cells on either side of it, getting bigger and bigger as if to infinity.'

Relationships – my parents split up when I was a year old. Mother re-married. I get on well with my stepdad.

Father – as a teenager I did anything to get his back up. He is critical of everybody; these days he is judgmental about my relationship with my husband. Talking about him my heart rate goes up and I get tense in my face and jaw, especially when I think about confronting him with what I really think of him. My brother completely dismisses my father for his ways with women – four wives in succession – and I am in the position of holding between him and my father. I'd like to tell my father what I think about him, but don't because it will hurt his feelings. I do feel sorry for him and love him.

Moods. The down side –

At university, depressed. Wanted to go travelling but went instead to uni to study. Got ill, down. Everything pointless.

Terminations aged 21 and 24, the first one at a time of self-loathing. Lot of judgement there. Generational guilt about pregnancy out of wedlock. Even now I don't feel worthy to have my daughter. First few weeks of her life, I struggled. Anti-depressant pills for ten months enabled me to enjoy her more.

Generally an outdoors person, so gets down moods in the winter. Remember having these moods as a young child.

I ask her what sensations she has, talking of these moods. 'A sinking feeling in my upper chest, a sad feeling, an emptiness around the sides of my head.'

Sensitive to criticism on a personal level: if criticised for how I never stop or that I am fastidious in my house, or about my weight in relation to what I ate; father was obsessed about this.

Guilt: that should be achieving things.

Always wanting something new, something to work towards, loved class teaching but after a while it was not that challenging. Loves to travel.

Highs –

As a child – happiness, loved and content at home, not real highs. Always very happy being with my friends, having a giggle.

In twenties, after meeting husband, took to mountain biking and loved it! Exhilarating, exciting, a feeling of achievement, of freedom being outside. Loves the speed, the wind in my face.

Considering death – a sense of infinity – things enlarging like a rolling snowball. What happens? What is it all about? Not scared of dying – spirit will go somewhere else. Scared a bit at the thought of nothingness.

The pointlessness of things – might suddenly feel this, or if down anyway.

Talking of these things she feels the same wrenching, pulling down in her upper chest.

Dreams – of falling into a dark hole, then don't know what happens next. Or, recently and recurring, of being chased by a weird gang. Being in a house and they are massacring people. Finding places to hide.

Mother and stepdad. They rely on me.

I try to do too much – as in keeping people happy, to stop them having a low opinion of me, and I don't want to let them down. This has an effect on my mental health.

Has the heavy feeling again talking about these things; at the same time feels calmer and relieved at this stage of the session.

Feels thirsty.

Get hot flushes, has had them since my twenties. Can be out of the blue, or if anxious, e.g. before being observed/assessed at work, or if cross or upset. Also heart rate goes up if anxious.

Gets very red with exercise. Blushes. This since childhood.

04.08.11 *Rx.* given in session *Amanita rubescens 30*

I ask if she has experiences of coincidences, recently or generally.

Yes, I go to the phone and the other person picks up the phone and calls me. Also, just this week, I was thinking about a person and then see them in the street.

Sensations and feelings after taking the tablet –

Heavy chest sensation releasing upwards.

Stomach (= abdomen) feels nice, calmer – with her hand she describes a small wheel spinning round. *(Chakra nicely activated?*

S.D.)

Face feels lighter – recently has felt numb on the left side, with anxiety and stress.

Pressure place mid-forehead is still there, but smaller. A sense of release.

The upwards releasing has reached as far as her neck.

Exhilarating feeling. Heart rate has gone up, but not in a bad way.

On my suggestion she takes a deep breath. 'I just want to laugh. The silliest things making me laugh.'

Chest/heart now much calmer.

Feet really cold since the tablet. Usually does get cold feet, but it's warm today.

Face: quite warm feeling.

She places the palm of her left hand on her right shoulder. 'It feels like a comfort, coming from behind.'

'I feel very calm.'

17.08.11

Second appointment

The first three days after last time – Elation. Giggling. Surreal. Bright red warm blushing face and cold feet. Got on very well with daughter, very loving. Laughing lots with her. Much less of 'I'm not a good mother and she's hard done by life because of that.'

Now, situations that would normally make her anxious didn't bother her. When she got wound up and anxious, she was able to let go of it. Had a row with her husband, but got over it quite quickly. It didn't seem to matter so much.

Now a calmness for the most part, finding times of just sitting on the sofa, without any feeling of should be achieving something. Previously always on the go.

None of the feeling of darkness – that tunnel vision with darkness on the outside.

Much less of the low self-esteem. Not thought about weight at all. Not wanting sugary carbs – puddings and chocolate.

Energy much better – able to get up and feel like I want to do stuff – like playing with my daughter or going for a swim.

All of us at home have colds.

Chest – not had the pulling down sensation at all.

Face – no numbness left side. Has had a nice tingly feeling.

Last two days – Bit more grumpy these last two days along with pressure in forehead building up. Yesterday, when sitting on the sofa, a moment of this pressure in forehead along with the thought, 'I should be achieving something.' Then, realizing that sitting here is doing me good, the pressure went.

Big hot flush again today, along with couldn't get her breath.

I ask if she has had any incidents of burning by leaving pans etc. on the cooker. Yes, yesterday I left the grill on by mistake, with the grill door closed. The grill panhandle began to smell of burning.

17.08.11 *Rx. Amanita rubescens 30* in session.

Mouth immediately dry on taking the tablet

Her own notes as presented to me in November 2011.

When I took the first remedy, (August 4th) I instantly got the giggles: something very simple and totally not funny made me laugh: a tree that had been recently been pruned.

That evening I drove home with a grin on my face, a hot cheek and freezing cold feet! I was relaxed and just found everything funny.

When I got home, my husband said I was different and wanted to know what the homoeopath had done to me as I was very giggly and couldn't stop grinning!

These are the notes I made from August to September 2011, and after that I have written in less detail about other experiences at home and work.

17.8 Second appointment. Remedy taken.

18.8 Huge argument with husband re how I handle stress. We

were getting ready for holiday and I was getting worked up and 'heightened'! raising voice, quicker pace of talking. He told me he had 'had enough.' My face and head felt like they were burning/on fire especially on left cheek.

Flew that day and had a nightmare journey! Our daughter (two year old) was difficult on the flight. She has always flown well and been very happy but this was the first time in her own seat and she did not like it – we weren't allowed to hold her for take off and landing and had to restrain her in her seat. (I found this awful and unnatural, but had no choice.) I got incredibly worked up in the car after flight as we got lost on way to hotel. She was distraught because she was exhausted. Again a very red/flushed face and anxious: tension was in cheeks and pressure in front of forehead (although much less than the symptoms I felt back in July when I first met with Stuart for my daughter).

19.8 and 20.8 Face began to feel hot and burning – came on very quickly and lasted about 20 minutes or so. Nothing noticeable triggered it. Was feeling generally calm and relaxed and all getting on really well.

21.8 Fine. Relaxed, calm. Exhausted (body felt lacking in energy and limp/weak).

22.8 Relaxed, happy and calm. No arguments. (Normally we all argue on holiday!)

26.8 Drank quite a bit of wine and went from not feeling at all drunk to feeling sick/ dizzy and very drunk in what felt like a minute! I have not felt that intoxicated for some years. Was not nice. My sister-in-law said I was fine one minute and suddenly declared that I needed to go home. She said she couldn't understand how I had got in that state, as I didn't drink that much!

27.8 So dizzy that it felt like the room was literally spinning and my head was going to fall off! Quite panicky/palpitations. Can't remember ever feeling that dizzy.

Flew home.

28.8 A little down (may have been an extended hangover) but not too bad. I was happy to stay at home today and take it easy. Normally I would be pressuring my husband to come out and do something, but was very happy to take it easy and relax at home ALL DAY!

29.8 Very fuzzy-headed and still incredibly tired. Had a glass of port in the evening and had an intense hot flush that came on quickly. Burning face and head. Headache, shivery and goose bumps.

30.8 Sore throat/huge ulcer on right hand side of throat. Wiped out/no energy. Pressure in head building up especially in centre of forehead between eyebrows. Feels like a pressure building up.

31.8 Feeling of exhaustion/head cloudy and confused. Simple tasks difficult to complete e.g. forget what I am doing/inability to think. Took remedy (no immediate reaction). In the evening had a big hot flush on head and face, especially cheek. Everywhere else was cold (had to sit in garden in shorts and T-shirts at 11 p.m. as head was so hot!)

1.9 Still sore throat and slight pressure between eyebrows but much less than it had been for the past few days.

2 + 3.9 Sore throat and ulcer still there and pressure and fuzzy-headedness/confused and again hot face (same symptoms as above).

3rd at night – Waking in the night so hot. Then couldn't get back to sleep.

Didn't feel this consciously but wonder if anxious about return to work and daughter starting nursery the next day

4.9 Still waking in night, very hot and uncomfortable/pressure in front of head and confused – difficulty concentrating although still far better than at the beginning of the summer when I felt desperately sad and depressed: (That feeling of wanting to drive into a brick wall! – they weren't suicidal thoughts but just a total frustration.)

5.9 Another bad night's sleep. Awake at 4.30 a.m. hot and restless.

6.9 Feeling foggy-headed and confused, and fed up with feeling ill but not depressed, just a little down! Quite a good night's sleep.

7.9 Woke again at 4.30 hot and restless. Had a weird dream about huge woodlice falling out of the ceiling at home. We have rather a lot of woodlice at home that become rather annoying! Felt good all day. No fogginess and an ability to get things done efficiently and effectively.

Can't put dates on the following as notes in my notebook but:

September

Wanted to give up teaching: said to husband, ' I just want to give it all up. Try something new' which pretty much came from nowhere… and I really meant it. I was going to go to school and hand my notice in. He convinced me to hold fire, which I am, but am really considering the options. I would have been (and probably still am) happy take up a spot of cleaning and a bit of supply teaching to keep the pennies coming in while I re-evaluate.

Began exercising again and enjoying it: loving running and cycling again but because I am not putting myself under pressure to diet and lose weight. It will happen when it happens.Also thinking about going abroad for a while and trying something different.

Generally much more efficient at home and work.Happy to sit and do nothing. One occasion where I just sat in the back bedroom on the sofa and did nothing. I literally just gazed at nothing – meditation that I hadn't planned on and wasn't really aware I was doing until I went downstairs and realized an hour or so had passed!

Also my husband is speaking up a lot more: 'I'm tired of taking this crap!' 'You can't behave like this' (If I am being overly dominant/expecting too much of him). This has made me take a breath a bit more often and take a step back and try and think! Doesn't work all the time but has been a small positive change.

School

We had quite a negative start to the academic year back in September regarding staff absence. We were told we were not entitled to time off with our sick children, and although I am a very honest person I normally speak more tactfully: I burst out with: 'What?! So when she is sick, I should just leave her outside on the street to be looked after?!' I spoke up for a single mum who has no one to help her out when her child gets ill. (She isn't a particularly likeable person, and has been known to take a lot of time off!) However, I still felt that what was being said was discriminatory and unfair.

The training day was an intense and negative one and it seemed the first few weeks of term, people were cross and negative. That doesn't normally happen in September.

Throughout September and October two members of management were very stressed about the threat of OFSTED coming in. *(Schools inspectors in the UK. Ed.)* Things were suddenly being put into place from nowhere and people were feeling, for the first time in a long time at our school, stressed and grumpy.

November

Sprinkled the plants in the staffroom and gave them a water with the remedy. (The 30 C.) Someone noticed me doing it and asked what I was doing. I just said I thought the plants needed a water but I started giggling quite a bit – which is unlike me especially at the moment (Gran has died and the grief has been very intense). 'What are you giving them?' she asked. So I quietly told her a little bit about the remedy.

During that same lunch hour, people's moods seemed lighter/more relaxed. One of my colleagues told me something very sad and personal about her depression. She also said that this year was the first year in many she hadn't gone back on anti-depressants for 'SAD'.

One colleague (who has always loved teaching, and still often does) is currently undergoing IVF, which has sadly failed. She told me she wants to leave teaching and do something else – she isn't depressed at all: a very positive, spiritual person. She just thinks life's too short and doesn't want to be spending her life working and not enjoying her spare time. That has come from nowhere.

In the same week another colleague said she is thinking of doing something else. She too has always loved teaching, but wants to try something else. She has had breast surgery to remove calcium spots and had biopsies to test for cancer – she says she has been re-evaluating her life.

People have been confiding in me. People are being more open about their feelings. That is new.

Colleagues at school seem to have calmed down over the past couple of weeks. People seem more relaxed and less grumpy and stressed. (Although I am less involved with people too – I haven't spent much time in the staffroom as have been getting things done instead.) I am focussing more on myself, selfishly and dealing with my grief and trying to concentrate more on my family, not work.

Case 7 P.B.
Female 61 yrs
D.O.B. 06.09.49

11.11.10
Takes on too much.

Nights of so much creativity – it's all going on in my mind all night long. Too exciting then overwhelming – ends up like a dish rag.

After break up of earlier relationships, filled every space – doing. As soon as had time to feel things, I would feel suicidal. I wasn't good enough, not loveable enough.

(A full narration of her childhood experiences and her relationship with her mother led to Plastic wrap 200 as her first remedy. It had a good effect. SD)

Hot flushes. Starts with the feeling of energy draining out of my body, then heat in upper body and head. At night get fizzy feet – as if all the blood is rushing around my feet very fast. Blood is as if boiling or on fire. Stands on the bathroom floor to get them cold. Can get this if I think about how much I have to do in the course of a day – feel under intense pressure.

(This big heat in her body lessened after Plastic wrap 200.)

Dreams: Busy. Chaos. Always very surreal. Being chased, but manage to get away. (These since eleven years old.) Also dreams of childhood house.

Too much doing – it's just like overeating. Tiredness, but busy – doing lots. I fill my life with stuff to do and think about – till there's no manoeuvre.

About her work – I feel inadequate. Stupid. Like a fraud. What do people think of me?

I feel disconnected, spaced out. Not touching ground. Don't feel here, not in my body. But at the same time I have a growing feeling of being guided and held. Not used to that. It's like beginning to plug into the mains.

Lots of synchronicity. Example: equilateral triangles appearing in clouds and at then in an outdoor ceremonial bonfire. *(The Star of David had some important associations for her.)*

Pain in right shoulder – like a toothache pain. Tight muscle.

Generally I'm not good at raising my arms. Can't get the strength to do it. It's like they are too heavy, leaden. If I try to raise them up I feel a constriction, like choking, and dizzy, as if I will pass out.

I give her a bottle of Am. rub. 30 to hold.

'I have a feeling of letting go. Dropping very deep.'

11.11.10 *Rx. taken: Am. rub. 30* and weekly for two weeks following.

After taking the tablet

Giggles. Laughter. 'As if I am being laughed, as sign of something cleared.'

Aware of tightness across sternum. A narrow band. 'It's like a chastity belt.'

Four weeks later

08.12.10 'It's been an exciting roller coaster of a ride.'

I feel more content.

Right shoulder excruciatingly painful for two days, then completely better and still is. Chiropractor's observation – I am clearing ancestral stuff and things to do with my first marriage.

Thirst. Can get unquenchable, raging thirst, but only at night.

'Everything else is wonderful: lots of things manifesting. Things just falling into my lap. The message is – I don't have to go looking to find it. Just put out a vision and imagine it as already here. It's all coming to me. No games, no egos, no manipulations to save face.'

Dream. Like Armageddon – to reconcile two warring parts of myself. A large round disk about an inch thick. Pink and dusky colour. It has the ability to kill us, if they had us backed up against a wall.

Waking image of Vesica Pisces – two parts of me coming into reconciliation. *(For Vesica Pisces see Part Six.)*

Took *Am. rub. 30* once again when energy was flagging; better for it.

Overall since taking this remedy I have felt more tuned in: everything that affects this world affects me. Now I am speaking the truth about personal things, being honest and coming from a place of integrity.

She tells me that from November 2010 to February 2011 in the Mayan calendar is a time associated with honesty and integrity. *(Compare with my story of my housemates during these months. Ed. Pages 54 to 60.)*

26.01.11

Why am I constantly delaying confrontation? Need to be more forthright and stand my ground, say what I feel and to hell with the consequences.

Always feeling things are my fault. In my childhood always trying to keep the peace for my mother. Guilt if don't. Sweep the pathway for mother.

I overeat when I am living a lie or not happy. When fired up and passionate it will go the other way and I forget to eat.

Holding the bottle of Am. rub. 200

As if it's a no win situation, whichever way I turn. The planetary situation – the task is so enormous. I try so hard. At times it feels like I'm drowning.

26.01.11 *Rx. taken: Am. rub. 200*

Report at next session, five weeks later.

02.03.11

Life. Joy. Connection. Happiness. Abundance. In the flow. Not trying to control. Nothing any big deal. Just getting on with everyday life.

Didn't think too much about others and my effect on them. Less self doubt.

New sense of grounding and being from my heart; was in head before. Spiritual things too. Things weaving themselves together, to a place of reconciliation, moving on. Like clearing the sludge from the bottom of a pool – the last few bits inside to be brushed away.

We talk about expanding the new 'heart' feeling with the breath.

She tells me that with any breath-work tears and fears always come up. The issue of saying YES to life. Couldn't cope with it – a sense and a memory of not wanting to be here. Resistance to breathing in the light. Resistance to do with a massive responsibility like a huge, heavy cross on my back, dragging myself up a hill; but since the remedy five weeks ago it's as if I've taken the cross off my back.

I have a sense of a left and right side. *(She has experiences with the symbols of the cross, the Vesica Pisces and the Star of David. See Part Six.)*

The left side – The dark shadow, safe and seductive, known so well. What I retreat into easily.

The right side – The light shadow, precious, on a pedestal but not experienced. Uneven, spinny and precarious. Out of my reach.

An email from her –

January 2011. You should have warned me about fire – I set fire to the laundry basket a couple of weeks ago, burning the kitchen floor and destroying loads of clothes!! No one was hurt and apart from the aforementioned, no other damage done!! My husband had left a cooker gas burner on slightly and I put the basket on top of the cooker and walked off! He continues to leave the gas on – but I don't put stuff on the cooker! *(Now when I give the remedy to clients I warn them to watch out for fire! S.D.)*

Her own review
September 2011. I was prescribed Amanita by Stuart Deeks, and having no prior understanding of the picture of this remedy, I had no idea that this would take me through the closing stages of a 19-year-old ongoing adventure – in preparation for my next 19-year cycle.

As he gave me the remedy he drew a diagram on a small white piece of paper – I gasped as he gave it to me. It was a six pointed star with a dot in the middle – a symbol that I had been given in an extraordinary vision in April 1992 when I was asked to take part in an earth energy balancing in and around Rennes le Chateau in southwest France. That vision has haunted my life ever since. It has been like a breadcrumb trail that has created a very rich tapestry along the way. In the successive months after Amanita, I was directed back on to the trail, still not allowed to reach either the final destination or see the complete picture, but given a big piece of the jigsaw.

The theme of 'as above, so below' has played itself out over and over – for example I was leading a full moon fire ceremony and a triangle appeared in the sky directly above the fire simultaneously with the fire collapsing into an identical triangle below! Synchronicity seems to be the name of the game, so much has it occurred in my life since taking the remedy, and all the things I have dreamed of doing for so long are beginning to materialize and come together. This remedy feels like the culmination of a very long search and journey taking me back home.

One of the themes has been not being afraid to speak my truth, and others around me doing the same – without falling out with each other! In fact in all the groups I belong to this is now becoming the norm. The knock-on effect to others seems to also be a theme of this remedy, much more so than with any other remedy I know. I have prescribed it for patients and seen this borne out. *(She is a homoeopath.)*

After the remedy I went through a massive upheaval with the direction of my life – I was so fed up with how it had been for ages but didn't know how to change it. The remedy gave me a new sense of direction and a determination to live more in the moment and do things I enjoy, rather than out of a sense of duty.

Creativity is something I always believed existed in others but not me. I had had a glimpse of my creative side earlier in the year, but after Amanita creative ideas were constantly pouring from me, much too much sometimes and hard to put a lid on because I had been waiting for this flow for so long, in fact never even believed it possible for me. And not only were they just ideas, but they actually came into being. I only had to think about something I wanted to do and the next minute the opportunity to do it presented itself! To be so in the flow is extraordinarily wonderful.

For example, I had always dreamed of having an allotment with a view (I had one forty years ago and yearned for this again for a long time) but knew this was not possible because we are away so much and there would be no one to look after it while we were gone. Within five days of taking the remedy I was offered a vegetable plot in the garden of a windmill on a hill overlooking the sea! I have now developed this into a community garden where we co-support each other and someone waters my plants when I am away!

At the same time I was asked if I wanted to join in with a woodland project – I have had a wood on my vision board for five years! Abundance was flowing in every direction.

Images I was seeing in meditation or shamanic journeying were showing up in ordinary reality and then linking into people, events, opportunities – it was as if my inner life was being reflected in the outer. Bees in particular began to play a big role. Symbols in my shamanic fires became reality, taking my breath away at times.

Flashbacks to childhood became common events after Amanita, with huge realizations about them. It's as if the remedy reconnected me to my past and allowed me to see it in perspective. Within two weeks of the remedy I had total recall of countless events, people, places, names from early childhood – it was as if a door to my psyche had opened making so much sense of things that had previously made no sense at all. I stayed in a friend's house that I had stayed in many times before and I had a flashback to my childhood because this house was exactly like my home as a kid – I felt like running around the house screaming my head off!

I took out a photo of myself as a baby and as I looked at it I saw the face of my grandson as a mirror image and I made friends with my inner child and understood for the first time her frustrations as she was growing up and my own frustrations with my daughter and family and the injustice of all of that. I grew up in a no-win situation and was still living in one now. The vivid image of constantly sweeping the path for others to smooth their way came to me, in order to avoid upset, conflict and to keep everyone happy and comfortable and how exhausting that was. I was trying so hard instead of leaving room for Grace to come in with another solution.

After Amanita 200 I felt like I was doing things from a place of choice. I had a terrible cough that lasted weeks, yet I felt like I was able to carry on regardless but coming from a different place to my usual reaction to things. Guilt had always featured large in my life, now I don't seem to feel so guilty if I say no or can't do things. I felt like I was in control of my life for the first time in a long time – busy but not chaotic.

The theme of fire is very strong with me – I run fire ceremonies every full moon so I love fire but exactly a month after taking the remedy I set fire to the kitchen and burnt all our laundry. I had huge outbursts of rage, very short lived – like the fire – but fierce. At times I felt like a dragon breathing fire from my mouth and scorching everyone in my path.

In the background of all of this happening to me, the group I set up two years ago – Earthkeepers – is evolving at the same rate as I am and incredible synchronicity is occurring for all its members. They had visions of a group coming together from Canada, Brittany, Wales and Malta in the shape of a Maltese Cross and the theme of dragon enters. Within a few months people we didn't even know ended up at my home in Brittany doing ceremony with each other from all over the globe – another dream come true for me. I wrote in my journal that I felt like I am in the third trimester of a pregnancy and I am waiting expectantly, on the edge of a new experience, a new way of being – I'm not there yet but it feels very close.

So many opportunities have opened up for me and my work is now going off in a completely different direction – much more in connection to the land, nature and sacred sites – an honouring of the ancestors and the old ways. I have been given opportunities I had never believed possible before – meeting people I have admired for so long, holding their hands, hugging them, singing with them, extraordinary gifts for which I am so grateful. Each day is now a joy to wake up to. I have had other remedies since the Amanita but I know that the turning point came with that prescription – it set me back on track, got me back into a flow that I lost 37 years ago when my mother died. I feel I have found myself again after a long detour that took me on an incredible journey. It's good to be home again.

I had these dreams:

1) Destruction, annihilation of species – all our relations – it has to stop – now! Geometric figures, patterns and colours that repeat in order to achieve balance. Meditation, preparing spaces for others but feeling on the outside of the group. Feeling inadequate, I don't belong; I don't know what I am doing. Seeing terrible destruction, the end of time for all things, so much pain and suffering – it

becomes unbearable, so overwhelming I die and move beyond it into stillness. Except I am not dead. Then it begins again – the last polar bear on earth, the pain is too great and I am sobbing, wailing, from my boots, I can't do this anymore, it has to stop. And then the symbols appear and I wake up and see in front of me a heart with a hole in the bottom and behind me a DNA symbol.

2) In a theatre where the seats don't face the stage! Realized we were in the wrong seats and were then shown to much better ones. There were many stages all running simultaneously with main stage all at different levels.

Then four of my usual recurring dreams within one week (unheard of before):

3) In an open but very dark pine forest. Being chased by two men and as I flee they throw giant pine cones at me that look like grenades, but they don't explode. A police car drives past with its siren on. They stop, it passes, they continue to pursue me. I scream, 'No, No!' and wake up.

4) Queuing for a toilet, someone jumps the queue and I let her because she is desperate. The toilet is filthy, smells terrible and I can't flush it. My husband comes to help me and burns his hand in the process because there is caustic stuff in there. I find another loo in a caravan but I can't use that either, because something is in the way, and my son comes to help me but says I have to read a note from someone before I use it.

5) My husband is trying to tell me that he has met someone else and she understands him and appreciates him far more than I do. I am devastated but not surprised because I don't always show how much I love him. I abuse his love and generosity too much. I realize that he actually loves her and that I have already lost him, his heart has already left me, he is already gone. And in my heart there is this deep, agonizing heaviness – a sorrow I know only too well, a leaden feeling, hopelessness, a depth of despair I have lived through and survived yet hoped I would never have to experience again. What can I do?

I go to find him, he is somewhere in a house we had hoped to buy. The bed has been lain on, is crumpled on his side where he has been lying. There is a note to me saying, 'Can we not find in our existing home what this one is offering?' I don't understand. If he wants to be with this woman, why are we even discussing this?

I wake hurt and confused, scared with a sense of that awful, profound pain from thirty years ago, the pain of being left, of not knowing what to do, where to go, how to heal, how to live, how to go on, how to survive, how to even take my next breath because I am choking from this excruciating sorrow. (Ending of an earlier relationship.) And I travel back in time to that deep numbing coldness, a chill nothing could warm, a heart that was so cracked, so shattered, so devastated, so utterly annihilated that it didn't even know it was ever possible to heal. There was no desire whatsoever to go on. And so I built a wall around my heart that no one has ever penetrated, and now he is gone, my wonderful man to someone whose heart is open.

And this cocoon, are we all in this place? Are we all so hurt, so afraid that the pain is too much to bear? Are we all marking time, waiting for release? Are we all filling our days with endless, meaningless stuff in order to compensate for what? For this?

Yet the dream has a glimmer of hope – the note on the bed…

This dream leaves me restless, expectant, wired, like in a bubble that is about to burst, a chrysalis that is about to explode and throw me out into something vast, expansive, unknown, or that this existence that I believed to be all there is was just a cocoon within which I have rested, waited to be reborn into something which is far more splendid, far more creative, far freer than anything I have ever known before, and yet it is who I have always been without realizing it, without the consciousness of its true potential.

What is happening to me? I feel out of control yet in control more than I have ever felt before. Endless possibilities present themselves daily now – like I am in the flow. Yet there is conversely this utter frustration of the daily grind.

6) I am in London at a choir performance. I return to my car afterwards and there is a big space where the car had been. Maybe I made a mistake. I walk round and round – no car. Panic, distress (I have had two cars stolen in real life, both of which I got back eventually), I don't know what to do. I wake up.

Case 8
From Pauline Black, homoeopath.

Amanita rubescens 200
Long-standing client – who had *Amanita 200*. Her brother who she was living with and who was an alcoholic never went anywhere for twenty years except to the betting shop and the shop across the road to get more alcohol and the paper. After the remedy he suddenly started talking about how he felt, stopped drinking, met an old flame from school on the Internet and moved to Spain with her. Her father, who she had a huge problem with, also started sharing how he felt and my client became so much more compassionate towards him as a result.

She had come to me because her home/family situation had become intolerable to her but she felt compelled to stick with it because she believed that there was a great healing opportunity for them all in it.

Case 9
Also from Pauline Black.

Amanita 1M
Another lLong-standing client who felt really down and unable to come back up – lots of family conflict with ex husband and son. Fear of becoming less able to care for herself with no support from anyone – 'No one is available for me, why can't I be allowed to be who I am?' Wanting to get in touch with her past and let it go. *(Having peeled away so much of my own past with this Rx I wondered if it*

would help her.)

After the Rx: 'I became furious with a client, felt huge rage inside. I realized it was because he was behaving towards his kids like my father used to with me.' She had a lot of realizations about her childhood and where her rage was stemming from (she has always been one angry lady) and for three months after the remedy she said, 'I feel SO good.'

I followed *Amanita* with *Plastic wrap 1M* because of a whole host of menopausal symptoms, and she had a series of childhood flash-backs (unknown before to her) that allowed her to see why her relationships with men had always been disastrous. Ever since then she feels her life and relationship with son, ex husband and male friend have taken on a different direction – one of respect and consideration (unheard of before). Everyone has said how different her ex-husband is now! Her genital herpes attacks that she has had for over twenty years have stopped since the Rx. She made an appointment for one and a half hours to come and explain to me how amazing her life now is and to express her extreme gratitude for these two remedies!

Case 10

From Roberta Young, one of the original provers, now a homoeopath.

26.07.11

This is the case of a lady aged 54 who came to me with feelings of being stuck in her life and not being where she should belong in herself. Due to this she has felt unmotivated and depressed for the last few months. She feels unsupported and unable to support herself. Money is problematic and she feels panic around this. She is a life coach enabling to help others but these skills are not working for her. She is physically strong, but smokes 15–20 roll-ups a day. Her partner also feels stuck in his life and they are avoiding issues with food/TV/wine and dope. She wants to become more conscious.

Six years ago she left her husband and is now feeling a huge loss around him and their family. She moved to the UK four years ago for something new, and feels that maybe her grief is holding her back from fully moving into the next stage of her life. She feels she is in transition but doesn't know how to move on. She feels knocked off course.

Rx. Amanita rubescens 100 ssd

01.09.11

She has been up and down emotionally, feeling that everything has become more extreme. She has been feeling very low with terrible insomnia. She went to a herbalist who told her that her system was not switching with the different times of year and gave her a herbal mixture to help this. She can't sleep until 3 or 4 a.m. or wakes at this time. She alternates from being energetic and positive to feeling tearful and hopeless. She doesn't feel like she's coming out of her situation. She has an underlying belief she has to do it all by herself and that she doesn't belong. Her ex-husband's wife has just had a baby, making her feel redundant, disconnected to her own children, and that she doesn't have a role any more in the family. There is nothing to confirm her in her life. Everything is bland, dulled, and her libido is low. Occasionally she has been getting heat flushes in bed, like when she went through menopause.

She feels gripped by fear – financial insecurity, not belonging to her society and family, and not having a role for her children. She has an expectation about her self and she's not there. She took risks to leave her husband, leave her country and change profession, now what is the way?

Rx. Buddleia 200 over 3 nights and to take as need for panic

Sulphur 1M 1 x weekly

13.10.11

Feeling a lot better, less fearful and more focussed. She feels like she's been going through an interesting process and she is back in her own shoes. When she first came to me she 'couldn't see the path, now I'm up on the hill and can see where to go.' She has become aware of belonging to a wider group with a social connectedness, a broader family. 'We're stretched to become wider, more embracing of the different constellations we call family.' She feels released from the grief of her ex and now has a sense of purpose.

Her sleep is better, her libido is a bit better, but is struggling with giving up smoking.

07.12.11

Continues to feel good. Aware that smoking is restrictive to her life, whereas she wants to expand and reach out in her life.

Rx. Amanita 200 ssd

17.01.12

The day after the last remedy a flu-type illness began and lasted for two weeks. For many years she has not been ill like that. Now she is a month into not smoking. She has begun to find it easy not to smoke. There has been a big shift from being depressed and finding the past very difficult. She continues to be well.

Case 11

Male D.O.B. 01.06.65

This review was written by him in November 2011.

I saw Stuart in 2007 having not seen him for several years after a move away from Brighton. In that time some difficulties had arisen between my parents, brother and me that had been long standing tensions which were difficult to name and seemed to have been embedded in past generations so that we were not entirely aware of the causes of the tension.

This had finally come to a visible head with some confrontation of the issues – the main ones seeming to be the rescuing of one family member who could not bear any disagreement or challenge. In not following the rescuer role as did my father and brother I would be cast as the persecutor. This model fits in with other similarities in my auntie and uncle's family also.

To keep the above structure there would be a scapegoating of me to avoid challenging the painful truth of rescuing to the extreme the family member who could not bear disagreement. This was old stuff for me as it had gone on through my teenage years to the point that I was asked to leave the family home as a young man. It had gone on into adulthood but less pronounced as independence had led to less potential flare up. Lots of love had existed in this time as before it is important to state.

The tension increased greatly when my wife and I had children and the expectations of closeness as grandparents did not match our preference and some of the old issues were brought back up more sharply.

I was upset but relieved that the grumbling of these old issues had come to a head but had no idea that Stuart had been around the remedy *Amanita rubescens* since the last time we had met. There was clearly a rejuvenation in him too which he later told me was partly as a result of the same remedy.

On taking the first remedy *(Am. rub. 30)* I felt an immediate inner reassurance that things would get better. In the next day or so I would feel a worsening of the sadness with a mental fug developing and I often noted that old physical recurrences would show themselves such as partial deafness in my right ear and dizziness.

On the advice of Stuart I took the doses at different times and became comforted by the familiarity of the process. This would be:

Initial reassurance of the emotional turmoil on taking the remedy.

A feeling that no stone was being left unturned in this ancient and complex multigenerational issue.

Deafness, fug state after 2–3 days.

Often copious diarrhoea that was sometimes 'hot' – this felt like the purging of old toxins.

Feeling as bad as I could about the situation for 1–3 days.

Then often feeling euphoric that the situation was being addressed, that I was no longer trapped by the confusion of this situation – that something was being sorted out.

On one occasion I felt so relieved and euphoric as I walked home from work that things were changing and that happiness and freedom would follow. I remember that walk home so clearly – it was a pivotal day.

I took the different strengths of the remedy as advised and incrementally the acute pain eased leaving no concrete answers but a reassurance that I was in the right process to work through this. *(The 30 was followed by the 100C potency. Ed.)*

Ultimately we emigrated for a while which was a wonderful experience in many ways, but I still felt that there was more work to be done with my family. We kept up some contact and after three years returned to our house in Sussex.

Something huge has happened in the connection with my parents and to a lesser extent my brother. There is a freshness and deep love without the tension at all – not just ignored but gone away. This is of course something to do with some physical space but I am convinced that the process of the remedy has taken me and all involved in the tension to a new level of peace, acceptance and warmth.

I have taken several remedies over the years but I feel that I know this one intuitively. It became a friend and comforter and I was glad to go through the tough stuff too as the remedy let me KNOW that it was useful.

There was a deep spiritual feeling connected to this remedy, one of knowing that it was the only catalyst to do the work that was needed for our extended family to go on well together. I strongly feel that it acted remotely on others.

It now makes sense that it would be me in the wider family who took the remedy and initially highlighted the old tensions. I have since had contact with extended family members who had a similar role in their family of origin. I also saw the similar profound effect it had on a friend.

Where there is a family impasse where the root cause is unknown or global or ancient I am sure that this remedy can assist in this deep but subtle and comforting way. The process whilst taking it can be harrowing and uplifting but in my case, I always felt that it was healing.

Case 12

November 2011

This account came in the form of an email from a woman in New Zealand who had been recommended *Amanita rubescens* by Graham of Case 11.

Hi Stuart,

Graham kindly introduced me to the remedy here in NZ (we worked together) at a time when I was going through huge life change and deep pain, emotional turmoil, stress etc. etc.

A quick background from where I was at when I took this remedy and actually when Graham actually presented in my life and also helped with my healing process (poor guy!).

Mother of 3 – turbulent teenage years – a lot of self-abuse – emotionally abusive relationship for 12 years – lies, infidelity etc.

Hit a turning point about 37. I needed to change me.

I respond well to remedies so being a little hesitant I took the plunge and never looked back. What an amazing life changing remedy this was for me.

Honestly I have never experienced a remedy so powerful as this remedy.

My progress has been slow in healing but this remedy helped move stuff along dramatically. It was some time ago now when I first took remedy one – it's been about 1.5 years from start to finish of using it.

Remedy 1 *Amanita rubescens 30*
I took this at an extremely traumatic – emotionally charged – time where – grief was also very present. I was exhausted (heavy fatigue) for at least three days to a week after taking the remedy. Felt hung over. This was the predominant feature for me with all the stages and dose of the remedy I took.

I used this remedy several times with gaps between each time and each time I felt a new layer needed shifting. Boy it shifted stuff. It almost got unbearable to take it as I was unpleasant for a week but the results became obvious and worth it. It helped me peel the layers one by one of issues that were deep and needed to be healed

I remember running through the bush literally vomiting up pain after taking the remedy in the initial stages. All the issues rose quickly. Sometimes even within minutes of taking the remedy they would escalate, then change would occur in my life. The effects on me flowed on to others. I often had to take time off work to recuperate at these times, as the feeling like being hit by a bus was huge.

Remedy 2 *Amanita rubescens 100*
I had several doses of this. I had the same fatigue and hangover state.

But after the 3–5 days with all the remedies I would become fresh and free and elated for a period of time. Life felt good until the next issue would arise and would deal with another trigger.

I have only just finished taking Remedy 3 *(Amanita rubescens 200).* This cleared the final residue. It now has no effect on me if I take it. The work has been done

I have combined taking this remedy along with energy healing and huge other personal work.

Today the result is an inner peace, which in the initial stages was chaos, turmoil, mental torture.

I am sorry I can't remember all the details of how this worked as I was living through it. The fatigue hangover state were the main things along with the issues presenting themselves immediately after taking it, issues that were mine, but someone was mirroring at me big time. It was amazing. Poor Graham had to live through most of it with me; he probably could describe how I was better than me.

I hope this helps

Rachel (NZ)

Case 13

From Ruth Radburn.

Female. Age 50

Presenting symptoms – Chronic fatigue since trauma 1979/80. Married with one child, aged 13.

Describes herself as intuitive, sensitive alert and open.

'Feel guided and protected. I have a stone shaped as a heart which is my helper.'

At difficult points in the conversation she held and stroked this large stone.

'Youngest of three children. Parents had difficulty expressing emotion and feeling. I was lonely and self sufficient. I thought it was my fault. Failed to fit in at school and left home at seventeen. Was unworldly but found friends in the city, found a tribe to belong too. One evening drink was spiked and was held prisoner for forty-eight hours, drugged and raped. I escaped but nobody knew, I shut myself away and holed up on my own. I finally reported it to police thirty years later. I tried later to explain the rape in 1990 to my parents but they couldn't hear it.

When I have flashbacks I want to lie down and pull the duvet round, it just falls on you. It's a sensation of heaviness, glands go up – armpits and throat. October to March are danger months < damp, wind. November acute chest pains: pleurisy left-sided.

Bed is a loving safe harbour, a bolt hole, I scurry back like a dormouse, to hole up in a little nest.

Crop circle experience: I felt compelled to lie on my front, I could feel the earth energy. Felt whole and alive.

Dreams – Link with great-granddad in WW1. Shot in a trench. I can feel the blood spread out across my chest. I carry the family sadness. It's in the blood line.

I fear for the future – 2012. It's like a runaway train.

I like to wear gentle, ethereal colours, blues, pinks, lilacs but I like to look upon bright colours.'

Prescription 1. Hedgehog spine 30. Dose a day for three days.

Follow up 1

Week 1 after remedy.

Lightness of spirit, it's my time, autumn. Grounded and good.

Dreams of father forgiving me.

Am very hungry, and need large comforting meals.

I feel strong, assertive, capable and happy. Energy and sleep good.

Week 2.

After day out, flattened. Glands up, loosing sparkle, sore throat.

Carried on working. Then massive head cold. Took to bed. Fluey, aching.

Menses stopped, just tiny drops of blood.

Memory of my father: He had a tough time, ramrod straight, but soft and sensitive underneath. Don't bother your father. I was in awe, fearful, I trod carefully. I sought an emotional response.

Feeling really close to husband, loving and tender. I soak up my son, aged thirteen, he's affectionate and huggy. Nice to feel needed as a mum. I'll milk it while I've got it.

Throat catarrh, want to bring something up. Migraine, distortion with sensation of flashing lights. Stool, mucusy, leaving my bottom sore,

Prescription 2. Chocolate 30 single dose, repeat as needed.

Follow up 2
Headache and cold symptoms much better. Physically in a good place.

Emerging quality of assertiveness, shocking people around me, asking for what I need. I like this new way of being. Husband was used to needy little me. Sexual energy better, empowerment on the feminine side of me.

I didn't get what I needed, I didn't want to go home but they love me now and I feel a pull to revisit places. Comfortable in my own skin. With my life experience I'm a springboard, am stripping back and here I am, wanting to share. Going to volunteer at local women's centre. It's like 2012 in me, coming into a new era. Things are shifting and moving.

Prescription 3. No remedy.

Follow up 3
Recurrence of previous physical and emotional symptoms. Sensation as if someone is sitting on my chest, as if run over by a truck. It's my father, the person who gave me life. Childhood was sad, lonely, loveless and cold. That was my father's stuff and it saddens me. I feel little me again, desperate for him to look at me, notice me. Feeling wobbly, nervy, I can feel the tectonic plates moving beneath me. Default place of comfort is my bedroom.

Prescription 4. Chocolate 30 single dose. Ignatia 12 as needed.

Follow up 4
Family stuff is sorted, a visitation from a ghost. Which felt like it was lying on top of me. Felt protected and comforted. Things in their rightful place, restful and peaceful.

Physically – Head cold. Bladder: frequent, couldn't hold it in. Breasts: tender like when pregnant. Menses: none for three months. Then bled and bled like a tap for seven days. Pure bright red, real clear out.

Had a holiday house sitting in forest, looking after animals, an affecting peace. I can feel the ancient energy of it. It was creative and basic. Heated by wood burner and candle lit.

I am not going to define myself by my illness any more. This is the me I've lost, creative and fun. This is who I am, I've forgotten. The me I haven't allowed to be. I want to get my hands dirty, I am not living the right lifestyle and life. It's not actually me, that's why I am so tired. I am coming back to the centre of the spiral, need to change job, live through my heart. Sometimes I feel the earth crying. Change is moving apace and I am feeling things acutely. I don't have energy I need to make the changes.

Prescription 5. Amanita rubescens 30 single dose.

Immediately felt much warmer. Could feel my aura glow like the Ready Brek ad.

No news after one month but a colleague who works alongside her tells me she has been well, with no time off work, energy and outlook good. Looking back I can see plenty that might have taken me to *Amanita rubescens* earlier, but this case has felt like a gradual sorting a layer at a time. There may yet be more. She does now have the energy she needs to do the work.

Part Five

Materia Medica. Here is a synthesis of features of the remedy – a bringing together of the strands. Also related remedies – those that may have been of benefit before or after the person has taken *Amanita rubescens*, or connected in other ways.

Towards a Materia Medica for *Amanita rubescens*
March 2008

The three strands –

1) From the proving. * Indicates a confirmed proving symptom. This is one that showed up first in the proving and then in a case.

2) From the cases. Initials refer to cases in which the remedy has been used to good effect, written up in the book. Some entries describe reactions shortly after taking the remedy.

3) Ed. = From my own experience.

Generalities

Energy and temperature fluctuations.

'Warmth from waist up, comes from middle of back' *(below lower heart centre.)* JC 'Huge rush of heat to head, from neck upwards.' JC

Feels icy cold at night. * IC

Libido increased. 'Instinctive, high energy. Trusting my instinct. The joy of that.' * JC *(After Rx.)*

'As if on a bike with poor brakes, going down hill.' (Ed.) Watch out!

Heat after exertion or anxiety (perhaps combining with guilt feeling.) * > fresh air.

Modalities

Time of day < 2 to 5 pm. *

Generally > open air.*

Locations and Direction of Remedy Action

Pulling down (below eyes). * JB

'Falling through air – dropping into the darkness, unknown territory.' * JC

'Energy moves upwards to third eye.' * AA *(After Rx.)*

'Warmth travels upwards from feet to knees.' * IC *(After Rx.)*

Solar plexus a prime centre of symptoms; also shoulders.

Solar plexus 'weak, watery and wobbly. No drive from that area.' * AA

Tension in heart area. Something stuck there. 'Unresolved matters held in the lower heart centre.' Ed. and Prover 8.

'Loosening starts from the centre, to shoulders and hands (feeling light.) IC *(After Rx.)*

'More solid around the heart centre and warmer.' IC *(After Rx.)*

Fire, Water and Electricity

Electric lights and switches blowing.*

Fire element. *Movement upwards as in flushes of heat.*

Burning. Forgets the boiling kettle. Cooking getting burnt.

Water element. *Movement downwards.* Spilling water and other drinks.

Other Particular Features and Symptoms

Suddenness.

Sensations: Lightness. Ungrounded, 'as if would be blown over by a puff of wind.' * JB

'Remedy makes me feel more solid. It grounds me, brings me back down to earth; gives an emotional sense of warmth, and feeling protected, a stronger compact stability and focus. A stable, restful place.' * IC

Heaviness * (head) JB. Slumping * JB (compare Prover 9 – concertina sensation.) Everything slowed down. * JB

'Energy drops.' * AA

Constriction – feelings of. Weight on chest. Hard to breathe.

Harsh. Rigorous, unrelenting remedy. Ed.

'I'm harsh to my body. Hard on myself.' * JC

Transformation. * AD/(Ed.)

'It felt like a block was moving, like snaking in my back *(he describes a figure of eight on its side)* before it left. Everything was moving as if something was looking for an exit.' * AD

'Spreading' or distant effect of the medicine. Coincidences. Telepathic (?) links. 'Journeying.'

Kingfishers and Kookaburras.

Psyche/Soma

Need for protection. Need to watch my back.

Feels protected 'by the universe.' * JB Protected feeling.

'Like a woolly layer over my back providing safety and comfort. Like a cape. Like a thick skin, not in the front at all.' * JC (*after taking Rx.)* 'With the protective layer I can trust that my decisions will be all right.' * JC

'It's like a security blanket. I don't have to watch my back.' * JC 'Like a shell.'

'Skin on my back is sore and sensitive, from my shoulders down to my waist. It feels raw. The rub of clothes is sore. This doesn't extend to the front.' * AA

'Feels knotted up – solar plexus and shoulders.' * JC

'Holding anger.' * JC He clenches fists by his sides (defended position) then (after the Rx.) releases arms down with hands in a cradling position. 'More of a whole feeling.' * JC

'In visualization – A cave in some woods; an old, priestess woman who was there to protect the place and take care of me, took my clothes and I got into the water. Everything was dark. She gave me some food.' * IC

'Strong winds agitate me. The Rx. gives protection and helps me stand firmer against the wind.' * IC

'Image of myself with a big harness on, trying to pull huge boulders in a bag with long handles. Physically everything feels heavy, slowing down, slumped, as if walking through treacle. A struggle to speak. Like an anaesthetic.' * JB

'Irritable, impatient anxiety attacks, with stomach cramps.' * IC

Mental/Emotional States

Excitement and exhilaration, uncontrollable or inappropriate giggling.

Giggles to himself in state of general happiness. * JC

Calm. * IC Relaxed, happy and secure, as if there are no time restraints. Defiant and reckless. Mentally alert and clear thinking. Fastidious. Able to get on with things and show feelings. 'Positive about starting all over again.' * IC

contrasted with

Insecurity and low confidence. Negativity and tearfulness. Joyless. *

Anger, kept in for a long time in a state of tension. > After finally speaking out. 'Began to feel cleansed and detached from this anger.' * IC (After Rx.)

'Impatience, anger and frustration.' * JC

Irritated with children – too noisy. * AA Eruptive anger. * AA

Anxiety. Restlessness.

Disorganized, unable to carry out tasks, clumsiness, bad writing and spelling errors.

'Not strong enough to move on' (e.g. from an unsatisfactory relationship). * JC

Forgetfulness, repetition of words. 'Mind goes blank, trying to hold on to thoughts, when under pressure, having to be in a certain way that I didn't want to be, associated with the fear of being judged.' * IC

Difficulties concentrating. 'Thoughts and memories clogging the mind.' * IC Irritability and wanting to be alone.

'Anger about not being understood.' * JC

'My fault.' 'Wants to be strong, firm and not to feel guilty.' * JC

Judgments. Anger and judgment. * AA Rigidity, superiority and critical of others. Instinct or 'need' to prove people wrong. Judging self and others. Ed.

The need to love self and others. Reconciliation, within the family – close family or a broader sense of family/group/nation.

Return of old symptoms. The need to sort out unresolved issues. Clearing out junk: 'yucky things'.

Anxiety about health. Negative attitude to illness. * AA

Fears. 'Fear of releasing how emotional I am'. * JC 'Learning how to hold anger.' 'Letting myself feel it.' *(After Rx.)*

Inability to stop smoking cannabis for fear being overwhelmed by strong feelings. * JC

Teenage resonances. * IC (several.)

Claustrophobia. < closed in places but also < bright light e.g. by the sea.

Sensitivity.

Body Parts and Functions

Head/Headaches. 'Pressure on skull behind ears.' * JC

Symptoms at back of head, lower part. * IC/JC

Tension in brow centre. * IC

Vertigo/light-headedness. Faint feeling when gets up from sitting in a sauna. * IC

Teeth and gums. Remedy seems to bring out latent teeth and gum problems; this in several provers and the cases too. Perhaps in teeth that are filled with mercury? It also helped with a patient's similar tooth pains at times of dental treatment. Sensitive gums and tense jaws. * IC Teeth sensitive to sweet foods, hot and cold things. * IC

Appetite and thirst.

Craving for sweets, especially biscuits, andchocolate e.g. KitKat.

Craving for sweets connected to emotional tensions. * AD

Effects of alcohol. Affected by drinking only a small quantity of alcohol.

Stomach, nausea and feelings of intoxication.

Abdominal discomforts associated with fear. * JC

Adrenalin felt in stomach. * AD

'Cold, hard feeling in abdomen, like ice, pointed icicles.' * IC

Noisy belly. * IC

Female. Menses: cramps. * IC

Throat. Swollen. Pain connects to ears as in ear infections, when swallowing. * IC

Cough.

Breathing. 'As if something is catching: instead of it being completely round like a straw, there are lots of things in the way like branches.' * JB

'I use the remedy to open up my chest and lungs. My breathing becomes wider, slower and deeper.' * IC

Skin 'Painful spots, (like teenage times) on face, ears, armpits, back. They stay for a long time.' * IC

Heart. Anxious heartbeats. * IC

Shoulders. Tension. 'Highly strung.' * JC 'Aggression held in shoulders.' * JC (With clenched fists.) Muscular knots. * JC 'Stiff everywhere.' AA 'Neck grinding/biting. Can't turn it.' * JC 'Tension accumulates in shoulders.' * AD 'Pain in left shoulder – feels tight, inflexible, trapped and vulnerable.' * AD

Nerves as if trapped. * AD

Back/neck. 'Back symptoms to do with arms and shoulder tension.' * JC

Extremities – limbs. 'Tingling down back of arms.' * JC

Cold hands and feet. * IC

Sleep. Rx. 'Allows really good sleep, esp. if tired or anxious.' * IC

Dreams – become more vivid after taking Rx.

of sifting through old stuff. * IC

Related Remedies

Yellow. Mercury. Lycopodium. Nux vomica. Sepia. Thuja. Phosphorus. Syphilinum. Natrum muriaticum (Salt). Staphisagria. Plastic wrap. Amethyst. Rose Quartz. Carcinosin. Sulphur. Argentum nitricum. Saccharum officinarum (Sugar).

Yellow. A remedy characterised by low self-esteem, confusion and ungroundedness; it also encourages the drainage of potential pathology from the system in those who have a past history of being excessively adrenally driven and who are still in a state of unquiet mind. (Colin Griffith. *The New Materia Medica,* Watkins 2007.)

Prover 2. *At college – the day we found out what the proving substance was.* Overwhelmed. Calm. Mind not clear. I had wondered if the remedy was yellow or connected to the colour yellow in some way (Day 48).

Supervisor of Prover 8. From her proving summary.

Whilst the proving was going on I went to see my homoeopath to continue my treatment with her. At this stage I did not know what the remedy was or a great deal about it, and neither did my homoeopath. She prescribed me a remedy. She did not tell me what it was at the time. Since then I have asked what the remedy was, knowing that it had played a positive part on the reduction of my fears. The remedy was *Yellow* – one of the colour remedies. The colour that resonated the most with the proving remedy was yellow. Again, this just shows me how far the proving 'stretched', and how it affects lots of people connected to it in one way or another on an energetic level.

Mercury. Several people who have taken *Amanita rubescens,* or been affected by being around it, have had symptoms of dental/amalgam problems. In the proving too. As we understand it the remedy exposes toxic states.

Prover 1. I couldn't switch my mind off; it was racing with thoughts about the remedy *Mercury* (Day 18).

Lycopodium. Prover 2. *Six days before the proving:* When Stuart was talking, I was thinking of *Lycopodium* (as an example of a remedy to note as having previously benefited from) and then he mentioned it.

Nux vomica. *During the proving:* A dream of *Nux vomica.* I dreamt I was with my Mum and brothers. We were trying to work out why my Dad had died. Somehow we discovered that he was one of twenty-nine people who died for a particular reason (which I cannot remember). It was something double top secret! At some point, we all woke up in the morning and one of my brothers had a hangover. I really wanted to give him *Nux vomica 200* but didn't have any with me. This troubled me greatly (Day 4).

(Easy intoxication from alcohol is a symptom of Am. rub. Ed.)

Proving effects? I took a *Nux vomica 30* for a hangover (pounding headache and nausea). It helped a bit. (I've not had much success with *Nux vomica* for previous hangovers.)

Later: *I took a Nux vomica 200* as the headache had returned full strength. All symptoms were gone within half an hour (Day 30).

Sepia. I went and met my supervisor to discuss the proving. I was feeling generally negative. I told her how I felt and realized I have felt like this once before. This was in December, now two months ago, starting about three weeks before Christmas (which I usually really enjoy) and up to New Year's Eve when I had a really good dance and felt better after that. During December my homoeopath prescribed *Sepia,* which helped my period a bit. I told my supervisor I thought I needed *Sepia* again. When I got home I apologised for being so negative and I explained I couldn't shake off this feeling (Day 26).

My supervisor rang me and said my negative feelings could be to do with the proving. I agreed it sounded similar to some experiences others had shared at college. I decided not to take *Sepia,* although I remain uncertain as the feelings are just like those I had in December before the proving commenced and even before the advance notice lecture at college the month before starting the proving (Day 27).

The proving co-ordinator phoned and I asked if I could resume the *Sepia.* He agreed, asking me to note what happens, as it is possible that the remedy we are proving may help other remedies act more effectively. I took it as soon as I came off the phone. (Subsequent addition: I have been feeling great since taking the *Sepia*; more loving towards my daughter, more patient and less tired (Day 40).

Sepia is a possible remedy for hot flushes – menopausal style (Ed.).

Prover 9. I feel very low, tired and like I can't cope with all the continual family stuff. Like the dream I feel like I've gone back to where I've already come from, I recognise this state from times when I have really struggled with my children and had little support in caring for them. *Sepia* was very helpful at those times.

I get a sense that this remedy affects the heart and sacral and crown chakras. The words amethyst and quartz come to mind, but I do not know about them for their possible relevance. I have a sense of calmness, love, and serenity (Day 11).

Thuja. I feel depressed, emotional and fragile. I feel that I'm always failing myself. I want to be nurtured and withdraw from practical matters. I feel disgust for myself. Recently I've had a strange movement in my abdomen, which reminds me of the sensation 'something alive in the stomach'. At the time I thought that this must be what *Thuja* has, but at the college weekend I picked up a fourth year project on *Thuja,* I felt led to it. I was also drawn to the sequoia tree in the gardens at college rather than to the large old oak (Day 25).

Syphilinum. Heart as central. Destructive or creative tendencies.

Prover 8. 'The proving brought out my syphilitic side very heavily and I have struggled, even with good homoeopathy, to move away from it.'

S.D. Editor. *Syphilinum 1M* was the necessary remedy for me at the critical time when my heart was playing up.

Natrum muriaticum – resentment and withdrawing. A heart/ emotional centre remedy.

Staphisagria – holding back the expression of anger at being treated badly, especially affecting the sacral, sex centre.

Phosphorus – affected by others, by energy fields. Need for grounding. Burnt out.

Lycopodium – critical and censorious.

Plastic wrap – healing of second chakra issues – sense of identity and place in the world. Hiding behind a mask.

Amethyst – 'is highly protective of the auric field and has been known to give patients a feeling of being more able to cope with pressures put on them by others who have a controlling or manipulative influence, or by personnel in institutions they work for.' From *The New Materia Medica,* Colin Griffith.

Rose Quartz – 'Opens up the heart chakra to the possibility of resolving emotional trauma that has been buried for far too long.' Ibid.

Carcinosin – cancerous tendencies, and much more besides.

Nux vomica – detoxification, effects of alcohol.

Sulphur – detoxification, grounding.

Argentum nitricum – anticipatory fears.

Thuja – self doubt. Split.

Saccharum Officinarum – conditioned responses. Conditioned to behave and respond in ways that perpetuate the status quo.

Cadmium, Chromium, Cuprum and **Plumbum** – elements that are readily absorbed by *Amanita rubescens* form the surrounding air, as is **Mercury.** *See Part Seven.*

Part Six

Notes and quotes from diverse sources – with relevance to the themes of *Amanita rubescens*. Also references to contemporary world events that have run in parallel with our work over these last six years.

Symbols that are referred to in the text.

Bibliography

Notes and Quotes

Contemporary events –

Since 2005, the year this connection with *Amanita rubescens* began for me, there were strikes by labour unions in Egypt, in protest at the Mubarak regime. These led eventually to the Tahrir Square uprising of February 2011.

As I came towards completing work on this book I was keenly aware of events running in parallel. This included the gradual and consistent improvement in my well-being. In the wider world context it was Libya's time for big changes.

The day I began to consider the title for the book was the day that Colonel Gaddafi died. The Arab Spring and other uprisings carry similarities with our remedy. People speaking out from a regained sense of personal will. Uprisings in relation to conditions of life and conditionings. As a nation feelings that had been held in are spoken out. Fiery courage. Long-held hurts. All facilitated by the speed of Internet and mobile phone connections between people.

My impression of the urban riots in England in August 2011 was of people in conditions and situations where their own vital personal will and fire found no integrated or creative expression. This energy then shows up in the streets. Looting and fire.

Also the Mayan calendar time frame and earth alignment to the centre of the galaxy. Accelerated change, revolutions, evolutions, moving towards 2012.

The web of interconnection –

The quantum effect – the work of physicists indicating the effect of the observer on what happens.

The Internet itself – an allegory and a physical representation of a growing awareness of interconnection in our times. That communications can be instantaneous, with or without the technology.

Quotes

November 2011, from a BBC Radio 4 news programme.

One of the Glasgow City Square 'occupation' campers was asked about the intentions of the protest. First he referred to the current banking/financial issues. Then he said, 'It's about looking deep inside yourself and changing for the better.' Awareness growing of personal responsibility, and the potential of internal change. Less talk of 'they' are doing it to us, those dreadful bankers.

From the book – *Heart*, 1932 (no named author). With thanks for permission to print. Publisher – Agni Yoga Society, Inc, USA.

This book comes from a previous time of upheaval – before World War Two. I notice parallels with the territory of *Amanita rubescens* as a homoeopathic remedy; also with the work of the HeartMath Institute's Global Coherence Initiative, and with the evolutionary impulses of our times. The text is presented in numbered sections.

62. Courage dwells in the warmth of the heart. This must be remembered. The appearance of the dark forces is like a frost to the sowing. Only the heart's warmth provides a glowing shield.

117. Intolerance is a sign of ignobility of spirit. Intolerance contains embryos of the most evil acts. There is no place for the manifestation of the growth of the spirit where intolerance breeds.

139. The significance of the all-embracing heart cannot be realized if, instead of cooperation, one dreams of various kinds of slavery. Thus, during the study of magnetic currents, let us determine that the realization of cooperation increases tenfold the might of all binding currents. It may seem strange that an ethical concept of cooperation should react on a physical concept of currents. Someone who is unaware of true science may think thus. But you are sufficiently aware of how inseparable is the domain of spirit from physical laws.

140. When you become aware of Infinity, then you must also become accustomed to its properties. Inexhaustibility is the very first property, which will make every courageous heart happy.

150. The summons to a unity of consciousness is necessary everywhere, because this is the simplest introduction to the life of the heart. This is not sorcery but a physical law that can weave a salutary net around the planet. Thus, everyone who follows the law of Being can justly consider himself a citizen of the Universe.

169. It happens that people are so savage of spirit that they can only live by condemning each other. This is not an inspection of another's armour with the view of helping; on the contrary, condemnation becomes the meaning of life. If one deprives such a condemner of his tongue, he will perish and wither like a plant without water... One can see in this condemnation a kind of obsessive vampirism, when the possession of more active vital fluids is needed to nourish the obsessed one.

179. You yourself know what courage is needed in order to cross by dangerous paths. One can offer a dangerous or a safe path, but the flaming heart will choose the first.

184. I affirm that the Great Battle is the renovation of Earth. The future must be understood not as a battle, but as an achievement. One can expect battles not only in their customary significance, but as a reconstruction of life. There may be various periods, but one can sense in them the strengthening of the tempo of life. You already sense this acceleration of the rhythm. Each one can sense its impact

according to his own nervous condition. But he will inevitably sense a new cosmic condensation. One can feel a direct, acute augmentation of the rays; one can feel alarm of striving into the distance. All these details will indicate the same new accelerated rhythm. One can understand how the intensification of energies builds a new step for the planet.

255. I affirm that the fire of the heart purifies the densest darkness. But along with purification the fire of the heart is impregnated with the qualities of a magnet, and thus it becomes the natural link with the Macrocosm.

261. Let us understand the heart as the focus of the physical laws and the highest laws as well. This centre was called the crossroad, and was represented by the *dorje*, like the swastika, indicated the rotation of the fire of the heart. Rotation and equilaterality are the signs of balance.

277. One can think with the brain or the heart. Time was, perhaps, when people forgot about the work of the heart, but now is the era of the heart, and we must concentrate our strivings in this direction. Thus, without relieving the brain of work, we are ready to recognize the heart as a moving power.

300. If thought itself contains creative energy, then how useful it is to direct good thought into space.

302. It is instructive to compile a book about the harm resulting from bad thoughts; for oneself, as well as others. These thoughts are the source of many sicknesses. Formerly, only psychic illnesses were connected with evil thoughts, but it is time to discern the multitude of the most varied physical illnesses that are born of thought. Not only diseases of the heart, but most of the stomach and skin diseases are the consequences of destructive thoughts.

339. One cannot conceive of the unity of humanity by way of the brain or the Kundalini, but the radiance of the heart can bring together the most seemingly varied organisms, even across remote distances. This experiment, of the unification of the heart across distance, awaits its workers.

446. One should firmly realize that the forces of the spirit which heretofore demanded decades, now, through the way of the heart, are accelerated to the highest degree.

462. You yourself see how events foregather. You also see that quantity has no significance and may be only a burden. You yourselves see that events are waxing, for the cosmic manifestations begin to astound even the short-sighted. But count the hours, for time is saturated like never before.

493. Is it not a wondrous experience to apply the heart's energy at great distances and to help the great cause? One can verify the dates and witness absolute precision. Therefore it is so imperative to write down the most important manifestations and sensations. Thus one can counteract absurdities which assert that there are only accidents and coincidences everywhere.

495. At times people are ready to admit the power of thought, but they do not apply this admission to themselves. They dream of great thoughts but will not discipline the small ones. They will ask how to transmute thought into action. One must begin by disciplining the smallest thoughts and then, only, create a thought that moves mountains. The advice about disciplining small thoughts is the inception of bringing health to the heart… Disorderly thoughts are like vermin, they injure the subtle substance. Often they carry deadly poison. Precisely the smallest thoughts are like madness, and they form the chief obstacle to the rapport of the subtle and dense worlds.

497. Let us again remember that this education (of the heart energy) should begin with the minutest sensations and the most usual actions. This circumstance complicates the situation, because people usually like to say, 'Let me fight a giant, but spare me from catching fleas.' Yet giants are rare, whereas fleas are innumerable. One must pass through these dark swarms. The house has to be protected from them. The venom carried by the giant is less than that of the flea. Furthermore, the appearance of the giant evokes unusual courage; yet courage is also needed against flies and fleas, and usually people suffer from flies rather than from giants.

506. First of all, it is necessary to have simple respect for psychic energy. It is necessary to respect an energy which, like fire, pervades all of space and condenses in the nerve centres. Even children should remember that this uniting energy is emanated in every handshake, every glance. Striving to respect it will also inspire care for this treasure of the heart.

535. The heart of humanity is sick. First of all, one must render healthy the sphere of the heart, certainly, if the people wish to avoid a catastrophe.

561. The great law is to transfer the heart from the category of ethical abstraction to a scientific motive force. The evolutionary step of understanding the heart has to begin in the days of Armageddon, as the sole salvation of humanity. Why are people unwilling to sense their own hearts? They are willing to seek within all vagaries, but reject the closest. Even though they call the heart a machine, let them observe all characteristics of this apparatus. We are not insisting on the moral significance of the heart – this is indisputable. But now the heart is needed as the bridge of salvation to the Subtle World. It should be affirmed that a realization of the qualities of the heart represents the most vital step for the world.

589. Many times I have warned against fear and treason; this must be remembered from an evolutionary point of view. All the substances of fear are contrary to Fire! All fruits of fear will be reduced to ashes by fire, hence striving to fiery energy signifies the renunciation of all fear. One must take as example those valiant hearts who not only do not flee from the fiery dragons but approach them fearlessly.

From the HeartMath website –

'The mission of the Institute of HeartMath is to help establish heart-based living and global coherence by inspiring people to connect with the intelligence and guidance of their own hearts.

The mission and vision of the scientifically based Global

Coherence Initiative is to unite millions of people, whatever their belief systems or cultures, to shift global consciousness from instability and chaos to balance and cooperation. This can be accomplished by increasing the potency of people's positive heart-directed intentions and by deploying a Global Coherence Monitoring System (GCMS) to scientifically measure the effects.

A key component of Global Coherence Initiative is the Global Coherence Monitoring System, developed in partnership with internationally renowned astrophysicist and nuclear scientist Elizabeth Rauscher and Institute of HeartMath researchers. In effect, the GCMS will be measuring the 'brain waves and heart rhythm' of the planet in real time. It will explore whether the earth's magnetic field is influenced by collective human emotional resonance resulting from heart-directed intention, or in response to major events, and whether the emotional energy generated by the collective intuition about major future events is measurable in this field.

Research has shown that 0.1 Hz is the human resonant frequency – the frequency at which spirit, heart, mind, emotions, and body are in resonant alignment with the planet. The term for this is heart coherence. The more heart coherent we are, the greater the resonant energetic connection we have with people, within ourselves, and with nature. This enhances individual and collective intuitive discernment for solving social, environmental and global problems.'

Considering resonance, tuning forks have been made to frequencies associated with earth and other planets' orbits, or other solar system cycles of time. See *The Cosmic Octave Tuning Forks* in the Bibliography.

Symbols and bodily movements

In relation to the **Y** and **X** forms referred to in my account *(Page 57)* I spoke with a Eurhythmy practitioner.

In that work associations and use of the Y shape with the arms reached upwards -

- To strengthen the capacity for wonder and interest. To create a space to receive cleansing. To overcome the animal in us. Hallelujah gesture.
- And the **X** shape (arms up as in the **Y**) with feet wide apart -
- Weight bears downwards and light streams upwards, and to hold the two triangles in balance. The two triangles meet in the solar plexus area.

And the prayer position – Up and down, connection to our star above and the earth below.

With thanks to Juliette Leighton, Eurhythmist.

Symbols

Drawings by Roberta Young to illustrate a sequence of movements.

Position 1. Horizontal meets vertical in the Indian style prayer position. Comparable with the Celtic cross. Palms together in front of the heart.

Part Six

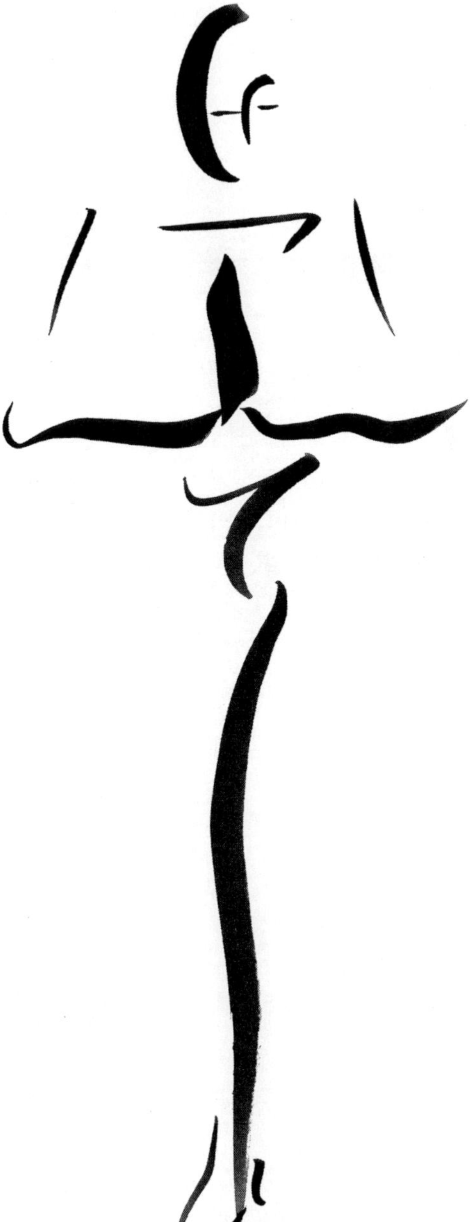

Position 2. Raising up to form the **I**. Earth to Heavens alignment, the sky to earth electrical charge.

Part Six

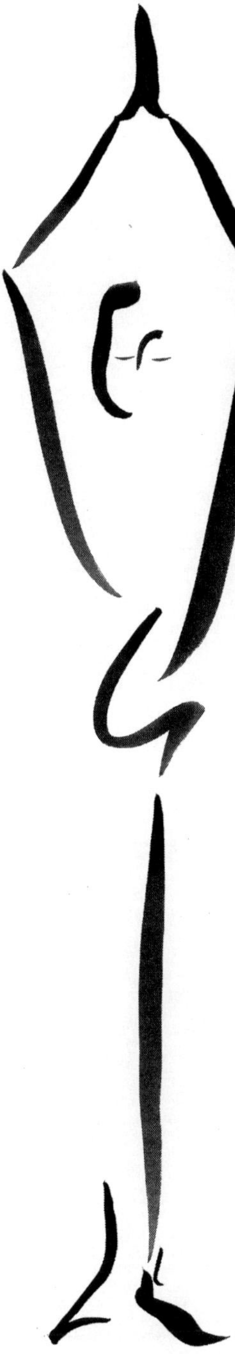

Position 3. Opening out to form the **Y**. Open to receive from above, opening to the 'higher' energies.

Part Six

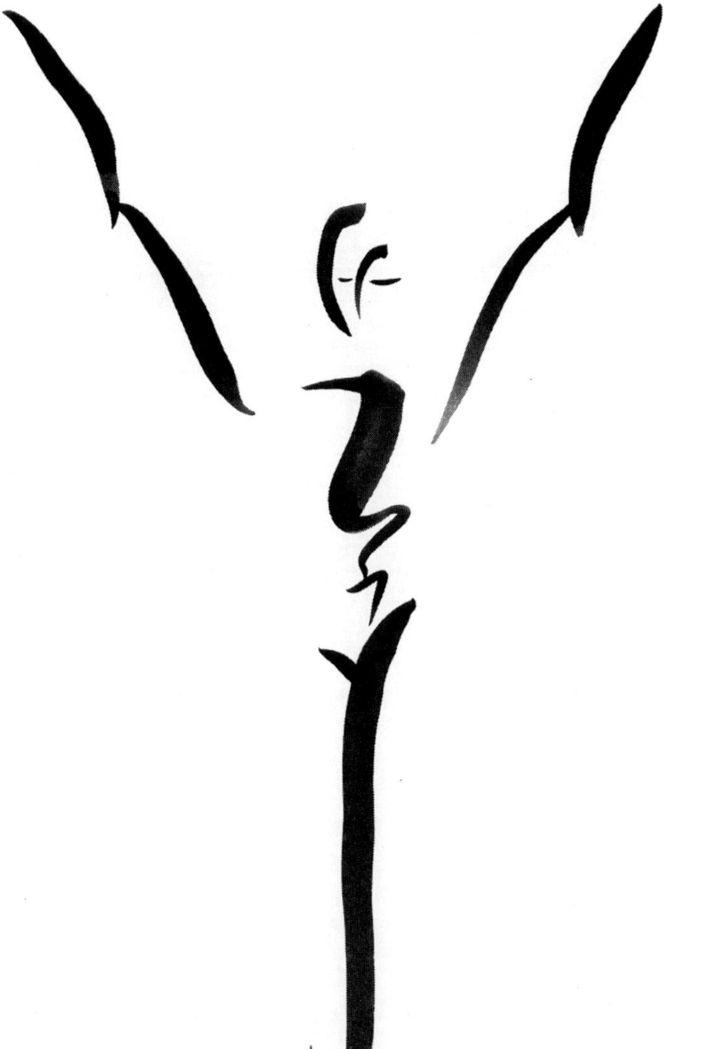

Position 4. Legs apart to form the **X**. Receiving from below too. Two triangles meeting. The meeting of above and below, from the earth up and from the heavens down. Heart as centre.

Part Six

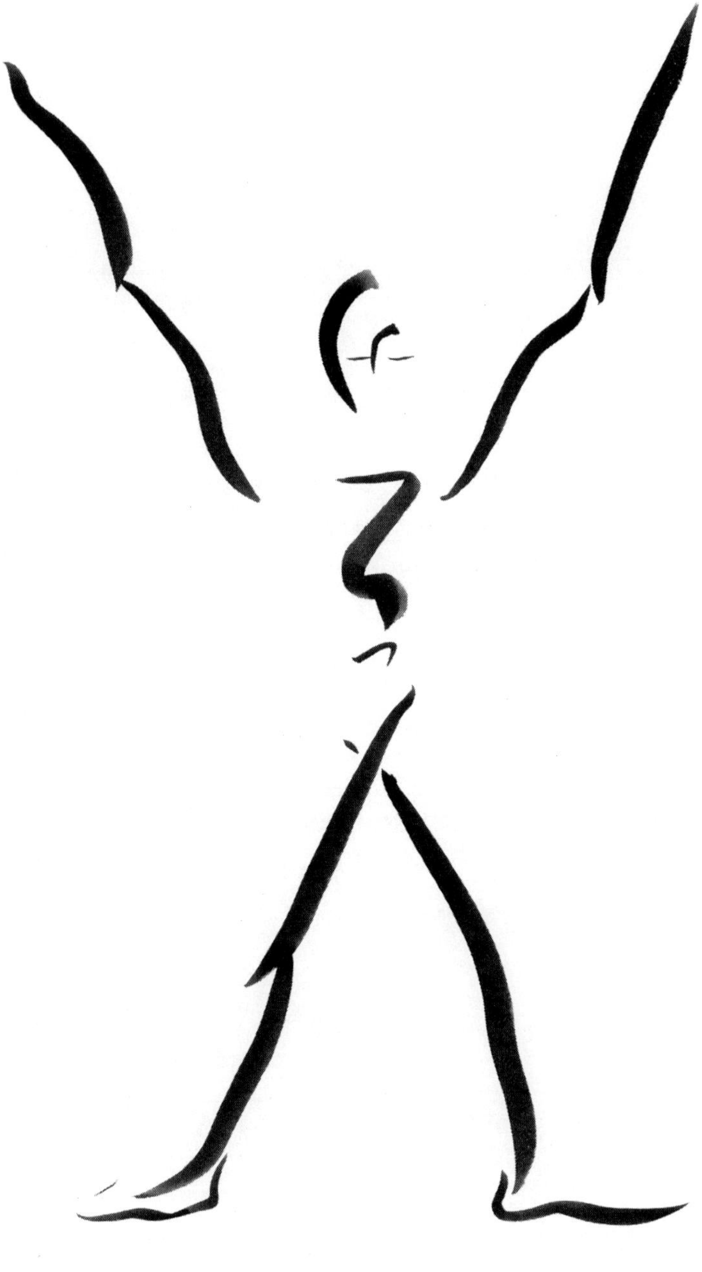

Return to Position 3, the **Y**.
Bring arms down along the diagonal back to Position 1.
Then lower arms for Position 5. The cradling **O**.

Part Six

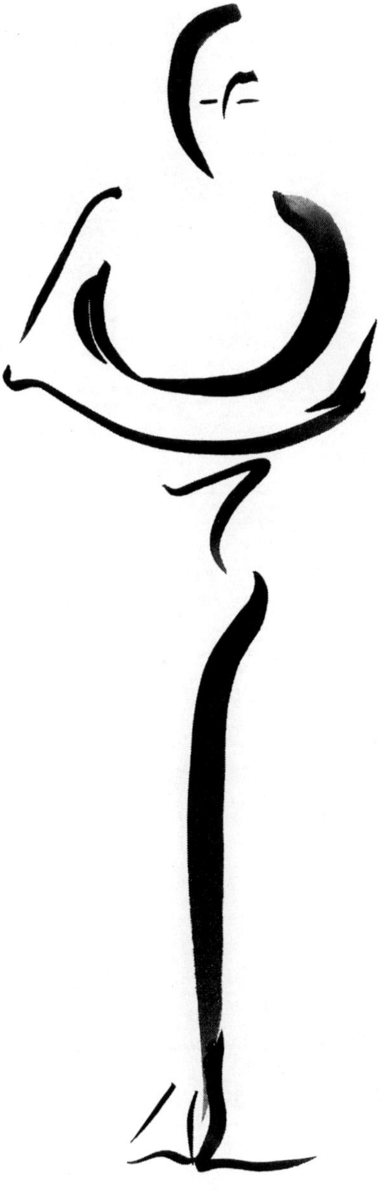

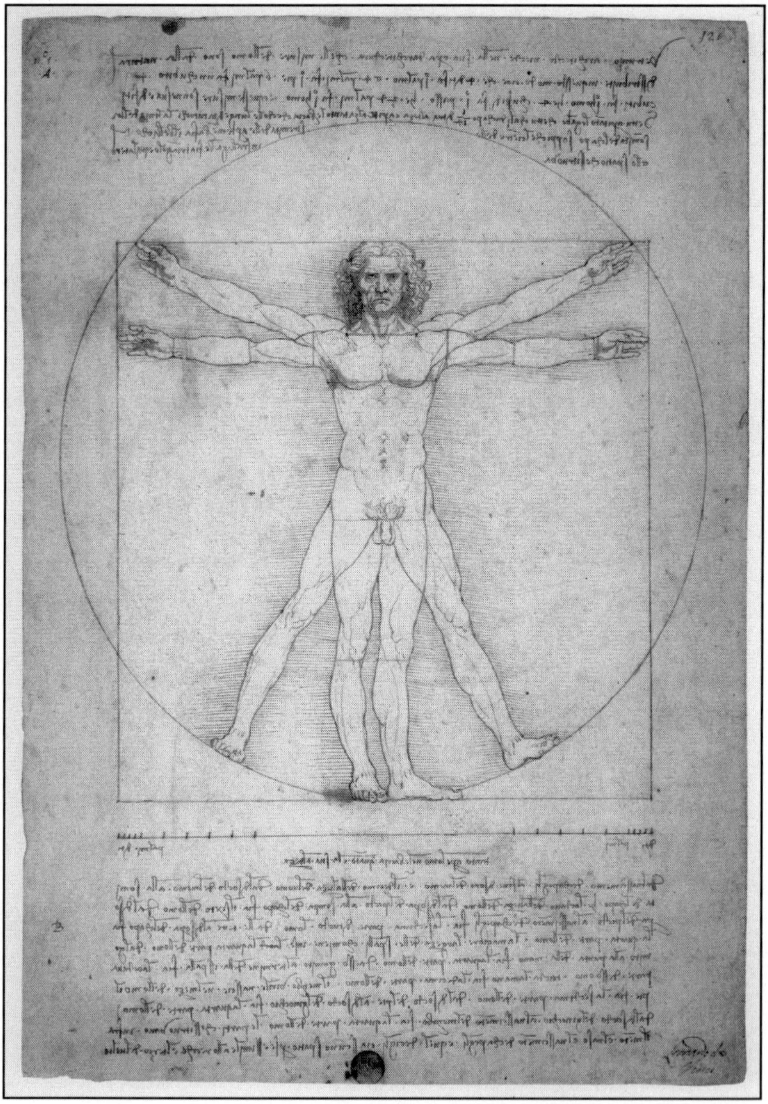

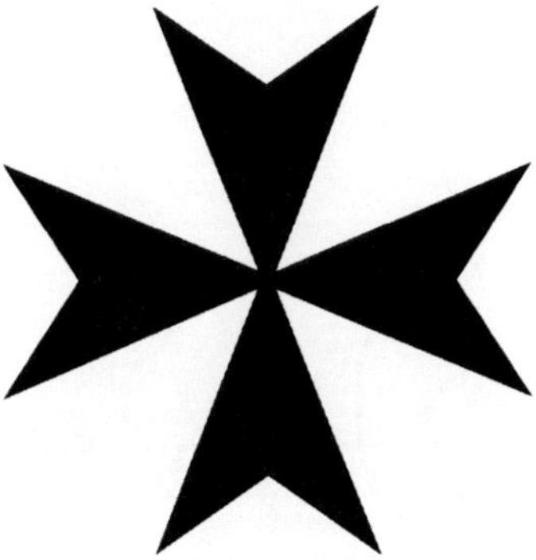

Maltese Cross

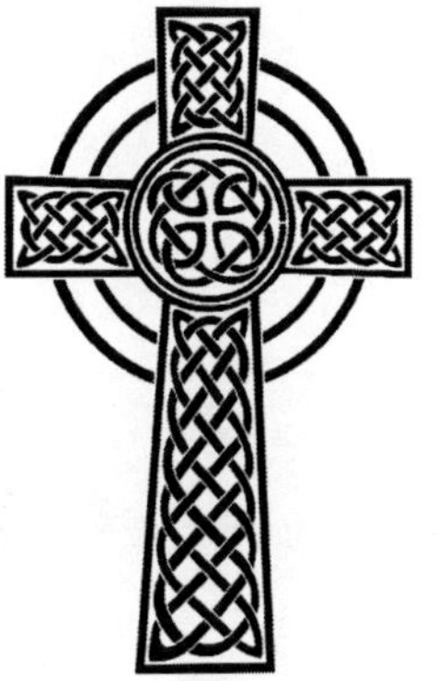

Celtic cross. Vertical meets horizontal.

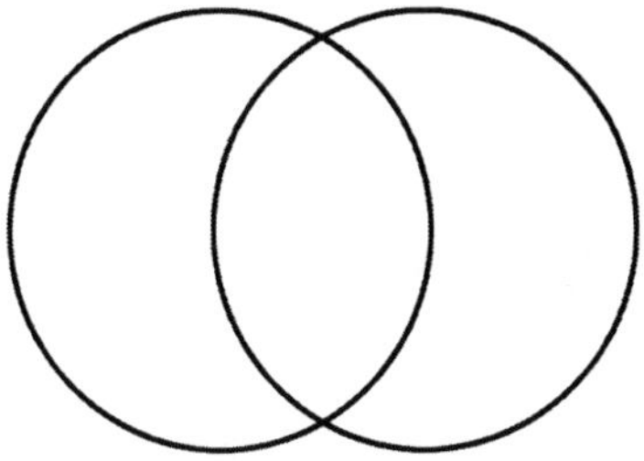

Vesica Pisces

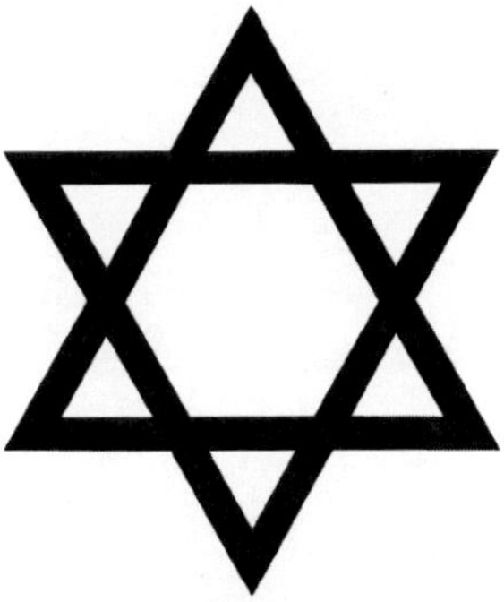

Star of David

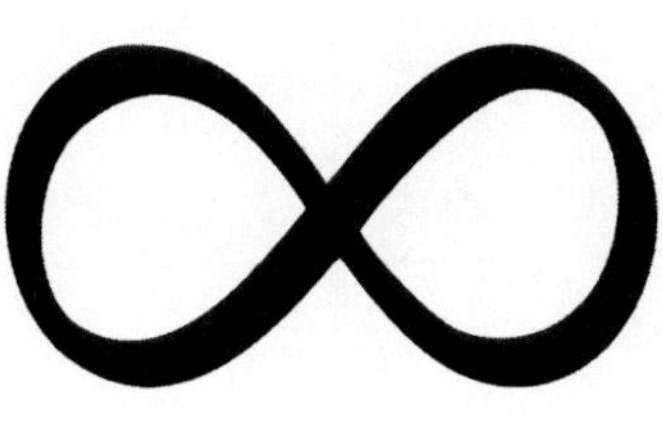

Infinity symbol

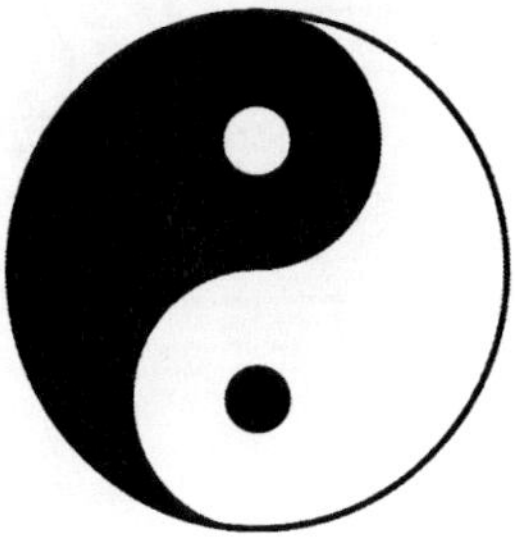

Yin yang symbol

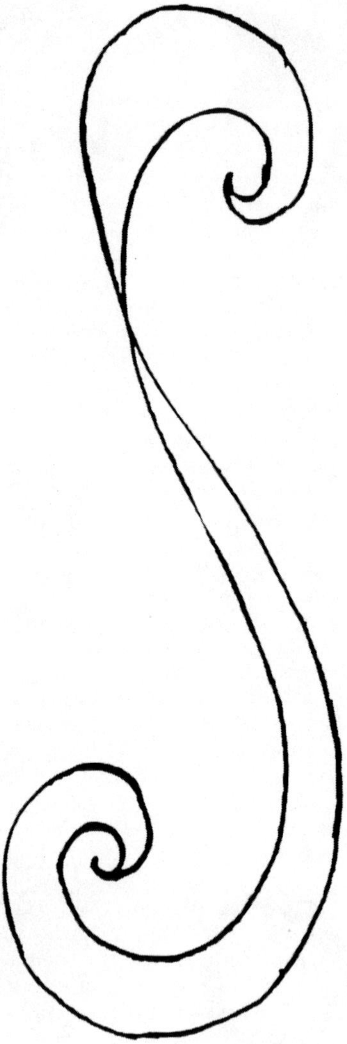

Spiral symbol.
Drawing by Roberta Young a prover.

Bibliography

Talking with Angels. Notated by Gitta Mallasz. Translated from the original Hungarian. Daimon Verlag. Einsiedeln, Switzerland, 1998

God is a Verb. Kabbalah and the Practice of Mystical Judaism. David A. Cooper. Riverhead Books, 1997

The Elements of the Chakras. Naomi Ozaniec. Element Books, 1996

The Eye of the I. David R. Hawkins. Veritas. USA, 2001

Matrix Energetics. Richard Bartlett. Atria Paperback, 2007

A New Earth. Eckhart Tolle. Michael Joseph, 2005

A Course in Miracles. New York. Viking. The Foundation for Inner Peace, 1996

Tuning the Diamonds: Electromagnetism and Spiritual Evolution. Susan Joy Rennison. Joyfire Publishing, 2008

Homoeopathy and Human Evolution. Martin Miles. Winter Press, 1992

Carcinosin: A Compendium of References. Compiled by RD Micklem, 1998

The New Materia Medica. Colin Griffith. Watkins, 2007

The Mad Hatter's Tea Party. Melissa Assilem. For an insight into sugar, as substance and homoeopathic remedy. 1994

Vibrational Medicine. Richard Gerber. 3rd Edition, Bear, 2001

The Divine Matrix. Gregg Braden. Hay House, 2007

Sand and Foam. Kahlil Gilbran. Heinemann, 1927

www.gizapyramid.com/russian/pyramids.htm

The Cosmic Octave Tuning Forks. Hans Cousto. Planetware, 2009. www.planetware.de

Plastic Wrapped – The Homoeopathic Proving of Cling Film. Stuart Deeks. The Well Books, 2009

Part Seven

Some general considerations about fungi. *Amanita rubescens* chemistry and toxicity.

The Capacity of Fungi To Clean Up Toxicity

From an article by Sarah Wilkinson in Positive News, Autumn 2010. With thanks for permission to include it.

Mushroom expert and author Paul Stamets has a viable solution for the long-term clean-up procedure after the oil spill in the Gulf of Mexico has been contained. Fungi were the first life forms to inhabit the land 1.3 billion years ago; 600 million years before plants evolved. After asteroid impacts darkened the skies, de-greened the Earth and caused mass extinctions 65 million years back, the only organisms to survive were the ones that 'paired up' with fungi and learnt how to be co-dependent.

'It's time for another re-greening,' Paul thinks, 'as Earth recoils from the ongoing catastrophes inflicted by our species.' And cleaning up after oil spills, pollution, storm damage, floods and volcanic clouds is just another day at the office for fungi. It's a process he calls mycoremediation and here's how it works.

Beneath the fruit – or mushroom, as we call it – fungal roots, known as Mycelia, spread outwards to create a vast mat of underground cells that permeate the soil. Now known to be the largest biological entities on the planet, a single colony can cover an area equal to 1,665 football fields and travel several inches a day. A massive network of whispering spaghetti, these 'neurological' tendrils intersect with neighbouring colonies and fuse with the roots of other species to share water, food and communicate vital information.

Paul explains: 'Mycelia are the Earth's natural internet – the essential wiring of the Gaian consciousness. The creation of the computer internet is merely an extension of a successful biological model that has evolved over billions of years.'

They produce enzymes that are excellent at disintegrating hydrocarbons – the base structure of all oils, petroleum products, pesticides and pollutants.

Through a series of trials. Paul's team at Battelle Laboratories, in the US, made some astonishing findings. Soil that had been heavily contaminated with oil and hydrocarbons was inoculated with oyster mushroom spawn. After a few weeks, it was bursting with fruit, while 99% of the hydrocarbons had been destroyed. Only non-toxic components remained and even the mushrooms themselves revealed no traces of petroleum.

'And then came another startling revelation,' Paul says. 'As the mushrooms rotted flies arrived. The flies laid eggs, which became larvae. The larvae, in turn, attracted birds, which apparently brought in seeds. Soon it was an oasis, teeming with life.'

Paul Stamets, *Mycelium Running: How Mushrooms Can Help Save the World.*

www.fungi.com

Some General Thoughts About Fungi from a Homoeopath

From Fungi – Kingdom Fungi (Spectrum Materia Medica Volume 2), by Frans Vermeulen, with thanks for permission to print.

The elements of penetration and expansion are keynotes of fungi. In each tube is a rushing torrent of the living contents, the protoplasm pressing towards the ever-expanding tip.

Affinities

Psyche, GI tract, liver, kidneys.

Expansion. Extension. Invasion. Penetration. Exploration. Colonization.

Pioneering. Ability to adapt to challenging conditions.
Beyond limits. Limitless. Rampant. Beyond control.
Uncontrollable. Lack/loss of control.
Space. Distorted sense of space.
Opportunistic. Commitment. Tentative. Flexibility.
Constant activity to maintain intimate relationship in environment.
Nothing ventured, nothing gained.
Invisible.
Symbiotic or saprophytic (recycling, transformation).
Exploitation.
Carbohydrates. Energy. Alcohol.
Strength.
Light photophobic or phototropic.
Moisture/dampness. Susceptible to drying. Dehydration.
Rapidity.
Death. Decay. Dissolution. Disintegration

Chemistry

(From my reading around the subject. Ed.)

The minerals and heavy metals play an important role in the metabolic processes, during the growth and development of mushrooms, when they are available in appreciable concentration. Chromium, Manganese, Iron, Nickel, Copper, Zinc, Selenium, Cadmium, Iron and Lead are found.

Research examples

Ovidius University, Romania. *Annals of Chemistry* Volume 21, Number 1, pp 9–14, 2010

Determination of heavy metals content in wild mushrooms and soil.

Mean concentration of heavy metals in fruiting body (cap and stipe) (mg/kg d.w.)

Zn Cu Fe Cd Mn Cr Ni Pb

Amanita rubescens (cap)

Zn 115.2±0.4	Cu 15.8±0.8	Fe 308.9±4.3	Cd 0.64±0.1
Mn36.7±0.4	Cr 1.66±0.3	Ni 0.92±0.4	Pb 1.12±1.3

Amanita rubescens (stipe)

Zn 98.3±0.2	Cu 12.9±0.7	Fe 289.4±3.5	Cd 0.39±0.2
Mn 33.4±0.5	Cr 0.33±0.2	Ni 0.43±0.8	Pb 0.68±2.2

The following three studies were found by going to www.ncbi.nlm.nih.gov/pubmed and entering Amanita rubescens.

1/ The Mercury connection.

Rocz Panstw Zakl Hig. 2008;59(2):139–46.

Content and bio-concentration of mercury by European Blusher (Amanita rubescens) from Northern Poland.

Rocz Panstw Zakl Hig. 2008;59(2):139–46.

Article in Polish. Source. Zaklad Chemii Srodowiska i Ekotoksykologii, Uniwersytet Gdański, 80-952 Gdańsk, ul. Sobieskiego 19.

Abstract

Total mercury content has been determined in 45 fruiting bodies of European Blusher (*Amanita rubescens*) and soil substrate collected from three spatially distant sites at the Pomorskie Voivodeship in 2006–2007. Mercury analysis carried out was by cold-vapour atomic absorption (CV-AAS) with amalgamation on golden wool. The European Blusher effectively accumulated mercury and median BCF values of this element ranged from 9.5 to 24 for the caps and from 6.1 to 15 for the stipes. For the areas surveyed mean concentration values of total mercury ranged from 0.46 to 0.93 (0.098–3.2) microg/g dw for the caps, from 0.27 to 0.65 (0.077–2.7) microg/g dw for the stipes and from 0.032 do 0.040 (0.0096–0.20) microg/g dw for soil substrate.

PMID: 18807911 [PubMed – indexed for MEDLINE]

2/ Cleaning up Lead and Cadmium. This research refers to the possibility of using *Amanita rubescens* to treat wastewater containing Pb(II) and Cd(II) ions.

J Hazard Mater. 2009 May 30;164(2–3):1004–11. Epub 2008 Sep 5.

Kinetic and equilibrium studies of biosorption of Pb(II) and Cd(II) from aqueous solution by macrofungus (Amanita rubescens) biomass. Sari A, Tuzen M.

Source: Department of Chemistry, Gaziosmanpasa University, Tokat, Turkey.

Abstract
The biosorption characteristics of Pb(II) and Cd(II) ions from aqueous solution using the macrofungus (*Amanita rubescens*) biomass were investigated as a function of pH, biomass dosage, contact time, and temperature. Langmuir, Freundlich and Dubinin-Radushkevich (D-R) models were applied to describe the biosorption isotherm of the metal ions by A. rubescens biomass. Langmuir model fitted the equilibrium data better than the Freundlich isotherm. The maximum biosorption capacity of A. rubescens for Pb(II) and Cd(II) was found to be 38.4 and 27.3mg/g, respectively, at optimum conditions of pH 5.0, contact time of 30 min, biomass dosage of 4 g/L, and temperature of 20 degrees C. The metal ions were desorbed from A. rubescens using both 1M HCl and 1M HNO(3). The recovery for both metal ions was found to be higher than 90%. The high stability of A. rubescens permitted ten times of adsorption-elution process along the studies without a decrease about 10% in recovery of both metal ions. The mean free energy values evaluated from the D-R model indicated that the biosorption of Pb(II) and Cd(II) onto A. rubescens biomass was taking place by chemical ion-exchange. The calculated thermodynamic parameters, DeltaG degrees , DeltaH degrees and DeltaS degrees showed that the biosorption of Pb(II) and Cd(II) ions

onto A. rubescens biomass was feasible, spontaneous and exothermic under examined conditions. Experimental data were also tested in terms of biosorption kinetics using pseudo-first-order and pseudo-second-order kinetic models. The results showed that the biosorption processes of both Pb(II) and Cd(II) followed well pseudo-second-order kinetics. Based on all results, It can be also concluded that it can be evaluated as an alternative biosorbent to treatment wastewater containing Pb(II) and Cd(II) ions, since A. rubescens is low-cost biomass and has a considerable high biosorption capacity.

PMID: 18845395 [PubMed – indexed for MEDLINE]

3/ Haemolytic toxic effects on rats and guinea pigs, and humans too.

Toxicon. 1982;20(4):765–81. Odenthal, KP, Seeger, R et al.

Damage in vitro to various organs and tissues by rubescenslysin from the edible mushroom *Amanita rubescens*. Odenthal, KP, Seeger, R et al.

Abstract
Rubescenslysin, a haemolytic protein from *Amanita rubescens,* disrupted the cytoplasmic membrane of human leucocytes which were more sensitive than erythrocytes. In the isolated hearts of rats and guinea pigs it caused systolic contracture, which was preceded by potassium outflow and sometimes by a transient positive inotropic effect. On the electrically stimulated guinea-pig left atrium it showed at first a positive, followed by a negative inotropic effect; on the spontaneously beating right atrium it produced transient positive followed by negative inotropic and chronotropic effects. Atria were less sensitive than intact hearts. In the isolated rat phrenic nerve-diaphragm preparation it produced a contracture, which was associated with reduction of indirect and direct contractility. In the isolated guinea-pig ileum it produced a slow contraction

followed by tachyphylaxis. As excitability declined due to rubescenslysin, so did excitability by acetylcholine and potassium. Atropine and pheniramine had only feeble antagonistic effects, but papaverine was more powerful. In isolated rat hepatocytes, rubescenslysin caused a rapid outflow of potassium and coarse cell protrusions while later the cells became stainable with trypan blue. In the isolated perfused rat liver it produced a rapid outflow of potassium and of cytoplasmic and mitochondrial enzymes, and a somewhat slower outflow of lysosomal beta-glucuronidase, accompanied by a rise in the lactate/pyruvate ratio and a decrease in bile production. In the isolated perfused rat kidney it caused an outflow of cytoplasmic and mitochondrial enzymes, together with massive proteinuria and serious restriction of sodium and potassium reabsorption and of urine output.

In all the tissues investigated the effects of rubescenslysin began within a few minutes, were dose-dependent and practically irreversible. There were only minor differences in sensitivity between various organs and species. The observations indicate that the toxin is relatively nonspecific in its attack on components of cell membranes.

PMID: 7135416 [PubMed - indexed for MEDLINE]

Further Notes

Toxic effects of *Amanita rubescens* experiments on rats.

- Lungs, Thorax, or Respiration – respiratory obstruction
- Blood – haemolysis with or without anaemia

Rubescenslysin from *Amanita rubescens* in vitro caused disruption of mast cells in rat mesentery. The mast-cell-degranulating potency of rubescenslysin roughly corresponded to its haemolytic potency; the dose-response curves were extremely steep and the cells were either completely destroyed or remained intact. The action of rubescenslysin was very fast: at 37° C 95 resp. 90% of the cells were disrupted within 5 min.

Zeatins.

Cytokinins are degradation products of DNA. They are made up of adenine nucleus and a furfural ring. This basic structure is known as furfurylaminopurine. Cytokinins stimulate cell division and enlargement of cells. The deficiency of cytokinins results in stunted growth in plants. Zeatin: It is a naturally occurring cytokinin in plants. Zeatin exists in two forms: One is cis-zeatin, and the other is trans-zeatin. Zeatins can be produced from *Amanita rubescens.*

Effects on the blood.

Experimental Oncology 23, 43–45, 2001 (March) Analysis of cytotoxicity of lectin and non-lectin proteins from *Amanita* mushrooms. Institute of Cell Biology, National Academy of Sciences of Ukraine.

Haemagglutinating lectins were found in *Amanita rubescens,* showing a weak agglutinating activity (200 mg/ml).

Contents of Carboxylic Acids and Two Phenolics and Antioxidant Activity of Dried Portuguese Wild Edible Mushrooms. Servicüo de Farmacognosia, Faculdade de Farma´cia, Universidade do Porto.

The organic acids and phenolics compositions of nine wild edible mushrooms species including, *Amanita rubescens,* were determined by HPLC-UV and HPLC-DAD, respectively. The antioxidant potential of these species was also assessed by using the DPPH scavenging assay. The results showed that all of the species presented a profile composed of at least five organic acids: oxalic, citric, malic, quinic, and fumaric acids. In a general way, the pair of malic plus quinic acids were the major compounds. Only very small amounts of two phenolic compounds were found in some of the analysed species: p-hydroxybenzoic acid (in *A. rubescens*). This acid has antioxidant properties.

All of the species exhibited a concentration-dependent

scavenging ability against DPPH.

Mushrooms are very appreciated, not only for their texture and flavour, but also for their nutritional properties. They have been described as therapeutic foods, useful in preventing diseases such as hypertension, hypercholesterolemia, and cancer. These functional characteristics are mainly due to their chemical composition. Previous studies of this food matrix revealed the presence of organic acids and phenolic compounds in several species. In addition, mushrooms' antioxidant potential has also been reported.

For *A. rubescens*, previous works concerned the phallotoxins, the accumulation of several heavy metals and lanthanides, and the toxic effects caused by a haemolytic protein from this species. In *A. rubescens*, it was possible to identify nine compounds: oxalic, aconitic, citric, ketoglutaric, malic, quinic, ascorbic, shikimic, and fumaric acids. Malic and quinic acids were the main compounds, representing ca. 68% of nonaromatic acids, whereas oxalic acid was detected only in vestigial amounts. This species presented a high total content of organic acids, reaching ca. 91 g/kg

The results obtained in this work indicate that the analysed mushroom species constitute a rich dietary source of organic acids. With regard to the antioxidant activity, these species can hardly provide an effective protection.

Some day,
after we have mastered the winds,
the waves, the tides and gravity,
we shall harness…
the energies of Love.
then, for the second time
in the history of the world,
man will have discovered fire.
Teilhard de Chardin

AYNI
BOOKS

"Ayni" is a Quechua word meaning "reciprocity" – sharing, giving and receiving - whatever you give out comes back to you. To be in Ayni is to be in balance, harmony and right relationship with oneself and nature, of which we are all an intrinsic part. Complementary and Alternative approaches to health and well-being essentially follow a holistic model, within which one is given support and encouragement to move towards a state of balance, true health and wholeness, ultimately leading to the awareness of one's unique place in the Universal jigsaw of life – Ayni, in fact.